Control of Transcription

BASIC LIFE SCIENCES

Alexander Hollaender, General Editor

Biology Division
Oak Ridge National Laboratory
and The University of Tennessee
Knoxville

Control of Transcription

Edited by

B. B. Biswas and R. K. Mandal

Bose Institute
Calcutta, India

and

A. Stevens and W. E. Cohn

Biology Division
Oak Ridge National Laboratory
Oak Ridge, Tennessee

PLENUM PRESS · NEW YORK – LONDON

Library of Congress Cataloging in Publication Data

Calcutta Symposium on Control of Transcription, 1973.
  Control of transcription; [proceedings]

  (Basic life sciences, v.3)
  Includes bibliographical references.
    1. Genetic transcription—Congresses. I. Biswas, B. B., ed. II. Title. [DNLM: 1.
Genetics, Microbial—Congresses. 2. Transcription, Genetic—Congresses. QH431 C144c
1973]
QH450.2.C34   1973   575.2'1   73-20166
ISBN 0-306-36503-0

Proceedings of the Calcutta Symposium on Control of Transcription,
February 12-15, 1973

© 1974 Plenum Press, New York
A Division of Plenum Publishing Corporation
227 West 17th Street, New York, N.Y. 10011

United Kingdom edition published by Plenum Press, London
A Division of Plenum Publishing Company, Ltd.
Davis House (4th Floor), 8 Scrubs Lane, Harlesden, London, NW10 6SE, England

ORGANIZING COMMITTEE

Alexander Hollaender—Oak Ridge National Laboratory, Oak Ridge, Tennessee,
     U.S.A., and University of Tennessee, Knoxville, Tennessee, U.S.A.
Sankar Mitra—Oak Ridge National Laboratory, Oak Ridge, Tennessee, U.S.A.
Salil K. Niyogi—Oak Ridge National Laboratory, Oak Ridge, Tennessee, U.S.A.
S. M. Sircar—Bose Institute, Calcutta, India.
R. K. Mandal—Bose Institute, Calcutta, India.
S. Ghosh—Bose Institute, Calcutta, India.
B. B. Biswas, Convener—Bose Institute, Calcutta, India.

SPONSORS

Bose Institute, Calcutta 700009, India.
Oak Ridge National Laboratory, Biology Division, Oak
     Ridge, Tennessee 37830, U.S.A.
United States National Science Foundation.
Ministry of Science and Technology, Government of India.

ACKNOWLEDGMENTS

The following institutions and firms have extended their generous collaboration
and assistance:

Rabindra Bharati University, Calcutta.
United States Consulate, Calcutta.
Toshniwal Brothers Pvt. Ltd., Calcutta.
Systronics, Calcutta.
Borosil Glass Works Ltd., Calcutta.

Foreword

In numerous conversations with our colleagues from India, it was suggested that we help to institute a series of symposia in India similar in nature to those that have been conducted by our Latin American colleagues for more than 10 years. We were fortunate to have with us in Oak Ridge Dr. Niyogi and Dr. Mitra from Indian universities. Their close ties with the Bose Institute in Calcutta and the resultant correspondence with the Institute Director, Dr. S. M. Sircar, provided the stimulus for organization of this first Indian symposium, which was held in Calcutta. Under the direction of Dr. Sircar, Dr. B. B. Biswas did an outstanding job of organizing this conference.

Financial support was arranged through Dr. R. R. Ronkin of the United States National Science Foundation, who smoothed the way for the use of PL 480 funds which were approved by the Indian Government for the organization and running of this most valuable symposium.

The many Indian scientists who contributed papers and enthusiastically and vigorously entered into the discussions demonstrated the strength of modern science in India. The topic, Control of Transcription, is a timely one, and considerable activity in this area is going on all over the world. The success of this symposium speaks well for the future of these Indian conferences and workshops being planned for the next few years.

Again, the worldwide "community of science" is clearly manifested by the close cooperation we have observed in this fruitful and successful symposium.

Alexander Hollaender

Biology Division
Oak Ridge National Laboratory
Oak Ridge, Tennessee
and
The University of Tennessee
Knoxville, Tennessee

Contents

ix

Introduction

In recent years, a revolution has occurred in biology—a revolution yielding breakthroughs in many fields. The breakthroughs commenced when biologists actually concentrated their attention on cells or cell organelles rather than on whole organisms. Studies at the molecular level yielded much information on the basic reactions of cells, and now studies are turning to the more complicated systems of differentiation and development. Certainly, a more unified molecular concept in biology has developed, and the barrier between physics and chemistry and biology has gradually become lessened, a situation foreseen by J. C. Bose, the founder of this Institute more than 50 years ago.

Several years ago, plans were initiated to hold an international symposium on modern biology at Bose Institute, Calcutta, India. In 1971, Drs. S. K. Niyogi and S. Mitra, who are at present working in the Oak Ridge National Laboratory, U.S.A., suggested to Professor A. Hollaender of the Oak Ridge National Laboratory and The University of Tennessee that meetings be held in India similar to those he so successfully organized in Latin America. Thereupon, Dr. S. M. Sircar, the Director of Bose Institute, contacted Professor Hollaender, who responded so quickly that in 1 year's time the Symposium on Control of Transcription was held in Calcutta (February 12–15, 1973). Professor Hollaender's untiring efforts and his experiences with the series of symposia in Latin America helped the organization of this symposium immeasurably. The National Science Foundation, U.S.A., was contacted for financing the symposium through the Department of Science and Technology, Government of India. Both the governments were agreeable to allocate money from tied-up United States funds in India.

A number of international symposia on different subjects had already been held in this country, but most of them were of wider interest and thus exchange of ideas between the scientists was rather limited. The specific aim of this meeting was to discuss a more narrow topic so that a number of Indian scientists from various disciplines could interact profitably. The purpose of the meeting was also to attract a large number of the young scientists who will be responsible for developing modern biological trends in India as well as in other countries. The topic, Control of Transcription, was chosen with special consideration of the work going on in this Institute.

DNA-dependent RNA polymerase, the enzyme involved in transcription, i.e., the copying of DNA molecules to yield RNA, was discovered more than a decade ago. Subsequent work showed many features of the reaction. However, when initiation and termination of specific RNA chains were looked into, additional protein factors were found to be involved. The mode of action and the precise control exerted by these factors on RNA synthesis are being studied at this time, and the overall process is certainly more complex than was envisaged. Studies of the role of transcription in DNA replication and the reverse transcriptase studies are also very exciting. The objective of arranging a Symposium on Control of Transcription and including topics on (a) viral transcription, both DNA and RNA dependent, (b) prokaryotic RNA polymerases with their controlling factors, (c) transcription in eukaryotic systems, and (d) transcriptional control of DNA replication was to discuss the present status and the future development of the field. The outcome of this discussion is embodied in this volume, prepared under the active advice of Drs. A. Hollaender, W. E. Cohn, A. Stevens, R. K. Mandal, and S. Ghosh.

The meeting left an excellent impression on the participants from India as well as on those from other countries. I am sure that new ideas on the process of transcription will evolve as a result of the meeting. It has been of tremendous value to the younger scientists from India who had never had a chance to attend the same kind of meeting elsewhere. The symposium also has had an effect on the public, because through the press and the radio the importance of transcription to medical and allied fields was emphasized. If symposia of this type are held in India every 2 years, it will surely strengthen science in this country and establish better human and scientific communication among scientists from all countries.

Lastly, I want to acknowledge the help of Professors Hollaender and Sircar, the National Science Foundation, U.S.A., the Government of India, and all members of the organizing committee as well as the participants in making the symposium a grand success. Plenum Publishing Corporation deserves special thanks for processing the publication so efficiently.

B. B. Biswas

Bose Institute
Calcutta, India

List of Participants

INTERNATIONAL SYMPOSIUM
ON CONTROL OF TRANSCRIPTION
Bose Institute, Calcutta, India
February 12–15, 1973

Contributors

Adhya, Sankar–Laboratory of Molecular Biology, National Cancer Institute, NIH, Bethesda, Maryland 20014, U.S.A.

Banerjee, A. K.–Roche Institute of Molecular Biology, Nutley, New Jersey 07110, U.S.A.

Bautz, E. K. F.–Molekulare Genetik der Universität Heidelberg, 69 Heidelberg, Germany.

Bhagwat, A. S.–Bhabha Atomic Research Centre, Trombay, Bombay-85, India.

Biswas, B. B.–Bose Institute, 93/1 Acharya Prafulla Chandra Road, Calcutta-9, India.

Butterworth, Peter H. W.–Department of Biochemistry, London University, London, England.

Chakrabarty, A. M.–Physical Chemistry Laboratory, General Electric Corporation, P.O. Box 8, Schenectady, New York 12301, U.S.A.

Chakravorty, Maharani–Department of Biochemistry, Institute of Medical Sciences, Banaras Hindu University, Varanasi-5, India.

Chambon, Pierre–Department of Biochemistry, Institut Chimie Biologique, Faculte de Medicine, Strasbourg, France.

Das, M. R.–Tata Institute of Fundamental Research, Bombay-5, India.

Dutta, S. K.–Department of Molecular Genetics, P.O. Box 105, Howard University, Washington, D.C. 20001, U.S.A.

Edmonds, Mary–Department of Biochemistry, Faculty of Arts and Sciences, University of Pittsburgh, Pittsburgh, Pennsylvania 15213, U.S.A.

Gallo, R. C.–National Cancer Institute, NIH, Bethesda, Maryland 20014, U.S.A.

Ghosh, S.–Bose Institute, 93/1 Acharya Prafulla Chandra Road, Calcutta-9, India.

Hamkalo, Barbara–Biology Division, Oak Ridge National Laboratory, Oak Ridge, Tennessee 37830, U.S.A.

Hollaender, Alexander–Biology Division, Oak Ridge National Laboratory, Oak Ridge, Tennessee, and The University of Tennessee, Knoxville, Tennessee 37830, U.S.A.

Kumar, Sushil–Indian Agricultural Research Institute, New Delhi-12, India.

Losick, R.—Biological Laboratories, Harvard University, Cambridge, Massachusetts 02138, U.S.A.

Lukanidin, E. M.—Institute of Molecular Biology, Academy of Sciences, Moscow B-312, USSR.

Maitra, U.—Department of Developmental Biology and Cancer, Albert Einstein College of Medicine, Bronx, New York 10461, U.S.A.

Mandal, R. K.—Bose Institute, 93/1 Acharya Prafulla Chandra Road, Calcutta-9, India.

Mitra, S.—Biology Division, Oak Ridge National Laboratory, Oak Ridge, Tennessee 37830, U.S.A.

Niyogi, S. K.—Biology Division, Oak Ridge National Laboratory, Oak Ridge, Tennessee 37830, U.S.A.

Paulus, H.—Department of Biological Chemistry, Harvard Medical School, Boston, Massachusetts 02115, U.S.A.

Poddar, R. K.—Biophysics Laboratory, Saha Institute of Nuclear Physics, Calcutta-37, India.

Rutter, W. J.—Department of Biochemistry and Biophysics, University of California, San Francisco, California 94122, U.S.A.

Sambrook, Joe—Cold Spring Harbor Laboratory, P.O. Box 100, Cold Spring Harbor, New York 11724, U.S.A.

Singh, U. N.—Molecular Biology Unit, Tata Institute of Fundamental Research, Bombay-5, India.

Stevens, Audrey—Biology Division, Oak Ridge National Laboratory, Oak Ridge, Tennessee 37830, U.S.A.

Szybalski, Waclaw—McArdle Laboratory, University of Wisconsin, Madison, Wisconsin 53706, U.S.A.

Takanami, M.—Institute for Chemical Research, Kyoto University, Kyoto, Japan.

Talwar, G. P.—All-India Institute of Medical Sciences, New Delhi-16, India.

Travers, A.—MRC Laboratory of Molecular Biology, Cambridge, England.

Verma, I. M.—Department of Biology, Massachusetts Institute of Technology, Cambridge, Massachusetts 02139, U.S.A.

Wickner, R. B.—Department of Developmental Biology and Cancer, Albert Einstein College of Medicine, Bronx, New York 10451, U.S.A.

Observers

Bagchi, Buddhadev—Department of Physics, Calcutta University, Calcutta-9, India.

Banerjee, A. B.—Department of Biochemistry, Calcutta University, Calcutta-19, India.

Banerjee, S.—Central Drug Laboratory, Calcutta-16, India.

Banerjee, Uma—Department of Physics, Calcutta University, Calcutta-9, India.

Barua, A. K.—Bose Institute, 93/1 Acharya Prafulla Chandra Road, Calcutta-9, India.

Basu, A. K.—Department of Chemistry, Bose Institute, 93/1 Acharya Prafulla Chandra Road, Calcutta-9, India.

Basu, Sandip—New York Public Health Research Institute, New York, New York 10011, U.S.A.

Bhadra, T. C.—Bose Institute, 93/1 Acharya Prafulla Chandra Road, Calcutta-9, India.

Bhaduri, Amar—Department of Pharmacy, Jadavpur University, Calcutta-32, India.

Bhargava, P. M.—Regional Research Laboratory, C.S.I.R., Hyderabad, India.

Bhattacharya, Asoke—Department of Biochemistry, Calcutta University, Calcutta-19, India.

Bhattacharya, S. B.—Biophysics Laboratory, Saha Institute of Nuclear Physics, Calcutta-37, India.

Biswas, (Mrs.) S.—Bose Institute, 93/1 Acharya Prafulla Chandra Road, Calcutta-9, India.

Bose, S.—Bose Institute, 93/1 Acharya Prafulla Chandra Road, Calcutta-9, India.

Bose, S. K. —Department of Biochemistry, Calcutta University, Calcutta-19, India.

Brahmachary, R. L. —Indian Statistical Institute, 203 Barrackpore Trunk Road, Calcutta-35, India.

Burma, D. P. —Banaras Hindu University, Varanasi-5, India.

Chakravorty, D. P. —Bose Institute, 93/1 Acharya Prafulla Chandra Road, Calcutta-9, India.

Chakravorty, P. —Massachusetts Institute of Technology, Cambridge, Massachusetts 02139, U.S.A.

Chanda, (Mrs.) Rita —University of Rochester, Rochester, New York 14627, U.S.A.

Chanda, S. K. —University of Rochester, Rochester, New York 14627, U.S.A.

Chanda, Sunirmal —Bose Institute, 93/1 Acharya Prafulla Chandra Road, Calcutta-9, India.

Chatterjee, Asis —Director's Laboratory, Bose Institute, 93/1 Acharya Prafulla Chandra Road, Calcutta-9, India.

Chatterjee, A. K. —Department of Physiology, Calcutta University, Calcutta-9, India.

Chatterjee, G. C. —Department of Biochemistry, Calcutta University, Calcutta-19, India.

Chatterjee, I. B. —Department of Biochemistry, Calcutta University, Calcutta-19, India.

Chatterjee, K. K. —Institute of Child Health, 95 Dilkhusa Street, Calcutta-17, India.

Chatterjee, M. L. —Bose Institute, 93/1 Acharya Prafulla Chandra Road, Calcutta-9, India.

Chatterjee, Rajyasree —Department of Microbiology, Bose Institute, 93/1 Acharya Prafulla Chandra Road, Calcutta-9, India.

Chatterjee, S. N. —Department of Zoology, Calcutta University, Calcutta-19, India.

Chatterjee, Smriti N. —Department of Biophysics, Calcutta School of Tropical Medicine, Calcutta-12, India.

Chatterjee, Subhendu —Department of Microbiology, Bose Institute, 93/1 Acharya Prafulla Chandra Road, Calcutta-9, India.

Chaudhury, D. K. —Department of Biochemistry, Calcutta University, Calcutta-19, India.

Chaudhury, Kanakendu —Chittaranjan National Cancer Research Centre, Calcutta-26, India.

Chaudhury, Utpal —Department of Physics, Calcutta University, Calcutta-9, India.

Choudhury, K. L. —Bose Institute, 93/1 Acharya Prafulla Chandra Road, Calcutta-9, India.

Choudhury, Manas —Department of Chemistry, Bose Institute, 93/1 Acharya Prafulla Chandra Road, Calcutta-9, India.

Das, Asis —Department of Botany, Bose Institute, 93/1 Acharya Prafulla Chandra Road, Calcutta-9, India.

Das, H. K. —Division of Biochemistry, Indian Agricultural Research Institute, New Delhi-12, India.

Das, J. —Department of Physics, Calcutta University, Calcutta-9, India.

Das, Sunil K. —Department of Chemistry, Bose Institute, 93/1 Acharya Prafulla Chandra Road, Calcutta-9, India.

Das, Susanta —Department of Chemistry, Bose Institute, 93/1 Acharya Prafulla Chandra Road, Calcutta-9, India.

Das Gupta, Chanchal —Biophysics Laboratory, Saha Institute of Nuclear Physics, Calcutta-37, India.

Das Gupta, Juthika —Department of Botany, Bose Institute, 93/1 Acharya Prafulla Chandra Road, Calcutta-9, India.

Das Gupta, Shantanu —Biophysics Laboratory, Saha Institute of Nuclear Physics, Calcutta-37, India.

Dass, C. M. S. —Delhi University, Department of Zoology, Delhi-7, India.

Datta, Asoke G. —Indian Institute of Experimental Medicine, Calcutta-32, India.

Datta, Lina —All-India Institute of Medical Science, New Delhi-16, India.

Datta, Sahana —Director's Laboratory, Bose Institute, 93/1 Acharya Prafulla Chandra Road, Calcutta-9, India.

Datta Gupta, A. K. —Department of Zoology, Calcutta University, Calcutta-19, India.
De, Dilip —Department of Biochemistry, Calcutta University, Calcutta-19, India.
Dutta, Asis K. —Division of Life Sciences, Jawaharlal Nehru University, New Delhi-53, India.
Dutta, J. —Bose Institute, 93/1 Acharya Prafulla Chandra Road, Calcutta-9, India.
Ganguly, Asok —Department of Botany, Bose Institute, 93/1 Acharya Prafulla Chandra Road, Calcutta-9, India.
Ganguly, Ranjan —Department of Zoology, Calcutta University, Calcutta-19, India.
Ganguly, Subhendu —Bose Institute, 93/1 Acharya Prafulla Chandra Road, Calcutta-9, India.
Ganguly, Subinoy —Department of Botany, Bose Institute, 93/1 Acharya Prafulla Chandra Road, Calcutta-9, India.
Gayen, Samir —Department of Chemistry, Bose Institute, 93/1 Acharya Prafulla Chandra Road, Calcutta-9, India.
Ghora, B. K. —Bose Institute, 93/1 Acharya Prafulla Chandra Road, Calcutta-9, India.
Ghose, A. M. —Bose Institute, 93/1 Acharya Prafulla Chandra Road, Calcutta-9, India.
Ghose, Bharati —Bose Institute, 93/1 Acharya Prafulla Chandra Road, Calcutta-9, India.
Ghosh, Amit —Biophysics Laboratory, Saha Institute of Nuclear Physics, Calcutta-37, India.
Ghosh, H. P. —Department of Biochemistry, McMaster University, Hamilton, Ontario, Canada.
Ghosh, J. J. —Department of Biochemistry, Calcutta University, Calcutta-19, India.
Ghosh, (Mrs.) K. —Department of Biochemistry, McMaster University, Hamilton, Ontario, Canada.
Ghosh, N. —Biophysics Laboratory, Saha Institute of Nuclear Physics, Calcutta-37, India.
Ghosh, P. K. —Department of Biochemistry, Calcutta University, Calcutta-19, India.
Ghosh, S. R. —Bose Institute, Calcutta-9, India.
Ghosh, T. N. —School of Tropical Medicine, Chittaranjan Avenue, Calcutta-12, India.
Ghoshal, Shamali —Department of Microbiology, Bose Institute, 93/1 Acharya Prafulla Chandra Road, Calcutta-9, India.
Guha, Chitrita —Indian Agricultural Research Institute, New Delhi-12, India.
Gupta, R. —Physics Department, Calcutta University, Calcutta-9, India.
Gurnani, Shantoo —Bhabha Atomic Research Centre, Trombay, Bombay-85, India.
Kahn, Regina C. —Institut de Biologie Moleculaire, 9 Quai Saint-Bernard, Paris Ve, France.
Kanungo, M. S. —Department of Zoology, Banaras Hindu University, Varanasi-5, India.
Khan, N. C. —Biophysics Laboratory, Saha Institute of Nuclear Physics, Calcutta-37, India.
Kundu, Asit —Director's Laboratory, Bose Institute, 93/1 Acharya Prafulla Chandra Road, India.
Lahiri Majumder, A. —Department of Botany, Biswa-Bharati, West Bengal, India.
Maitra, (Mrs.) Shila —Department of Biochemistry, Calcutta University, Calcutta-19, India.
Maity, I. B. —Department of Botany, Bose Institute, 93/1 Acharya Prafulla Chandra Road, Calcutta-9, India.
Mazumder, B. —Bose Institute, 93/1 Acharya Prafulla Chandra Road, Calcutta-9, India.
Mazumder, Hemanta K. —Bose Institute, 93/1 Acharya Prafulla Chandra Road, Calcutta-9, India.
Mazumder, P. —Saha Institute of Nuclear Physics, Calcutta-37, India.
Mehrotra, N. N. —All-India Institute of Medical Science, New Delhi-16, India.
Mishra, A. K. —Bose Institute, 93/1 Acharya Prafulla Chandra Road, Calcutta-9, India.
Mishra, Tapan —Department of Microbiology, Bose Institute, 93/1 Acharya Prafulla Chandra Road, Calcutta-9, India.
Mitra, B. —Bose Institute, 93/1 Acharya Prafulla Chandra Road, Calcutta-9, India.
Mitra, Nivedita —Department of Zoology, Calcutta University, Calcutta-19, India.
Mitra, Santosh —Chittaranjan National Cancer Research Center, Calcutta-26, India.
Mondal, S. —Department of Zoology, Calcutta University, Calcutta-19, India.

Mondal, Sisir—Department of Zoology, Calcutta University, Calcutta-19, India.

Mukherjee, B.B.—Bose Institute, 93/1 Acharya Prafulla Chandra Road, Calcutta-9, India.

Mukherjee, K. L.—Institute of Child Health, Calcutta-17, India.

Mukherjee, (Mrs.) Manju—Department of Biochemistry, Calcutta University, Calcutta-19, India.

Mukherjee, Pranab—Department of Chemistry, Bose Institute, 93/1 Acharya Prafulla Chandra Road, Calcutta-9, India.

Mukherjee, Subhas—Nil Ratan Sarkar Medical College, Calcutta-14, India.

Murthy, Leelavati—Bhabha Atomic Research Centre, Trombay, Bombay-85, India.

Nandi, P.—Bose Institute, 93/1 Acharya Prafulla Chandra Road, Calcutta-9, India.

Neogy, R.—Chittaranjan National Cancer Research Centre, Calcutta-26, India.

Netrawali, M. S.—Bhabha Atomic Research Centre, Trombay, Bombay-85, India.

Palit, Pratip—Director's Laboratory, Bose Institute, 93/1 Acharya Prafulla Chandra Road, Calcutta-9, India.

Palta, H. K.—Department of Botany, Panjab University, Chandigarh-8, India.

Pradhan, D.S.—Bhabha Atomic Research Centre, Trombay, Bombay-85, India.

Ranade, S. S.—Cancer Research Centre, Bombay-12, India.

Roy, Deb Dutta—Department of Biochemistry and Biophysics, School of Medicine, University of California, San Francisco, California 94122, U.S.A.

Roy, Gouranga—Bose Institute, 93/1 Acharya Prafulla Chandra Road, Calcutta-9, India.

Roy, Jashodhara—Department of Chemistry, Bose Institute, 93/1 Acharya Prafulla Chandra Road, Calcutta-9, India.

Roy, Pampa—Department of Microbiology, Bose Institute, 93/1 Acharya Prafulla Chandra Road, Calcutta-9, India.

Roy, S. C.—Department of Biochemistry, Calcutta University, Calcutta-19, India.

Roy, Tapati—Director's Laboratory, Bose Institute, 93/1 Acharya Prafulla Chandra Road, Calcutta-9, India.

Roychoudhury, R.—Indian Institute of Experimental Medicine, Calcutta-32, India.

Sadhukhan, P.—Department of Physics, Calcutta University, Calcutta-9, India.

Salahuddin, A.—Aligarh Muslim University, Aligarh, India.

Samanta, H.—Saha Institute of Nuclear Physics, Calcutta-37, India.

Sarkar, P. K.—Department of Botany, Bose Institute, 93/1 Acharya Prafulla Chandra Road, Calcutta-9, India.

Sarkar, (Mrs.) Nilima—Department of Biological Chemistry, Harvard Medical School, Boston, Massachusetts 02115, U.S.A.

Sarkar, S.—Institute of Muscle Research, Boston, Massachusetts 02109, U.S.A.

Sen, A.—Bose Institute, 93/1 Acharya Prafulla Chandra Road, Calcutta-9, India.

Sharma, A. K.—Department of Botany, Calcutta University, Calcutta-19, India.

Siddiqi, O.—Tata Institute of Fundamental Research, Homi Bhabha Road, Bombay-5, India.

Singh, Lalji—Department of Zoology, Calcutta University, Calcutta-19, India.

Singh, S. K.—Department of Microbiology, Bose Institute, 93/1 Acharya Prafulla Chandra Road, Calcutta-9, India.

Sinha, N. B.—Department of Microbiology, Bose Institute, 93/1 Acharya Prafulla Chandra Road, Calcutta-9, India.

Sircar, S. M.—Bose Institute, 93/1 Acharya Prafulla Chandra Road, Calcutta-9, India.

Sirsat, S.—Cancer Research Center, Bombay-12, India.

Srivastava, L. M.—All-India Institute of Medical Sciences, New Delhi-16, India.

Sreenivasan, A.—Bhabha Atomic Research Center, Trombay, Bombay-85, India.

Subrahmanyam, C. S.—Indian Agricultural Research Institute, New Delhi-12, India.

Thakur, Asok—Department of Physics, Calcutta University, Calcutta-9, India.

Control of Transcription

1

Fine Structure of Active Genes in Prokaryotes and Eukaryotes

Barbara A. Hamkalo* and O. L. Miller, Jr.[+]

Biology Division
Oak Ridge National Laboratory
Oak Ridge, Tennessee, U.S.A.

Use of the novel but simple preparative techniques developed by Miller and coworkers (1-5) for electron microscopy of nuclear and cytoplasmic material provides preparations suitable for ultrastructural analysis of active genes in a variety of systems. These direct observations, complemented by biochemical and genetic analysis, provide a new approach to the problems of molecular genetics. This chapter compares electron microscopic studies of active genomes in representatives of prokaryotic and eukaryotic cell types.

PROKARYOTES

Since transcription and translation are normally closely coupled in prokaryotes (6), electron microscopic study of active bacterial genomes permits simultaneous visualization of the two processes. Logarithmically growing bacterial cultures rendered osmotically sensitive by a brief treatment with T4 lysozyme (Calbiochem) can be osmotically shocked by dilution into distilled water, and prepared for electron microscopy (7).

Figure 1 is an electron micrograph of the material extruded from an *Escherichia coli* cell after the treatment described above. The fibrillar network consists of bacterial chromosomes, and the material attached to the genome represents sites of genetic activity. Active structural genes are identifiable as regions of the chromosome with attached polyribosomes that were translating

---

*Present address: Department of Molecular Biology and Biochemistry, University of California, Irvine, California.

[+]Present address: Department of Biology, University of Virginia, Charlottesville, Virginia.

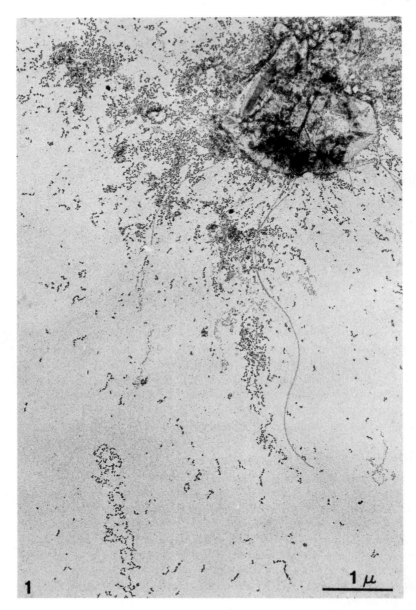

Fig. 1. Osmotically shocked Escherichia coli *from rapidly growing culture.* Shocked
spheroplasts are deposited on a carbon-coated, glow-discharged electron microscope grid by
low-speed centrifugation (2350 × g, 6 min) through a 10% formalin – 0.1 M sucrose
cushion; grids are rinsed in water containing 0.3% Kodak Photo-flo, air-dried, and stained
for 30 sec in a 1% ethanolic solution of phosphotungstic acid, rinsed in 95% ethanol, and
air-dried. Details in Miller and Bakken (5).

nascent messenger RNA (mRNA) molecules into protein. Under optimal growth conditions, active ribosomal RNA (rRNA) genes also are identifiable, because many RNA polymerases simultaneously transcribe each gene, and proteins rather than ribosome associate with the nascent rRNA chains (8), generating short-to-long gradients of ribonucleoprotein (RNP) fibrils.

Figure 2 shows higher magnifications of portions of an *E. coli* chromosome at sites of active structural genes (Fig. 2a,b) and active rRNA cistrons (Fig. 2c). The transcription unit in Fig. 2a, as delimited by the single short-to-long polyribosome gradient, measures approximately 3.1 μ. Since isolated lactose operon DNA that codes for three proteins measures about 1.4 μ (9), the region shown is presumably an active, although unidentified, polycistronic operon.

Adjacent polyribosomes on active genes are unequally spaced. If RNA polymerases transcribe all sequences at about the same rate, then this observation suggests aperiodic initiation of transcription. Occasionally, several adjacent polyribosomes are very close to each other along the genome, possibly the result of a wave of initiation activity.

The fact that free polyribosomes usually are not seen in these preparations indicates that mRNAs are degraded while still attached to the genome. This requires the direction of degradation to be from the 5'-phosphate to the 3'-hydroxyl end of the molecule, as suggested by several groups (10-12). The number of ribosomes in the polyribosomes of a given gradient typically increases in a regular fashion, an observation that can be used as evidence for a nonrandom process of mRNA degradation. This problem could be studied more readily by analysis of polyribosome gradient patterns on specific active genes where the initiation and termination sites can be identified.

When polyribosomes are stretched somewhat during preparation, a small granule (80 Å in diameter) is visible at the site of attachment of the first ribosome of a polyribosome to the genome (Fig. 2a). Although definitive evidence is lacking, these granules most probably are RNA polymerase molecules that were transcribing the genome at the time of preparation. These putative polymerases are more conspicuous in negatively stained preparations, where they are seen as granules that are smaller and less densely stained than the ribosomes (Fig. 2b). Extrapolation from a polyribosome gradient to the approximate initiation site of transcription frequently reveals a granule that may also be an RNA polymerase (Fig. 2a).

The double fibril gradient shown in Fig. 2c is an active rRNA region composed of one 16S and one 23S rRNA cistron. Identification of such regions as rRNA genes is based on predictions of their structural configurations from biochemical and genetic data and the use of a conditional lethal mutant of *E. coli.*

16S and 23S rRNA cistrons are closely linked in many microorganisms (13,14), and the molecular weights of the rRNAs (0.55×10^6 and 1.1×10^6) (15) provide an estimate of the length of B-conformation DNA required to code

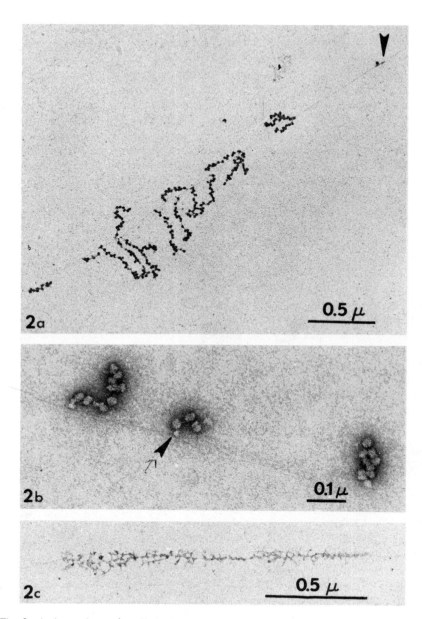

Fig. 2. Active regions of an Escherichia coli *chromosome.* (a) Active polycistronic structural operon; the arrow indicates approximate transcription initiation site. (b) Polyribosomes attached to the genome at RNA polymerases (arrow); negatively stained with 4% aqueous uranyl acetate. (c) Single 16S–23S rRNA doublet from rapidly growing cell.

for each rRNA region (approximately 1.65 μ). Manor *et al.* (16) have calculated that, since there are few rRNA regions per *E. coli* chromosome (approximately 0.3% of the genome) (17), under optimal growth conditions each region must be transcribed simultaneously by 80–90 closely spaced RNA polymerases. The proteins associated with nascent rRNA chains (9) allow visualization of the nascent chains as RNP fibrils. Taken together, these data predict a conformation for active bacterial rRNA regions essentially identical to that shown in Fig. 2c.

Positive identification of these regions as rRNA genes was obtained with a temperature-sensitive mutant of *E. coli*. Although the mutation is in the gene for fructose-1,6-bisphosphate aldolase (A. G. Atherly, personal communication), under appropriate growth conditions the strain shows temperature-sensitive synthesis of rRNA. Cells grown at 30°C, the permissive temperature, show normal fibril gradients, but these gradients disappear after cells are shifted to 42°C, the nonpermissive temperature. No noticeable change is seen in the polyribosome configurations or rRNA fibril gradients of wild-type cells grown at 42°C (B. A. Hamkalo and O. L. Miller, Jr., unpublished data).

The first RNP fibril gradient in Fig. 2c is about one-half the length of the second, in agreement with the difference in molecular weight of the 16S and 23S rRNAs. Each region is about 1.3 μ, somewhat shorter than predicted from molecular weight figures; however, local denaturation of the DNA at the many closely spaced sites of transcription could cause foreshortening of the DNA from its B conformation.

Although two distinct fibril gradients are seen, there is only one site at the proximal end of the 16S cistron at which RNA polymerase initiates. This conclusion is derived from the patterns of disappearance of fibril gradients when initiation of transcription is inhibited by the drug rifampin (7). That is, only after the 16S fibril gradient disappears does the 23S gradient begin to shorten from the proximal end. Pato and von Meyenburg (18), Doolittle and Pace (14), and Kossman *et al.* (19) also have provided biochemical data for the existence of a single polymerase initiation site.

As growth rate is reduced by shifting cells to a less rich medium, active rRNA regions become exceedingly difficult to recognize, because the number of RNA polymerases transcribing each region is drastically reduced (7). This observation is direct evidence that the rate of initiation of transcription is a function of growth rate at constant temperature, as concluded by Mosteller *et al.* (20) from biochemical analysis of tryptophan operon transcription.

The rRNA regions in Fig. 1 appear to be randomly scattered in the extruded contents of the cell, so it is unlikely that these redundant genes are closely clustered as they are in many eukaryotes (see below) and as has been suggested for *E. coli* by Yu *et al.* (21). It has not yet been possible to measure unambiguously the minimum length of DNA between two adjacent rRNA regions. However, it is not unusual to observe single rRNA regions bracketed by structural gene activity (7).

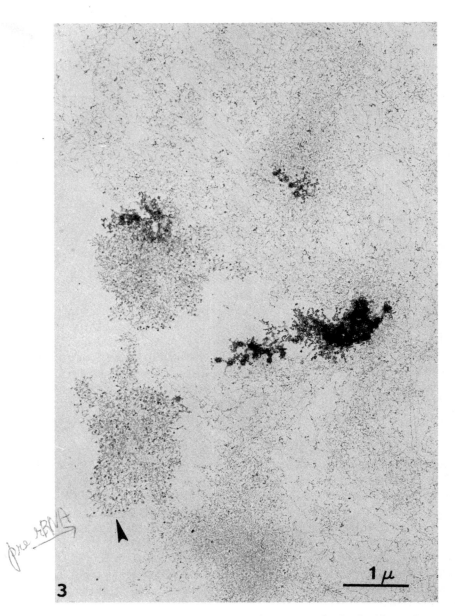

Fig. 3. *Portion of nuclear material liberated after osmotic shock of* Schizosaccharomyces pombe *spheroplasts.* Putative active pre-rRNA genes are at arrow.

EUKARYOTES

Yeast

Cells of a lower-order eukaryote such as *Saccharomyces cerevisiae,* a budding yeast, or *Schizosaccharomyces pombe,* a fission yeast, can be rendered osmotically sensitive by treatment with Glusalase (Endo Laboratories). The spheroplasts will then restart RNA and protein synthesis in growth medium supplemented with an osmotic stabilizing agent such as sorbitol (22). This procedure was followed by Udem and Warner (23) to study ribosome biogenesis in yeast, and spheroplasts also can be used for structural studies of both nuclear and mitochondrial genetic activities.

Figure 3 shows a portion of nuclear material liberated after osmotic shock of yeast spheroplasts, prepared for electron microscopy as described in the caption of Fig. 1. Fragments of nuclear envelope with distinct pores and some cytoplasmic polyribosomes can be seen in the midst of the deoxyribonucleoprotein (DNP) fibers. Unlike bacterial genomes, which are fairly smooth, uniform fibers, the yeast genome is studded with protein granules of various sizes. The arrow (Fig. 3) points to a region of DNP with attached, short, closely spaced fibrils. Such regions are similar in appearance to partially unwound nucleolar cores of higher eukaryotes, sites of ribosomal precursor RNA (pre-rRNA) synthesis.

Finkelstein *et al.* (24) found that all the ribosomal DNA (rDNA) of *S. cerevisiae* is included in two size classes of DNA and that the majority of the DNA of chromosome one consists of rDNA. Cramer *et al.* (25) have presented data suggesting that the redundant (more than 100 per haploid genome) yeast pre-rRNA genes are arranged as sets of 10–32 genes closely clustered within each set but separated from neighboring sets by long stretches of nonribosomal DNA. Refinement of preparations such as that shown in Fig. 3 should provide substantive evidence for or against such an arrangement.

Amphibian Oocytes

Developing oocytes of amphibians such as *Triturus viridescens,* the common spotted newt of North America, and *Xenopus laevis,* the South African clawed toad, have been used extensively for both structural and biochemical studies of transcription, especially of the redundant pre-rRNA genes. Oocyte maturation occurs over several months to years, during which time cells and nuclei grow to dimensions that permit rapid manual isolation of single nuclei. Early in oogenesis, after chromosomal DNA duplication is completed, there is synthesis of a large amount of DNA that has a greater buoyant density than main-band DNA and that hybridizes to 18S and 28S rRNAs (26). This DNA is localized in the

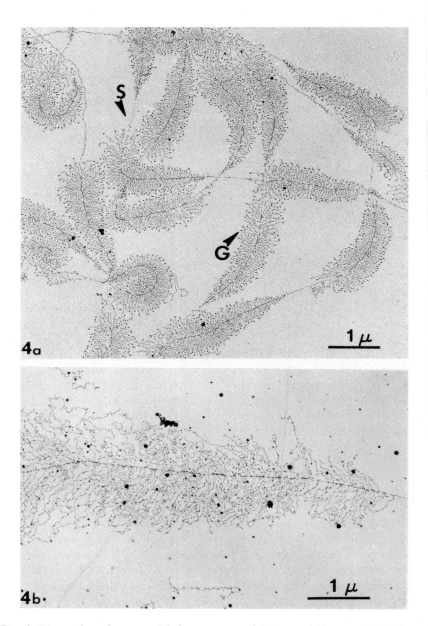

Fig. 4. Dispersed nuclear material from oocyte of Triturus viridescens. (a) Portion of dispersed nucleolar core showing pre-rRNA genes (G) and matrix-free spacers (S). (b) Portion of lampbrush chromosome loop actively synthesizing RNA.

hundreds of extrachromosomal nucleoli that appear in each oocyte nucleus (27). Each nucleolus is composed of two separable components, a dense core and a surrounding granular cortex. Several lines of evidence (28) suggest that pre-rRNA genes reside in nucleolar cores and that nucleolar cortices are sites of pre-rRNA processing.

Miller and Beatty (1,2) developed procedures for the rapid isolation and preparation of unwound nucleolar cores from oocyte nuclei for electron microscopic visualization. Figure 4a shows a portion of an unwound core. The axial fiber is composed of DNA and protein, and the laterally attached fibrils that make up closely spaced fibril gradients are composed of RNA and protein. Each fibril gradient in a given core exhibits the same polarity of short-to-long RNP fibrils and is separated from adjacent gradients by matrix-free DNA, typically about one-third the length of a matrix unit.

Electron microscopic autoradiography localizes RNA synthesis to matrix units, and combined autoradiographic and biochemical data indicate that 40S pre-rRNA is the material synthesized (1, 2, 29). Based on an estimate of approximately 2.6×10^6 for the molecular weight of the amphibian precursor molecule (30), approximately 2.6μ of B-conformation DNA is required to code for a 40S molecule; each matrix unit shown in Fig. 4a is about 2.3μ, somewhat shorter than the expected length. However, as suggested for active bacterial rRNA genes, transcription by many closely spaced RNA polymerases again might foreshorten the DNA from its B-conformation length. From the above data, Miller and Beatty (1,2) concluded that each matrix unit is a gene actively synthesizing 80–100 pre-rRNA molecules simultaneously and that each nascent RMP fibril is attached to a 125-Å-diameter granule on the DNA axis, presumably RNA polymerase. The fact that mature pre-rRNP fibrils are only one-tenth the length expected from the molecular weight of a 40S pre-rRNA suggests extensive foreshortening of RNA within RNP fibrils as a result of RNA-protein interactions.

Oocyte chromosomes also actively synthesize RNA during oogenesis, and the ultrastructure of such transcription is visible in the same preparations used for studying active nucleolar genes. Active sites on oocyte lampbrush chromosomes are seen at the light microscope level as series of extended lateral loops with thin-to-thick matrices along each loop axis (31). The matrix gradient reflects increasing lengths of nascent RNP fibrils, proceeding from the thin to the thick end of the loop. Figure 4b shows a representative electron micrograph of transcription of a portion of a lampbrush chromosome lateral loop. As with active pre-rRNA genes, putative RNA polymerases are seen along the DNP axis at each attachment site of an RNP fibril. However, the RNP fibrils on lampbrush chromosomes grow to many times the length of mature pre-rRNAs, suggesting synthesis of relatively large RNAs. At present, it is not possible to identify specific genetic loci among these active sites.

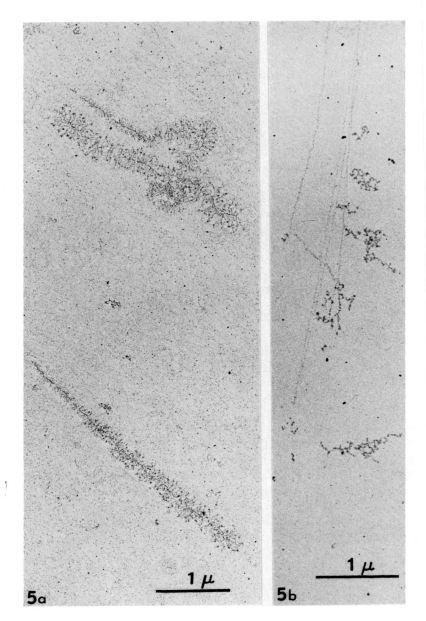

Fig. 5. Nuclear material from lysed HeLa nuclei. (a) Putative pre-rRNA genes. (b) RNP fibrils attached to genome and free in nucleoplasm, possibly heterogenous nuclear RNA synthesis.

HeLa Cells

HeLa cells and nuclei can be lysed by brief treatment with a mild dish detergent, Joy (Procter and Gamble), at 4°C (5). Electron microscopic preparations of such material reveal large amounts of apparently genetically silent DNP, with some regions of high transcriptive activity (Fig. 5a). The fibril matrices are quite similar in conformation to active amphibian pre-rRNA genes. Based on a molecular weight of 4.5×10^6 for the HeLa precursor (32), each gene in B conformation would be about 4.5 μ; each matrix in Fig. 5a is about 3.5 μ, but such loci again may be foreshortened due to the exceedingly high transcription activity at these sites. Mature fibrils are only about one-thirtieth the length anticipated from the molecular weight of pre-rRNA; there may be extensive folding of the RNA within RNP fibrils, similar to the situation in the amphibian oocyte.

Although clusters of these matrices are seen, the number of matrices in a cluster does not approach the number of genes in humans (about 1100 per HeLa cell) (33). However, Henderson et al. (34) used in situ hybridization to localize rDNA to five human chromosomes, providing direct evidence for the existence of several rRNA loci.

Measurement of "spacer" DNA between adjacent putative pre-rRNA genes in HeLa cells is difficult because of the large amount of DNP in the background of preparations. When such a measurement is possible, however, spacers separating neighboring active loci are as long as the putative pre-rRNA genes themselves, whereas the spacer length in amphibian oocytes is much shorter in comparison to the length of the genes. The differences in spacer length in different organisms may well be significant, but their functional role is not known at present.

At other sites of activity (Fig. 5b), the structural aspects of transcription are quite different from those on the lateral loops of amphibian oocyte lampbrush chromosomes. In HeLa cells, short, randomly spaced RNP fibrils are seen attached to the genome and free in the nucleoplasm. There are no obvious fibril gradients, and the long spaces between adjacent fibrils probably indicate infrequent initiation of transcription. At present, it is not possible to estimate the amount of RNA in these RNP fibrils, but most of them presumably represent sites of synthesis of the labile large heterogeneous nuclear RNA that makes up 95% of the RNA synthesized in these cells (35).

CONCLUSIONS

The development of simple and rapid preparative techniques for electron microscopy permits the direct visualization of active genetic material. In bacterial preparations, both active structural genes and rRNA genes are identifiable. Development of appropriate techniques, in conjunction with those used in these studies, should provide the necessary tools for the study of specific genes and operons in order to probe the mechanisms of such processes as mRNA degradation, control of initiation of transcription, and polarity-induced reduction in transcription of genes distal to those harboring mutations. Active pre-rRNA genes have been identified tentatively in several eukaryotic cell systems. Refinements in current technology should provide the potential to study the activity of selected eukaryotic genes, as well as interactions between host and viral genomes during the processes of productive infection and transformation.

ACKNOWLEDGMENT

Oak Ridge National Laboratory is operated by the Union Carbide Corporation for the U.S. Atomic Energy Commission.

REFERENCES

1. O. L. Miller, Jr., and B. R. Beatty. *Science* **164**:955 (1969).
2. O. L. Miller, Jr., and B. R. Beatty. *Genetics* **61**:1 (1969).
3. O. L. Miller, Jr., B. A. Hamkalo, and C. A. Thomas, Jr. *Science* **169**:392 (1970).
4. O. L. Miller, Jr., B. R. Beatty, B. A. Hamkalo, and C. A. Thomas, Jr. *Cold Spring Harbor Symp. Quant. Biol.* **35**:505 (1970).
5. O. L. Miller, Jr., and A. H. Bakken. *Acta Endocrinol.* **168**:155 (1972).
6. G. S. Stent. In M. Kohoutova and J. Hubacek (eds.), *The Physiology of Gene and Mutation Expression,* Academia, Prague (1967), p. 267.
7. B. A. Hamkalo, and O. L. Miller, Jr. In F. T. Kenney, B. A. Hamkalo, G. Favelukes, and J. T. August (eds.), *Gene Expression and Its Regulation,* Plenum Press, New York (1973), p. 63.
8. G. Mangiarotti, D. Apirion, D. Schlessinger, and L. Silengo. *Biochemistry* **7**:456 (1968).
9. J. Shapiro, L. MacHattie, L. Eron, G. Ihler, K. Ippen, and J. Beckwith. *Nature* **224**: 768 (1969).
10. M. Kuwano, C. N. Kwan, D. Apirion, and D. Schlessinger. *Lepetit Colloq. Biol. Med.* **1**:222 (1969).
11. N. Morikawa, and F. Imamoto. *Nature* **223**:37 (1969).
12. D. Morse, R. Mosteller, R. Baker, and C. Yanofsky. *Nature* **223**:40 (1969).
13. W. Colli, and M. Oishi. *Proc. Natl. Acad. Sci. (USA)* **64**:642 (1969).
14. W. F. Doolittle, and N. R. Pace. *Proc. Natl. Acad. Sci. (USA)* **68**:1786 (1971).
15. C. G. Kurland. *J. Mol. Biol.* **2**:83 (1960).
16. H. Manor, D. Goodman, and G. S. Stent. *J. Mol. Biol.* **39**:1 (1969).
17. S. A. Yankofsky, and S. Spiegelman. *Proc. Natl. Acad. Sci. (USA)* **48**: 1466 (1962).
18. M. L. Pato, and K. von Meyenburg. *Cold Spring Harbor Symp. Quant. Biol.* **35**:497 (1970).
19. C. R. Kossman, T. D. Stamato, and D. E. Pettijohn. *Nature New Biol.* **234**: 102 (1971).
20. R. D. Mosteller, J. K. Rose, and C. Yanofsky. *Cold Spring Harbor Symp. Quant. Biol.* **35**:461 (1970).
21. M. T. Yu, C. W. Vermeulen, and K. C. Atwood. *Proc. Natl. Acad. Sci. (USA)* **67**:26 (1970).
22. H. T. Hutchison, and L. H. Hartwell. *J. Bacteriol.* **94**:1697 (1967).

23. S. A. Udem, and J. R. Warner. *J. Mol. Biol.* **65**:227 (1972).
24. D. B. Finkelstein, J. Blamire, and J. Marmur. *Nature New Biol.* **240**:281 (1972).
25. J. H. Cramer, M. M. Bhargava, and H. O. Halvorson. *J. Mol. Biol.* **71**:11 (1972).
26. D. D. Brown, and I. B. Dawid. *Science* **160**:272 (1968).
27. D. Evans, and M. L. Birnstiel. *Biochim. Biophys. Acta* **166**:274 (1968).
28. O. L. Miller, Jr., B. R. Beatty, and B. A. Hamkalo. In J. D. Biggers and A. W. Schuetz (eds.), *Oogenesis,* University Park Press, Baltimore (1972), p. 119.
29. J. G. Gall. *Natl. Cancer Inst. Monogr.* **23**:575 (1966).
30. U. E. Loening, K. W. Jones, and M. L. Birnstiel. *J. Mol. Biol.* **45**:353 (1969).
31. J. G. Gall. In W. D. McElroy and B. Glass (eds.), *The Chemical Basis of Development,* Johns Hopkins Press, Baltimore (1958), p. 103.
32. U. E. Loening. *Symp. Soc. Gen. Microbiol.* **20**:77 (1970).
33. Ph. Jeanteur, and G. Attardi. *J. Mol. Biol.* **45**:305 (1969).
34. A. S. Henderson, D. Warburton, and K. C. Atwood. *Proc. Natl. Acad. Sci. (USA)* **69**:3394 (1972).
35. J. E. Darnell. *Bacteriol. Rev.* **32**:262 (1968).

DISCUSSION

Question (Ghosh): Is there any poly(A) present in the T7 polysome associated with membrane?

Answer: At present, there is no evidence of poly(A) associated with any prokaryotic messenger RNAs.

Question (Sarkar): What percentage of the total polysomes in your HeLa cell preparations are the large polysomes that you consider as polycistronic?

Answer: We haven't made such estimates, except to say that exceedingly long polyribosomes are not rare.

Question (Sarkar): What criterion did you use to assign these polysomes as polycistronic?

Answer: We aren't certain they are polycistronic, but they are larger than polysomes synthesizing average-sized proteins. We would like to keep the possibility of the existence of polycistronic messengers in eukaryotic cells open.

Comment (Sarkar): There are cell types which, although they are not muscle cells, synthesize very large polypeptides such as myosin heavy chain (mol wt 200,000) on large polysomes (60–90 ribosomes) very similar to those observed by you. The large polysomes which you have observed in your HeLa cell preparations fit into these classes of monocistronic large polysomes. It will be of particular interest to characterize the products of these polycistronic messages before a final assignment is made.

Question (Pradhan): Can you see any difference in the electron microscopic pictures of transcribing and nontrascribing chromosomes of the eukaryotes?

Answer: The obvious difference is the lack of nascent ribonucleoprotein fibrils attached to nontranscribing regions. Otherwise, there are no obvious structural differences between the two types of chromatin, although the level of resolution we are working at is fairly low.

Question (Szybalski): What is the size of transcribing RNA polymerase in the negatively stained preparations?

Answer: Approximately 80 Å.

Question (Szybalski): Is there any RNA synthesized in the spacer regions when two transcriptional units (arranged in tandem with a spacer between them) are initiated by one promoter?

Answer: By electron microscopic autoradiography of amphibian oocyte material, there is no obvious RNA synthesis in the spacer regions.

Question (Chambon): Did you try to characterize the granules which are present at the region of the RNA fibrils seen on *E. coli* chromosomes using labeled antibody against *E. coli* RNA polymerase? Are these granules the same as those which are seen in the spacer regions?

Answer: We are attempting to use ferritin-conjugated antibody for that very purpose.

Question (Adhya): Have you tested successfully any *in vitro* transcribing system?

Answer: Preparations from Geoff Zubay's coupled transcription-translation system revealed extensive meshworks (presumably as a result of the high concentration of protein in the reaction mixture) in which DNA and attached polyribosomes were entrapped; it wasn't possible to follow along long enough stretches of the DNA as a result of this. Although not as severe, a similar meshwork was seen in the *in vitro* transcription system as utilized in Ira Pastan's lab.

Question (Das): Can the proportion of polysomes on mRNA still bound to DNA to that on completed and free mRNA be quantitatively estimated?

Answer: At present, we would only be able to make qualitative estimates, but we have not seen free polyribosomes in normal preparations under conditions that we know will sediment them if present. Therefore, we feel that virtually all polyribosomes are bound to the bacterial genome.

Question (Sambrook): In HeLa cell lysates, do you see any mitochondrial transcription complexes?

Answer: Since a mitochondrial DNA molecule has a contour length of only 5 μ, it is unlikely that it would be liberated from the organelle with a high enough frequency to visualize it.

Question (Sambrook): Does cordycepin or α-amanitin affect the pattern that you see?

Answer: We have not tested these inhibitors.

Question (Sambrook): In the prokaryotic system, can you see areas of denaturation of the DNA around the site of attachment of RNA polymerase?

Answer: Presumably, the local denaturation occurs over such a short length of the DNA that RNA polymerases hide it from view.

2

Changes in the Subunit Structure of *Bacillus subtilis* RNA Polymerase During Sporulation

Richard Losick

The Biological Laboratories
Harvard University
Cambridge, Massachusetts, U.S.A.

Sporulating *bacilli* undergo a series of dramatic changes in morphology and physiology. During the first hours of sporulation, the bacterial cell is partitioned into a forespore and a sporangium or mother cell. Next, the sporangium engulfs the forespore. Engulfment is followed by the synthesis of the cortex and coat components of the spore and, finally, by the release of the mature spore from the mother cell. These morphological events are accompanied by changes in gene transcription. New classes of messenger RNA appear during sporulation (1), while the synthesis of ribosomal RNA is turned off in *Bacillus subtilis* (2) and *Bacillus cereus* (3).

RNA polymerase holoenzyme from *B. subtilis* contains a σ subunit having a mass of 55,000 daltons (Fig. 1). During the first hour of sporulation, the loss of vegetative σ-factor activity causes a change in the template specificity of RNA polymerase (4,5). RNA polymerase purified at later stages of sporulation contains a polypeptide of mass = 110,000 daltons in place of one of the β subunits of the core enzyme and does not respond to σ (5) or bind σ (11). Recent experiments in our laboratory (12) in which RNA polymerase was purified from a mixture of vegetative and sporulating cells separately labeled with two different radioisotopes indicate that this alteration of β is due to *in vitro* proteolysis and that most if not all of the RNA polymerase in sporulating *B. subtilis* is not proteolytically cleaved.

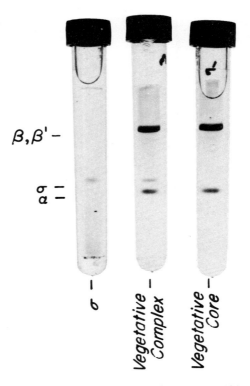

Fig. 1. *Sodium dodecylsulfate gel electrophoresis of vegetative RNA polymerase.* Vegetative RNA polymerase holoenzyme was purified and fractionated into core and σ components as described by Shorenstein and Losick (11). The gels were 5% acrylamide and were stained with Coomassie brilliant blue.

   The loss of σ-factor activity early during sporulation has offered a possible explanation for the turnoff of ribosomal RNA synthesis (2) and the failure of *B. subtilis* phage φe to grow in sporulating cells (6), since the σ polypeptide is required for the transcription of ribosomal RNA genes (7) and φe DNA (5) *in vitro.* Furthermore, certain sporulation-defective mutants that prevent the complete loss of σ activity permit the continued synthesis of ribosomal RNA and the growth of phage φe during stationary phase (8).

   These findings prompted us to examine sporulating *B. subtilis* for factors that might replace σ and that could direct the transcription of sporulation genes. Such polypeptides might be expected to bind to RNA polymerase and could be isolated by virtue of this binding. To search for such polypeptides, RNA polymerase was precipitated from extracts of radioactively labeled vegetative and sporulating *B. subtilis* by precipitation with antiserum prepared against

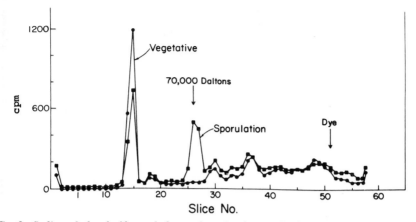

Fig. 2. *Sodium dodecylsulfate gel electrophoresis of an antibody precipitate of radioactive RNA polymerase.* Vegetative and sporulating cells of *Bacillus subtilis* were radioactively labeled separately with [^{3}H] trytophan and [^{14}C] tryptophan, respectively. RNA polymerase was precipitated from the extract of a mixture of the cells with antiserum prepared against pure vegetative core polymerase as described in Greenleaf *et al.* (9). The precipitate was solubilized and subjected to disc electrophoresis through a dodecylsulfate gel of 5% acrylamide. The gel was cut into slices and each slice solubilized and the radioactivity measured. ●, ^{3}H; ■, ^{14}C.

vegetative core polymerase (9). The precipitates were solubilized and analyzed by sodium dodecylsulfate polyacrylamide gel electrophoresis. Antiserum added to an extract of vegetative *B. subtilis* precipitated only the known subunits of core polymerase, but antiserum added to an extract of sporulating cells precipitated a new polypeptide of mass = 70,000 daltons in addition to the subunits of core enzyme. The experiment of Fig. 2 shows that the 70,000-dalton polypeptide precipitated from an extract of a mixture of vegetative and sporulating *B. subtilis* separately labeled with two different radioisotopes contained only the radioisotope characteristic of the sporulating cells.

The 70,000-dalton protein was freed of core RNA polymerase and extensively purified by chromatography on phosphocellulose (9). Precipitation of the purified 70,000-dalton protein by the anti − polymerase serum requires the prior addition of vegetative or sporulation core RNA polymerase. Thus the 70,000-dalton protein apparently binds to RNA polymerase. The reaction is specific since the purified protein is not precipitated during antibody precipitation of either phage λ repressor or bovine serum albumin.

The binding protein first appears from the first to third hour of sporulation and is synthesized by mutants blocked at intermediate stages of spore formation (*spo*II and *spo*IV). However, the binding protein does not appear in mutants blocked early in sporulation (*rfr* 10, *spo*OA, *spo*OB, and *spo*OC) (13).

The σ subunit of vegetative polymerase directs asymmetrical transcription of *B. subtilis* DNA *in vitro* (Pero cited in 10) and the synthesis of ribosomal RNA *in vitro* (7). Attempts to demonstrate a role for the 70,000-dalton binding protein in the transcription of sporulation genes have not yet been successful.

REFERENCES

1. T. Yamakawa, and R. Doi. *J. Bacteriol.* **106**:305-310 (1971).
2. C. Hussey, R. Losick, and A. L. Sonenshein. *J. Mol. Biol.* **57**:59-70 (1971).
3. J. Wise and D. Fraser. *Spores* **5**:203-211 (1972).
4. R. Losick and A. L. Sonenshein. *Nature* **224**:35-37 (1969).
5. R. Losick, R. G. Shorenstein, and A. L. Sonenshein. *Nature* **227**:910-913 (1970).
6. A. L. Sonenshein and D. H. Roscoe. *Virology* **39**:265-276 (1969).
7. C. Hussey, J. Pero, R. G. Shorenstein, and R. Losick. *Proc. Natl. Acad. Sci. USA* **69**:407-411 (1972).
8. A. L. Sonenshein and R. Losick. *Nature* **227**:906-909 (1970).
9. A. Greenleaf, T. Linn, and R. Losick. *Proc. Natl. Acad. Sci. USA* **70**: 490-494 (1973).
10. R. Losick. *Ann. Rev. Biochem.* **41**: 409-446 (1972).
11. R. G. Shorenstein and R. Losick. *J. Biol. Chem.* **248**: 6163-6169 (1973).
12. T. Linn, A. Greenleaf, R. Shorenstein, and R. Losick. *Proc. Natl. Acad. Sci. USA* **70**: 1865-1869 (1973).
13. A. Greenleaf and R. Losick, *J. Bacteriol.* in press (1973).

DISCUSSION

Question (Bose): What happens to σ factor in asporogenous mutants?
Answer: Sigma is retained in mutants blocked early in sporulation.

Question (Szybalski): Could the chain of events be summarized as follows: (a) RNA polymerase loses σ (this does not happen if RNA polymerase has a *rif*-resistant β subunit); (b) resulting core enzyme transcribes 70K protein operon, and 70K protein is synthesized; (c) 70K protein binds to the core enzyme; (d) new 70S + core enzyme does something new and important for the sporulation process.
Answer: Yes, that is a possible scheme.

Question (Biswas): Regarding the protein which appears during sporulation, is it a DNA binding protein?
Answer: Yes.

Question (Subrahmanyam): What are the comparative efficiencies of the vegetative and sporulation enzymes *in vitro* with *B. subtilis* DNA?
Answer: Enzyme from sporulating cells is less active with *B. subtilis* DNA than vegetative RNA polymerase.

Question (Sarkar): Since RNA polymerase from sporulating cells as well as the new 70,000-dalton protein has been extensively purified, did you do any binding studies using the conditions for *in vitro* RNA synthesis? If so, do you have any idea about the K_m of the new protein for RNA polymerase from sporulating cells?
Answer: No.

Question (Sarkar): Is the time course of appearance of your 70,000-dalton protein compatible with the hypothesis that it is translated only during the time when cells are *committed to sporulation?* The time course suggests that this protein may be synthesized rather late when sporulation has already started.

Answer: The appearance of the binding protein is an early event in sporulation. However, its appearance is certainly not the earliest event in the sporulation process.

Question (Sarkar): What is the stoichiometry of the 70,000-dalton protein in the sporulating RNA polymerase?

Answer: About one per polymerase.

Question (Bautz): Does the rifampicin-resistant mutant which is sporulation negative fail to bind the protein, or does it not make it?

Answer: The rfr 10 mutant apparently does not synthesize the binding protein since the 70,000-dalton protein does not appear even if old-type polymerase is included in the precipitation reaction.

Question (Das): Can the 70,000-dalton protein be detected in mature spores? What happens to it on spore germination?

Answer: Yes, the binding protein is present in spores, but we have not tested for its presence during germination.

3

Control of Transcription in *Bacillus brevis* by Small Molecules

Henry Paulus and Nilima Sarkar

Department of Biological Chemistry
Harvard Medical School
Boston, Massachusetts, U.S.A.

Bacterial sporulation consists of a progression of biochemical changes whose orderly sequence seems to be effected primarily by the regulation of specific gene transcription (1). In order to understand the control mechanisms involved in this process, we have concentrated our attention on the ways by which RNA synthesis in *Bacillus brevis* may be modulated by low molecular weight substances.

INHIBITION OF RNA POLYMERASE BY PEPTIDE ANTIBIOTICS

Peptide antibiotics are produced by sporulating but not by other bacterial species, and genetic studies (8) as well as physiological correlations (5) have implicated these substances in the sporulation process. A possible regulatory function is suggested by the observation that peptide antibiotics, when added at concentrations at which they are produced early in sporulation, inhibit vegetatively growing cultures of the producing organism (6,9-11). The fact that peptide antibiotics inhibit a process that is essential for growth but not for sporulation would be consistent with a regulatory role during the transition from vegetative to sporulation metabolism. We have investigated this possibility in *B. brevis,* which produces the tyrothricin complex of antibiotics that includes the tyrocidines, a family of cyclic decapeptides, and the gramicidins, linear pentadecapeptides whose end groups are masked by a formyl and an ethanolamine moiety.

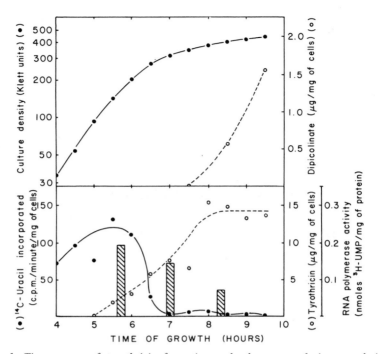

Figure 1. Time course of tyrothricin formation and other events during sporulation of Bacillus brevis *ATCC 8185.* The organism was cultured as described by Sarkar and Paulus (6). Tyrothricin was assayed in ethanol extracts of culture samples using the plate-filter paper disc method with *B. subtilis* ATCC 6051 as the indicator organism. Dipicolinate was determined colorimetrically in boiling-water extracts of the cells. The incorporation of [^{14}C] uracil into RNA was measured by incubating samples (1 ml) of the culture with 0.1 μc of [^{14}C] uracil (0.16 c/mole) for 10 min at 37°C, followed by precipitation and washing with 0.6 N trichloroacetic acid. RNA polymerase activity (hatched bars) was estimated in sonic extracts of cells after centrifugation at 100,000 × g for 1 hr and precipitation with ammonium sulfate between 35 and 60% saturation as described by Sarkar and Paulus (7).

Figure 1 illustrates some of the events that occur in *B. brevis* during the transition from growth to sporulation. The end of exponential growth was accompanied by the abrupt cessation of *net* RNA synthesis, measured by the incorporation of [^{14}C] uracil. Significant RNA synthesis occurred, however, throughout sporulation, and the formation of heat-stable spores was inhibited by the addition of rifampicin until the very late stages of sporulation. The decline in *net* synthesis of RNA was not accompanied by a reduction in the level of RNA polymerase, which occurred only slowly and may have been an artifact due to degradation by proteases that are produced early in sporulation. The formation of tyrothricin began near the end of exponential growth, and the antibiotic reached a maximum level of nearly 10% of the dry weight a few hours later. All antibiotic activity was associated with the cell material and was absent from the culture fluid. Unlike tyrothricin, other sporulation-specific products such as dipicolinic acid were formed considerably later.

The time course of tyrothricin production is thus consistent with a role very

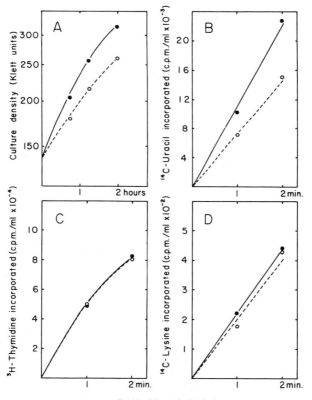

TIME OF INCUBATION

Fig. 2. Effect of tyrothricin on exponentially growing cultures of Bacillus brevis *ATCC 8185.* Tyrothricin (100 µg/ml) was added to cultures at a cell density of 140 Klett units, and the growth (○) was compared with that of a control culture without tyrothricin (●) in a Klett-Summerson photoelectric colorimeter (A). Exponentially growing cultures, with (○) or without (●) tyrothricin (100 µg/ml), were also incubated, 5 min after addition of the antibiotic, with (B) 0.1 µc/ml of [^{14}C]uracil (7 c/mol), (C) 1 µc/ml of [^{3}H]thymidine (2 c/mmol), or (D) 0.2 µc/ml of L[^{14}C]lysine (222 c/mol). At the times indicated, samples were transferred to an equal volume of cold 0.6 N trichloroacetic acid. The precipitates were collected on glass fiber filter paper (Whatman GF/C), washed with 0.3 N trichloroacetic acid and alcohol, and dried, and their radioactivity was determined in a liquid scintillation spectrometer.

early during sporulation, such as the turnoff of vegetative functions, and we therefore examined the effect of the antibiotic on growth. As shown in Fig. 2, tyrothricin (100 µg/ml) inhibited the growth of vegetative cells by about 30%, and this growth inhibition was accompanied by a similar inhibition of the initial rate of [^{14}C]uracil incorporation into RNA, while the initial rate of the incorporation of precursors into DNA and protein was unaffected. This suggests that growth inhibition by tyrothricin is due to a direct effect on RNA synthesis.

To identify the site of action of the antibiotic, we studied its effect on RNA polymerase, highly purified from vegetatively growing cultures of *B. brevis* (7). Tyrothricin was found to inhibit the enzyme by nearly 50% at a concentration of 5 µg/ml, and its constituent antibiotics, tyrocidine and gramicidin, were equally effective inhibitors (Table I). In contrast, gramicidin S, a cyclic decapeptide produced by a different strain of *B. brevis,* had a much smaller effect on the enzyme. The observed inhibition bore no relationship to the surfactant nature of the antibiotics (the linear gramicidins are only very weak surface-active agents, while gramicidin S is an even stronger detergent than the tyrocidines) and therefore was probably not due to denaturation. This conclusion was supported by the observation that the inhibition of RNA polymerase could be readily reversed by the dilution of the antibiotics.

Tyrothricin is thus seen to act as a specific inhibitor of RNA synthesis *in vitro* and *in vivo.* Since the production of the antibiotic begins near the end of exponential growth, its intracellular concentration must be already quite high at the time when the net synthesis of RNA begins to decline. It would be surprising if, under these conditions, RNA polymerase activity were not substantially inhibited, and we propose that this inhibition serves the specific function of terminating the transcription of genes that are expressed only during vegetative growth. In this context, it is interesting that a eukaryotic RNA polymerase is specifically inhibited by α-amanitin, a cyclic peptide produced by a sporulating fungus (3).

**Table I. Inhibition of RNA Polymerase by
Peptide Antibiotics[a]**

Antibiotic	Percent inhibition by antibiotic	
	At 5 µg/ml	At 50 µg/ml
Tyrothricin	40	96
Tyrocidine	44	100
Gramicidin	50	90
Gramicidin S	—	23

[a]RNA polymerase (holoenzyme) was purified and assayed with *B. brevis* DNA as described by Sarkar and Paulus (7).

EFFECT OF CYCLIC GMP ON RNA SYNTHESIS

In order to examine more systematically the changes in RNA synthesis that occur at the onset of sporulation, we turned to the study of washed cells of *B. brevis* that were made permeable to small molecules by treatment with toluene. The incorporation of [³H]UTP into RNA in permeable cells of this type was totally dependent on the presence of the four nucleoside triphosphates and was completely abolished by the addition of rifampicin or streptolydigin. Figure 3 shows the synthesis of RNA in toluenized cells obtained from cultures at various stages of growth and sporulation. A considerable reduction in the incorporation of [³H]UTP was observed early during sporulation. This seemed to parallel the marked reduction in the net synthesis of RNA that accompanies the onset of sporulation and suggested that transcription in toluenized cells reflects the changes that occur in the intact organism. Another striking feature of RNA synthesis in toluenized cells was its apparent stimulation by cyclic 3′,5′-nucleo-

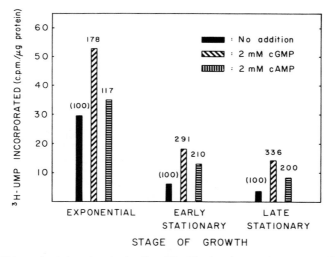

Fig. 3. *RNA synthesis in toluenized cells of* Bacillus brevis *at various stages of growth. B. brevis* was grown as described previously (6). Samples (30 ml) were removed from the culture at cell densities of 149 (exponential), 248 (early stationary), and 375 Klett units (late stationary) and centrifuged at 5000 × g for 5 min at 25°C. The cells were resuspended in 0.5 ml of 0.1 *M* triethanolamine buffer, *p*H 7.5, and toluene (0.005 ml) was added. The mixtures were gently agitated at 25°C for 10 min, chilled to 4°C for 5 min, and then centrifuged at 5000 × g for 5 min at 25°C. The sedimented material was suspended in 0.05 *M* triethanolamine, *p*H 7.5, containing 50% glycerol, and stored at −20°C. RNA polymerase activity in toluenized cells was assayed at 37°C for 30 min as described previously (7) in the absence and presence of cyclic nucleotides as indicated. The numbers above the bars represent the incorporation of [³H]UMP relative to the values observed in the absence of cyclic nucleotides.

side monophosphates. Cyclic GMP (2 mM) enhanced the incorporation of [^{3}H]UTP by 50–100% in vegetative cells and three- to fourfold during sporulation, while cyclic AMP had a smaller effect and GDP and GMP were ineffective. As shown in Fig. 4, half-maximal stimulation of RNA synthesis was obtained with 2 mM cyclic GMP. Cyclic AMP was much less effective, even at higher concentrations. That the observed changes were related to sporulation and not merely to cessation of growth was demonstrated by results obtained with cells

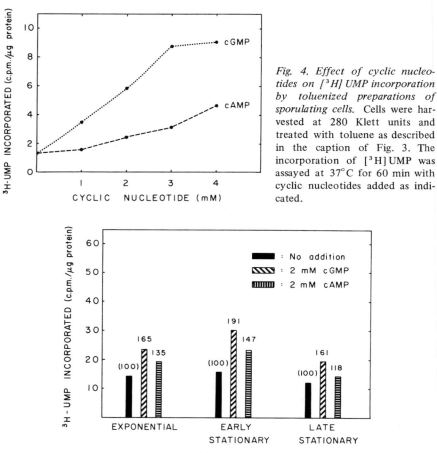

Fig. 4. Effect of cyclic nucleotides on [^{3}H] UMP incorporation by toluenized preparations of sporulating cells. Cells were harvested at 280 Klett units and treated with toluene as described in the caption of Fig. 3. The incorporation of [^{3}H]UMP was assayed at 37°C for 60 min with cyclic nucleotides added as indicated.

Fig. 5. RNA synthesis in toluenized cells of Bacillus brevis grown under nonsporulating conditions. B. brevis was grown in Penassay broth, and samples were removed at 124 (exponential), 200 (early stationary), and 236 Klett units (late stationary) for treatment with toluene and assay of RNA synthesis as described in the caption of Fig. 3, except that [^{3}H] UMP incorporation was measured after an incubation of 60 min.

that were grown in Penassay broth, a medium that does not support the sporulation of *B. brevis* (Fig. 5). Even in late stationary phase, RNA synthesis did not decline, and the effect of cyclic nucleotides remained at the level characteristic of vegetative growth.

A possible basis for the decline in RNA synthesis and increased stimulation by cyclic GMP during sporulation was suggested by the examination of the time course of [³H] UTP incorporation in toluenized preparations of vegetative and sporulating cells (Fig. 6). In the former, the accumulation of radioactivity reached a constant level after about 45 min, and the stimulation by cyclic GMP was independent of time. In sporulating cells, however, the incorporation of labeled precursor reached a maximum in 10 min and then declined sharply, suggesting a rapid degradation of the product. The effect of cyclic GMP seemed to be primarily a reduction of RNA hydrolysis, for its apparent stimulation of RNA accumulation was most pronounced at later times. In fact, the initial rates of RNA synthesis were quite similar in growing and in sporulating cells and were little affected by cyclic nucleotides. The degradation of RNA could be directly examined in toluenized cells that had been briefly incubated with [³H] UTP and then treated with streptolydigin to prevent further RNA synthesis. Figure 7 shows that the half-life of RNA synthesized by toluenized cells was only 10 min, but was prolonged to 20 min in the presence of cyclic GMP, while cyclic AMP had a lesser effect. A similar inhibition of RNA hydrolysis by cyclic GMP was

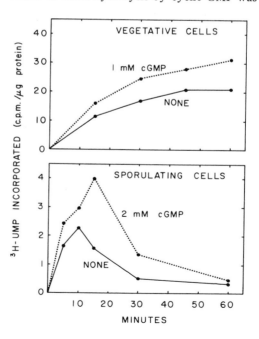

Fig. 6. Time course of [³H] UMP incorporation in toluenized cells of Bacillus brevis. *Toluenized cells were prepared from cultures harvested at 115 (vegetative cells) and 380 Klett units (sporulating cells), and the incorporation of [³H] UMP was assayed for various times in the absence and presence of cyclic GMP, as described in the caption of Fig. 3.*

observed in cell-free extracts, using [^{14}C]poly(A,C) as substrate (Fig. 8). These results indicated that *B. brevis* contains an intracellular ribonuclease whose activity is inhibited by cyclic GMP and, to a smaller extent, by cyclic AMP. Since no significant hydrolysis of cyclic GMP was observed under the conditions of these experiments, the inhibition of ribonuclease activity by the cyclic nucleotide was not simply due to action as a competing substrate; rather, it must represent a more specific kind of regulation.

The apparent reduction of RNA synthesis and the stimulation by cyclic GMP in toluenized preparations of sporulating cells seem therefore to be due to the presence of a ribonuclease whose activity is regulated by cyclic nucleotides, a conclusion supported by the similarity of the relative effects of cyclic GMP and cyclic AMP on nuclease activity and RNA synthesis. On the other hand, the observed differences between growing and sporulating cells cannot be solely due to the action of the nuclease, since neither its level nor its sensitivity to inhibition by cyclic GMP changes significantly during sporulation (Figs. 7 and 8). Additional factors must thus exist that are responsible for the different behavior of vegetative and sporulating cells.

It is difficult to discuss the physiological roles of the ribonuclease and cyclic GMP in relation to sporulation because we have not yet measured the changes in cyclic nucleotide levels during the growth cycle of *B. brevis*. Unpublished experiments by N. Goldberg (quoted in ref. 2) suggest that vegetative cells of

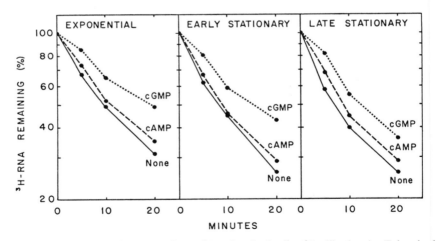

Figure 7. Degradation of RNA synthesized in toluenized cells of Bacillus brevis. Toluenized cells prepared from cultures harvested at 149 (exponential), 248 (early stationary), and 375 Klett units (late stationary) were incubated with [^{3}H]UTP for 10 min at 37°C in the absence of cyclic nucleotides under conditions used for measurement of RNA synthesis (7). Streptolydigin (2 μg/ml) was then added, and incubation was continued for the times shown with and without cyclic nucleotides (2 mM) as indicated.

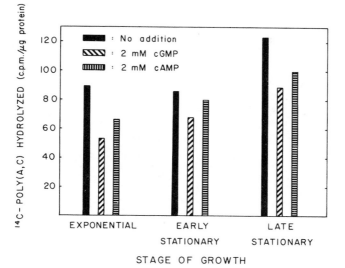

Fig. 8. Effect of cyclic nucleotides on the hydrolysis of poly(A,C) in cell-free extracts of Bacillus brevis. Cells were harvested at 139 (exponential), 246 (early stationary), and 365 Klett units (late stationary), disrupted by grinding at 4°C with levigated alumina, suspended in 10 vol of buffer A (10 mM tris, pH 8.4, 10 mMMgCl$_2$, 10 mM 2-mercaptoethanol, 1 mM EDTA, 0.2 M KCl, and 5% glycerol), and centrifuged at 12,000 × g for 10 min. The supernatant fraction (0.02 ml) was incubated at 37°C for 30 min, in a final volume of 0.1 ml, with 1 mM [*adenosine*-8-^{14}C] poly(A,C) (0.1 c/mole, prepared with polynucleotide phosphorylase from equimolar amounts of [8-^{14}C] ADP and CDP), 10 mM MgCl$_2$, 2 mM MnCl$_2$, and 10 mM 2-mercaptoethanol. The reaction was terminated by the addition of cold 70% ethanol (1.9 ml), the precipitate was removed by centrifugation, and the radioactivity remaining in the supernatant fraction was measured in a liquid scintillation spectrometer.

Bacillus licheniformis have low levels of cyclic AMP and high levels of cyclic GMP, while the reverse is the case in sporulating cells. If a similar situation prevails in *B. brevis*, the ribonuclease in question would be inhibited during vegetative growth but be active during sporulation, and its role might be the rapid turnover of RNA during sporulation. However, one must be cautious in making speculations of this kind until the levels of cyclic GMP in *B. brevis* have actually been measured.

NUCLEOTIDE-DEPENDENT INACTIVATION OF RNA POLYMERASE

In this discussion of the effects of small molecules on transcription, we must consider one more phenomenon even though its physiological role is not at all understood. In the course of the purification of RNA polymerase from *B. brevis*, it was observed that the addition of ATP (1 mM) to preparations of the enzyme led to complete and irreversible loss of activity in less than 1 hr at $0°$C. Figure 9 shows the characteristics of the inactivation process at $25°$C. In the presence of 2 mM ATP and 10 mM MgCl$_2$, RNA polymerase had a half-life of less than 1 min under conditions where in the absence of nucleotides it was quite stable. The dependence of inactivation on the concentration of ATP was highly sigmoid and required the presence of Mg^{2+} ion. Inactivation of RNA polymerase could also be promoted by low concentrations of dATP and NAD$^+$ (Table II), while CTP, NADP$^+$, and NMN had a smaller effect and GTP, UTP, NADH, ADP, AMP, and cyclic AMP were ineffective. The nucleotide specificity suggested that inactivation was not due to the formation of polyadenylate by polynucleotide phosphorylase, a conclusion that was supported by the observation that highly purified preparations of RNA polymerase "core," completely free of polynucleotide phosphorylase activity (7), also underwent inactivation in the presence of ATP. Another interesting feature of the inactivation process, illustrated in Table II, is its prevention by orthophosphate and arsenate. This represents a protective effect and not the reversal of inactivation, for the later addition of orthophosphate did not lead to reactivation. In fact, orthophosphate itself is a potent inhibitor of the RNA polymerase from *B. brevis*. The concentration of orthophosphate required for the protection of RNA polymerase was highly dependent on the concentration of the inactivating nucleotide. DNA also protected RNA polymerase from inactivation, even in the absence of σ factor, a fact that explains why RNA polymerase is not inactivated under the conditions of its assay.

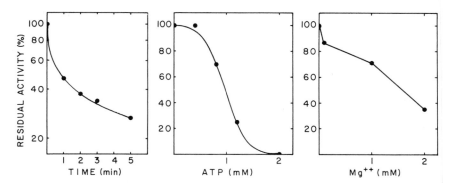

Fig. 9. ATP-dependent inactivation of RNA polymerase. (A) Rate of inactivation in the presence of 2 mM ATP and 10 mM MgCl$_2$. (B) Effect of ATP concentration in the presence of 10 mM MgCl$_2$. (C) Effect of MgCl$_2$ concentration in the presence of 2 mM ATP. Purified RNA polymerase holoenzyme (7) was incubated at $25°$C for the times indicated (A) or for 5 min (B and C), as described in the footnote to Table II, and assayed for residual RNA polymerase activity.

Table II. Effect of Nucleotides and Orthophosphate on the Inactivation of RNA Polymerase[a]

Enzyme	Additions	Residual activity (%)
Holoenzyme	1 mM ATP	54
"	1 mM ATP + 1 mM P_i	100
"	1 mM dATP	42
"	1 mM dATP + 1 mM P_i	72
"	2 mM NAD$^+$	22
"	2 mM NAD$^+$ + 1 mM P_i	47
"	1 mM ATP	38
"	1 mM ATP + 1 mM As_i	84
Core enzyme	1 mM ATP	42
"	1 mM ATP + 1 mM P_i	85

[a]RNA polymerase holoenzyme or core enzyme purified as described by Sarkar and Paulus (7) was incubated at 25°C for 5 or 20 min, respectively, with 10 mM $MgCl_2$, 9% glycerol, bovine serum albumin (0.4 mg/ml), and other additions as indicated, in a final volume of 0.05 ml. The samples were then assayed for RNA polymerase activity and compared with control mixtures from which nucleotides and orthophosphate had been omitted.

The nucleotide specificity of the inactivation process might suggest that adenylylation of the enzyme is involved as in the case of glutamine synthetase (4). However, the fact that CTP and NMN are also weak inactivators makes this possibility unlikely. Moreover, gel filtration of the enzyme after inactivation with radioactively labeled ATP showed that neither the adenylyl moiety nor the terminal phosphate of ATP was covalently linked to the enzyme during the inactivation process. The same experiments also showed that polyadenylate was not formed under the conditions of inactivation. Since covalent modification of RNA polymerase or the production of polyadenylate thus cannot be involved in its inactivation, the most plausible mechanism is a conformational change. Indeed, the sigmoid dependence of inactivation on nucleotide concentration is suggestive of an allosteric effect. Such a mechanism is supported by the effect of the solvent on nucleotide-dependent inactivation. As shown in Fig. 10, inactivation of RNA polymerase by ATP and NAD$^+$ was not observed in the presence of 20% glycerol under conditions where nearly complete inactivation occurred in 5% glycerol. Since the most likely effect of glycerol is on protein conformation, this implicates a conformational transition to a more stable but inactive form, promoted by adenine nucleotides, as the mechanism of the inactivation process.

We cannot yet speculate on the physiological role of nucleotide-dependent inactivation of RNA polymerase in *B. brevis*. However, we have observed that a similar type of inactivation occurs with the RNA polymerases of *Bacillus subtilis*

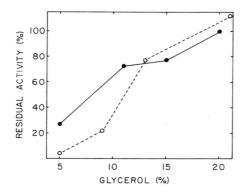

Figure 10. Effect of glycerol on nucleo-tide-dependent inactivation of RNA polymerase. Purified RNA polymerase holoenzyme was incubated for 5 min at 25°C, as described in the footnote to Table II, at the glycerol concentrations indicated in the presence of 2 mM ATP (•) or 2 mM NAD⁺ (○), and the residual activity was assayed.

and *Bacillus polymyxa,* while such a process has not been found in *Escherichia coli.* If this phenomenon is characteristic of *Bacilli* and absent from other bacterial species, it may perhaps have a special function in spore formers.

CONCLUSIONS

It appears that many different ways exist by which small molecules can modulate transcription in *B. brevis.* Thus RNA polymerase is inhibited by specific small peptides, a process that may perhaps represent one of the earliest regulatory events during the transition from vegetative growth to sporulation. In addition, an apparent stimulation of RNA synthesis during sporulation by cyclic GMP is observed, which appears to be due to the inhibition of an intracellular ribonuclease by the cyclic nucleotide, a rather unorthodox but not unreasonable function for cyclic GMP. Finally, RNA polymerase of several *Bacilli* is subject to inactivation by specific nucleotides, which seem to promote a conformational transition of the enzyme to an inactive state. Admittedly, it has not been proved that any of these phenomena represent primary events in sporulation; neverthe-less, the recognition of the many ways in which transcription can be regulated in *Bacilli* is important if we wish to unravel the complex series of steps that occur in the transition of a growing cell into a heat-stable spore, a process that undoubtedly involves the interaction of many different types of control mecha-nisms.

ACKNOWLEDGMENTS

We thank Dr. G. B. Whitfield of the Upjohn Company for a generous gift of streptolydigin. This work was supported by Grant GM-9396 from the National Institute of General Medical Sciences. H. P. is the recipient of Career Develop-ment Award 1-K3-GM-9848 from the U.S. Public Health Service.

REFERENCES

1. G. Balassa. The genetic control of spore formation in bacilli. *Curr. Top. Microbiol.* 56:99 (1971).
2. V. L. Clark and R. W. Bernlohr. Catabolite repression and the enzymes regulating cyclic adenosine 3',5'-monophosphate and cyclic guanosine 3',5'-monophosphate levels in *Bacillus licheniformis*. In H. O. Halvorson, R. Hanson, and L. L. Campbell (eds.), *Spores V* (1972), p. 167, American Society for Microbiology, Washington, D.C.
3. S. T. Jacob, E. M. Sajdel, and H. N. Munro. Specific action of α-amanitin on mammalian RNA polymerase protein. *Nature* 225:60 (1970).
4. H. S. Kingdon, B. M. Shapiro, and E. R. Stadtman. Regulation of glutamine synthetase. VIII. ATP:glutamyl synthetase adenylyl transferase, an enzyme that catalyzes alterations in the regulatory properties of glutamine synthetase. *Proc. Natl. Acad. Sci. (USA)* 58:1703 (1967).
5. H. Paulus. Polymyxins. In D. Gottlieb and P. D. Shaw (eds.), *Antibiotics,* Vol. II, Springer, Berlin (1967), p. 254.
6. N. Sarkar and H. Paulus. Function of peptide antibiotics in sporulation. *Nature New Biol.* 239:228 (1972).
7. N. Sarkar and H. Paulus. Nucleotide-dependent inactivation of RNA polymerase from *Bacillus brevis. Proc. Natl. Acad. Sci. (USA)* 69:3570 (1972).
8. P. Schaeffer. Sporulation and the production of antibiotics, exoenzymes and exotoxins. *Bacteriol. Rev.* 33:48 (1969).
9. R. Schmitt and E. Freese. Curing of a sporulation mutant and antibiotic activity of *Bacillus subtilis. J. Bacteriol.* 96:1255 (1968).
10. J. E. Snoke and N. Cornell. Protoplast lysis and inhibition of growth of *Bacillus licheniformis* by bacitracin. *J. Bacteriol.* 89:415 (1965).
11. T. Yoshida, H. Weissbach, and E. Katz. Inhibitory effect of actinomycin upon the producing organism. *Arch. Biochem. Biophys.* 114:252 (1966).

DISCUSSION

Comment (Sarkar): The effect of cyclic GMP on stimulation of transcription in sporulating cells could actually be due to a combination of two factors. One is stabilization of newly synthesized RNA by inhibiting a specific nuclease with cyclic GMP. The other could be the action of cyclic GMP as a positive control factor of transcription during sporulation, analogous to the cyclic AMP story with catabolite-repressible genes. At present, however, we have conclusive evidence only for the first mode of action; the other remains to be elucidated.

Question (Bose): What is the type of relationship that exists between Sp^+ and Sp^- mutants and antibiotic synthesis?

Answer: We have not studied asporogenic mutants of *B. brevis,* but our earlier work on *B. polymyxa* has revealed a strict correlation between the abilities to sporulate and to produce polymyxin. Also, the very interesting studies of Dr. S. K. Bose at Calcutta University have shown that mutants of *B. subtilis* unable to produce the peptide antibiotic mycobacillin are defective in the ability to sporulate.

Question (Bautz): Have you considered the inactivation by ATP to be due to polyphosphate kinase?

Answer: This is unlikely because we would have observed polyphosphate formation in our gel filtration experiments and because we observed inactivation also with NAD^+.

Question (Adhya): I believe the question of decreased rate of synthesis or degradation RNA may be answered by using shorter pulses of radioactive precursors of RNA. Have you done this experiment?

Answer: The incorporation of [^{3}H]UMP into RNA is a linear function of time for about 5 min in toluenized preparations of both vegetative and sporulating cells. The initial rates of RNA synthesis are very similar in the two cell types. This suggests that the differences observed between vegetative and sporulating cells are mainly due to RNA degradation.

Question (Burma): So far as I understood, you mentioned that rate of degradation of RNA by *B. subtilis* varies at different stages of vegetative growth and sporulation but gross RNase level is not affected. Did you look at specific nucleases? This is interesting because then we can get an idea about the enzyme responsible for the degradation of RNA. If not, have you at least looked at the products formed (oligonuclotides or nucleotides) in order to detect any change in level of exonuclease or endonuclease?

Answer: We are now in the process of purifying the cGMP-sensitive ribonuclease from *B. brevis* to study its properties and mode of action.

Question (Wickner): Does tyrocidine or gramicidin inhibit RNA synthesis by purified sporulation RNA polymerase?

Answer: We have been mainly interested in the changes that occur during the transition from vegetative growth to sporulation and have therefore not purified RNA polymerase from sporulating cells. However, the questions you raise is an interesting one which should be investigated.

Question (Salahuddin): You said that cyclic peptides cause denaturation of RNA polymerase. Did you use any physical parameter to show that indeed there is a conformation change which is caused by the antibiotics? Have you only used inactivation of the enzyme by the antibiotics as a criterion for denaturation?

Answer: Denaturation occurs only at high antibiotic concentrations. To avoid such non-specific effects, we have confined our studies to low concentrations of antibiotics where inhibition is freely reversible by dilution and therefore is not due to denaturation but must represent a more specific phenomenon.

Question (Chakravorty): During the early phase of sporulation, you find that incorporation of uracil into RNA is inhibited. If I understood you correctly, you mean to say the cyclic peptide antibiotic synthesized during this period is inhibiting RNA polymerase. But there are other reasons for which one may get less incorporation of labeled uracil, e.g., a change in permeability or a sudden expansion of the cellular pool of nucleoside or nucleotide. Did you look into those possibilities?

Answer: We have not directly measured permeability to small molecules or nucleotide pools during the early stages of sporulation. However, we have noted no change in the incorporation of [^{14}C]leucine into protein and only a small decline in the incorporation of [^{14}C]adenine into DNA under conditions where the incorporation of [^{14}C]uracil into RNA is greatly reduced. This suggests that the decline in the incorporation of radioactive precursor into RNA is not due to changes in permeability or intracellular pools.

4

Control of Transcription in Phage P22 Infected Host

Maharani Chakravorty, P. S. Khandekar, G. R. Koteswara Rao,* and Sushil Taneja

Molecular Biology Unit
Department of Biochemistry
Institute of Medical Sciences
Banaras Hindu University
Varanasi, India

Phage P22, a temperate phage of *Salmonella typhimurium,* upon infection induces either of two types of response in the host: lytic or lysogenic. In the lytic response, the phage multiplies inside the host and the progeny particles come out after lysing the cell. Sometimes the bacteria survive the infection; the virus DNA integrates with the host DNA and gives rise to lysogenic cells. The lysogenic bacteria are immune to superinfection by homoimmune phages. The immunity to superinfection is due to the presence of repressor protein in the cytoplasm of the lysogenic cell. Being a temperate phage, P22 possesses more complicated regulatory processes than the virulent phages, which produce only one kind of response leading to lysis of the cells.

Whether a bacterium will be lysed or lysogenized following infection with wild-type phage, $P22C^+$, depends on the multiplicity of infection (6). To establish lysogeny, it is essential that the vegetative development of the phage be stopped first. This initial phase of repression, known as "reduction" (24), is controlled by three closely linked genes, C_1, C_2, and C_3. Mutation in C_1 or C_2 results in 100% lytic response, but somewhat less in C_3. All three are termed

*Present address: National Institute of Arthritis and Metabolic Diseases, National Institutes of Health, Bethesda, Maryland, U.S.A.

"clear mutants," as they produce clear plaques in contrast to the turbid plaques produced by the wild-type, P22C$^+$.

The two genes C_1 and C_2 function sequentially to repress phage replication. Infection with the clear mutants represses host protein synthesis, and phage-specific protein synthesis starts very early (around 4 min following infection) and continues thereafter (12). But even in the case of infections leading to

Table I. Description of Genes of Phage P22 Shown in Fig. 1[a]

Gene	Mutant phenotype	Reference
19	Lysis defective, no lysozyme	Botstein et al., cited by Levine (19)
h_{21}	Plaque morphology	Levine (17), Levine and Curtiss (21)
13	Lysis defective	Botstein et al., cited by Levine (19)
12	DNA synthesis defective, integration defective	Gough and Levine (14), Levine and Schott (22)
18	"	Levine and Schott (22)
C_1, C_2, C_3	Clear plaques	Levine (17), Levine and Curtiss (21)
K_s, V_x	Operator constitutive mutants	Bronson and Levine (8)
int	Integration defective	Smith and Levine (30), Smith (28)
sie	Failure to exclude superinfecting phage	Rao (25)
mnt	Lysogeny defective, maintenance defective	Zinder (32), Gough (13)
25	DNA synthesis defective, no association of DNA with intermediate I	Bezdek and Soska (1), Levine et al. (20)
m_3	Plaque morphology	Levine (17), Levine and Curtiss (21)

[a]att is the site at which the phage chromosome is opened during insertion into bacterial chromosomes (28).

lysogeny, a lytic situation exists at the very first phase, although the situation is subsequently overcome. For example, phage-specific protein synthesis continues for some time (12), and synthesis of L-arabinose isomerase, a host-specific protein, is temporarily repressed (10); there is also a burst of phage DNA synthesis with simultaneous inhibition of that of the host (29). All these events are discernible between 4 and 8 min after infection. Even the association of the parental DNA with the membrane complex, which is the site of phage DNA replication (3-5), does not start before 5 min or so.

We shall first discuss the phage-induced events that happen before the so-called early events discussed above. These will be termed "pre-early events." The regulation of the pre-early events as well as the control of late transcription is dealt with in detail. The brief description and the relative map position of the mutants used for the study are listed in Table I and Fig. 1, respectively.

PRE-EARLY EVENTS FOLLOWING INFECTION

One of the first discernible changes following infection is transient depression of macromolecular synthesis (11). The rates of overall RNA and protein synthesis, followed by pulsing the cells with labeled precursors, decline immediately after infection and reach a minimum between 3 and 5 min and then begin to recover (Fig. 2). The extent of inhibition as well as the time of recovery

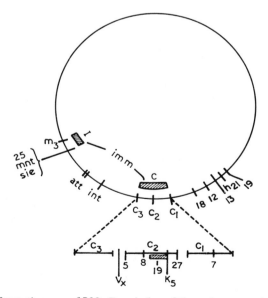

Fig. 1. Vegetative map of P22. Description of the various genes is in Table I.

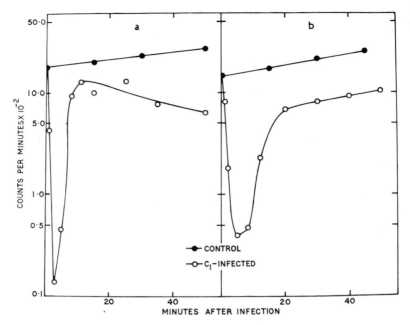

Fig. 2. Effect of $C_1 h_{21}$ infection on the rate of RNA (a) and protein (b) synthesis in Salmonella typhimurium. Cells growing exponentially in unsupplemented minimal medium (generation time in this medium is 60 min at 37°C) were infected at a m.o.i. of 20 and kept at 37°C with constant shaking. Infection was done at a cell density of 2.5×10^8 c/ml. At different times following infection, 1 ml of cell suspension was transferred into tubes containing [^{14}C] uracil (3.3 nmoles; 5×10^4 cpm) and incubated at 37°C with constant shaking. The reaction was stopped after 1 min by adding 1 ml of ice-cold 10% trichloroacetic acid. Acid-insoluble counts were determined after collecting and washing the trichloroacetic acid insoluble material on Millipore filters. The rate of protein synthesis was measured by labeling the cells with L-[^{14}C] leucine in much the same way as described for [^{14}C] uracil. The volume of the cell suspension for each sample was 0.5 ml; L-[^{14}C] leucine, 0.22 nmole containing 8×10^3 cpm, was present in each incubation mixture during pulsing, and the pulsing was done for 30 sec. From Chakravorty and Bhattacharya (11).

depends on the multiplicity of infection (m.o.i.). Chloramphenicol has no effect on the depression in the rate of RNA synthesis. It is quite possible that the pre-early protein involved in host depression is chloramphenicol insensitive.

At this point, it was essential to know whether or not phage gene expression is a prerequisite for such drastic repression of macromolecular synthesis. The product of gene 25 is required very early after infection for the association of parental DNA with the membrane complex (1,20). Hence this particular mutant would give us an idea whether the expression of the gene(s) needed to depress the macromolecular synthesis takes place before that of gene 25. Interestingly enough, infection with *ts25* causes no depression in the rate of protein synthesis and only partial depression in the rate of RNA synthesis, which recovers very slowly (11).

Superinfecting P22 cannot grow in a lysogen even if the immunity repressor is destroyed. It is only the prophage that multiplies, and the superinfecting phage is excluded. Growth of superinfecting P22 in a lysogen is prevented not only due to the presence of immunity repressor but also due to the exclusion phenomenon controlled by the *sie* locus of P22. Heteroimmune phages such as L, MG178, and MG40 (related to P22) also cannot grow on the wild-type lysogen, called *sie*$^+$ lysogen. *Sie*$^-$ lysogens, in which the *sie* gene of the prophage is mutated, support the growth of heteroimmune phages. The expression of the superinfecting phage genome is not expected in lysogens. Therefore, it was of interest to measure the rates of macromolecular synthesis in *sie*$^+$ and *sie*$^-$ lysogens after superinfection with the clear mutants of P22 (Fig. 3). As expected, there is no depression in the rate of RNA and protein synthesis in *sie*$^+$ lysogen. By contrast, RNA and protein synthesis undergo transient depression in *sie*$^-$ lysogen. It seems that the *sie* gene, like the C_2 gene, produces some regulatory protein that controls the expression of the gene(s) necessary for the inhibition of macromolecular synthesis.

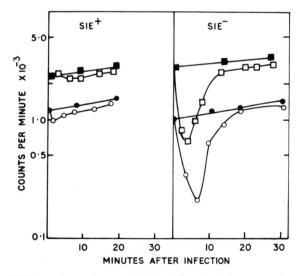

Fig. 3. Rates of RNA and protein synthesis in sie$^+$ and sie$^-$ lysogens after superinfection with C_1 mutant. Infection was carried out with the same C_1 mutant as in Fig. 2 at a m.o.i. of 10. The rates of RNA synthesis (●, uninfected; ○, infected) as well as protein synthesis (■, uninfected; □, infected) were followed. From Chakravorty and Bhattacharya (11).

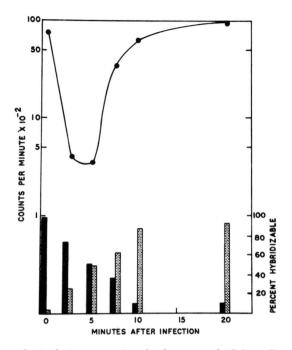

Fig. 4. RNA synthesis during vegetative development of $C_1 h_{21}$. *Growing cells of S. typhimurium were infected with* $C_1 h_{21}$ *at a m.o.i. of 10. The upper portion of the figure represents the rate of RNA synthesis in infected host at different times after infection. Experimental conditions for determination of rate of RNA synthesis are as described for Fig. 2. The lower portion of the figure represents relative amounts of host- and phage-specific RNAs determined with the help of a DNA·RNA hybridization technique (15). Solid bars, host-specific RNA; dotted bars, phage-specific RNA.*

Such depression in the rates of macromolecular synthesis was eventually found to be due to a transient alteration in the active transport process across the membrane of the host (27).

TRANSCRIPTION DURING THE DEVELOPMENT OF P22

The question arises whether the phage genome is expressed during the period of drastic inhibition of macromolecular synthesis immediately following infection. It would also be of interest to know how much host transcription takes place during the period of recovery. Hence the phage- and host-specific transcriptions were measured by isolating labeled mRNAs produced at various stages of infection with different mutants and subsequently annealed with phage and host DNAs.

Transcription Following Infection with Clear Mutants of P22

As shown earlier (Fig. 2), infection of sensitive cells with $C_1 h_{21}$, a clear mutant, results in a transient depression of macromolecular synthesis. During this period of depression, the host-specific transcription is decreased and phage-specific transcription is discernible even from 3 min after infection (Fig. 4). The switchover from host- to phage-specific transcription starts during this period.

When the transient depression in macromolecular synthesis was studied with another clear mutant, $m_3 C_2 h_{21}$, the drastic repression of RNA synthesis was observed, but subsequently there was not much recovery (Fig. 5). It has already been observed that in $C_1 h_{21}$ infection phage-specific transcription is quite significant from 3 min onward and continues almost at an exponential rate

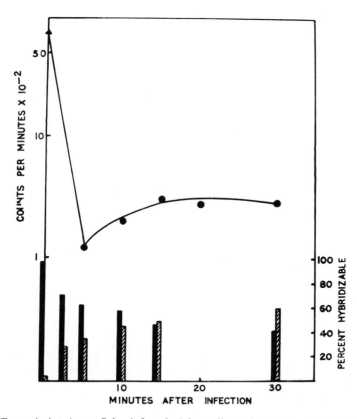

Fig. 5. Transcription in $m_3 C_2 h_{21}$-infected Salmonella typhimurium. Conditions of the experiment were as described in Fig. 2. Presentation of figure the same as for Fig. 4. Solid bars, host-specific RNA; shaded bars, phage-specific RNA.

during the quick recovery from the transient depression of total RNA synthesis. In $m_3 C_2 h_{21}$ infection, the host- and phage-specific transcriptions are comparable to those following $C_1 h_{21}$ infection up to 3 min. Later, both host- and phage-specific mRNA syntheses remain inhibited. Active transport processes across the host membrane also never recover, and the infected cell loses viability.

Membrane-Bound Transcription of P22

Within about 5 min following infection, the input phage DNA starts associating with the membrane of the host. This membrane complex has been designated

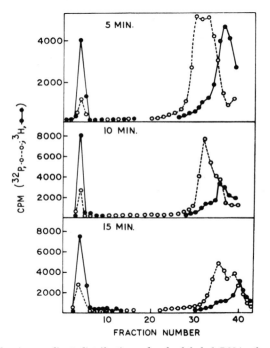

Fig. 6. Sucrose density gradient distribution of pulse-labeled RNA after phage infection. Exponentially growing cells (10^8/ml) were infected with ^{32}P-labeled phage ($C_1 h_{21}$ mutant) at a m.o.i. of 20. At 5, 10, and 15 min following infection, samples (0.5 ml) were pipetted into tubes containing 25 μc of [^{3}H]uridine (20 c/mmole); after 1 min, the reaction was stopped as usual with unlabeled uridine and lysis mixture. The lysate was prepared according to the method of Botstein (3), and a sample (0.2 ml) was layered on 5–20% neutral sucrose, centrifuged for 60 min at 35,000 rpm at 20°C in a Spinco rotor SW39. Recovery of ^{32}P was more than 90%. Samples (5 drops) were collected by piercing the tube at the bottom and processed for determination of trichloroacetic acid precipitable counts as described by Botstein (3).

"intermediate I" and is found to be the site for replication of phage DNA (3-5,20). Although the assumption has been made that, under normal physiological conditions, replication, transcription, and translation take place in a coupled system (7,9), not much information is available regarding the role of the replication complex in the transcription process. In order to check whether any transcription takes place in the replication complex, the cells were infected with ^{32}P-labeled $C_1 h_{21}$ phage. Samples were collected at different times, lysed gently, and analyzed on a sucrose density gradient (Fig. 6). A fraction of the pulse-labeled RNA is found to be membrane bound, sedimenting along with the intermediate I, and the rest is seen as free RNA. As infection proceeds, more and more of the pulse-labeled RNA is found in the replication complex. This may be due to the availability of more template in the complex, as the ratio of input DNA and the amount of RNA synthesized remains constant. That the radioactivity is incorporated into RNA was quite evident from the alkali lability of the labeled material. To elucidate whether the membrane-bound RNA in the phage-infected host was transcribed from the phage genome, DNA · RNA hybridization of purified preparations of both the membrane-bound and the free cytoplas-

Table II. Hybridization of Membrane-Bound and Free RNA with Phage or Host DNA[a]

Cpm of input RNA	DNA	Amount of DNA on filter (μg)	Cpm hybridized	Percent hybridized
A. Membrane-bound RNA				
1. 13,260	Phage	8	6,700	50
2. 13,260	Host	6	142	1.07
3. 6,200	Phage	8	3,371	54
4. 6,200	Host	6	80	1.2
B. Free RNA				
1. 6,000	Phage	5	800	13.
2. 6,000	Host	8.7	38	0.6
3. 9,000	Phage	50	3,281	36
4. 9,000	Host	50	1,314	14
C. Host mRNA				
1. 17,640	Phage	30	130	0.7
2. 20,000	Host	40	16,000	80

[a]mRNA was isolated from infected cells exposed to [^{3}H]uridine for 24 sec. DNA-RNA hybridization was carried out on a nitrocellulose membrane filter by the method of Gillespie and Spiegelman (15).

mic RNAs of the infected host was carried out with host and phage DNAs. The results presented in Table II show that membrane-bound RNA hybridizes exclusively with phage DNA. This indicates that after phage infection only phage DNA is transcribed in the complex. Although the major fraction of the cytoplasmic RNA is found to be phage specific, it contains host-specific RNA as well. Thus it confirms that host transcription is not completely shut off even in case of infection leading to lysis. The above experiments definitely indicate that the intermediate I or replication complex is also a site for transcription and that the transcription of the phage DNA alone takes place in the complex after phage infection. The fraction of phage genome transcribed in intermediate I was determined by hybridization experiments in which the maximum amount of DNA · RNA hybrid formed with a fixed amount of DNA was measured. The saturation curve (Fig. 7) indicates that for saturation of all the sites of DNA available for hybridization the amount of RNA required is approximately half the amount of DNA loaded on the filter. Thus within the limits of detection the entire phage genome is transcribed in the replication complex. It is quite possible that this transcription at the membrane site is required for replication and is not involved in the gene expression, suggesting that replication and transcription are coupled under physiological conditions.

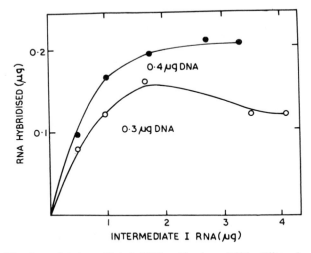

Fig. 7. Hybridization of intermediate-I RNA with phage DNA. Filters loaded with denatured phage DNA were punched to make smaller circular discs (7-mm diameter). Two sets of hybridizations were carried out. One set contained 0.4 μg DNA, the other set 0.3 μg DNA per filter. Amount of RNA added is as indicated. Hybridization was carried out as described by Gillespie and Spiegelman (15).

CONTROL OF LATE TRANSCRIPTION

It has already been shown that the clear mutant $m_3 C_2 h_{21}$ produces permanent depression in macromolecular synthesis (Fig. 5). Usually, the infections are carried out at a m.o.i. of 20 because the multiplicity-dependent transient depression is very significant at this m.o.i. It was observed that the mutant $m_3 C_2 h_{21}$ never yields lysates with reasonable PFU/ml unless the infection is carried out at a very low m.o.i. Even at a m.o.i. of 10, the burst size is much lower than that of $C_1 h_{21}$. Careful pulsing experiments revealed that the permanent depression observed in $m_3 C_2 h_{21}$ is multiplicity dependent. At lower m.o.i. (e.g., 5), there is recovery in the rate of macromolecular synthesis.

Effects of M.o.i. on the Multiplication of $C_1 h_{21}$ and $m_3 C_2 h_{21}$

As mentioned above, the depression in macromolecular synthesis following $m_3 C_2 h_{21}$ infection is transient at low m.o.i. but permanent at high. If phage transcription is repressed at high m.o.i., it should be reflected in the development of phage particles. Hence the physiology of development of the mutant

Table III. Effect of M.o.i. on the Multiplication of $C_1 h_{21}$ and $m_3 C_2 h_{21}$[a]

M.o.i.	$C_1 h_{21}$		$m_3 C_2 h_{21}$	
	Infective centers (PFU/ml)	Burst size	Infective centers (PFU/ml)	Burst size
2	1.3×10^8	177	1.8×10^8	240
5	2.5×10^8	220	2.4×10^8	183
10	2.5×10^8	400	2.5×10^8	144
20	2.6×10^8	380	2.4×10^8	8
50	2.5×10^8	200	6.8×10^7	2
100	2.9×10^8	186	1.1×10^7	1

[a]LT2 cells were grown in minimal medium up to a cell density of 2.6×10^8/ml and infected with either $C_1 h_{21}$ or $m_3 C_2 h_{21}$ at the indicated m.o.i. in presence of 1 mM NaCN. After allowing 5 min for absorption, 0.1 ml of the infected cell suspension was diluted with 0.9 ml medium containing P22 antiserum (final $K = 2$). The antiserum treatment was done for 5 min, and infective centers were measured by plating the antiserum-treated suspension after suitable dilution. Properly diluted samples of the infected cells were incubated at 37°C for 2 hr and treated with chloroform, suitably diluted, and plated to determine the final phage yield. Burst size was calculated from the infective centers irrespective of the number of cells used for infection.

was studied using burst size as an index. These results (Table III) also support the multiplicity repression phenomenon observed with the C_2 mutant ($m_3C_2h_{21}$). The burst size of C_1h_{21} varies within a range of about 200–400, which has no direct relationship with m.o.i. The infective centers produced are also fairly constant except at low m.o.i. (m.o.i. = 2), which is expected. In $m_3C_2h_{21}$ infection, however, an entirely different situation is observed. Although the infective centers remain fairly constant at m.o.i.s between 2 and 20, their number is considerably reduced at high m.o.i.s. Apparently, most of the cells lose their capacity to produce the phage under these conditions. This is also reflected in the burst size calculated on the basis of the infective centers obtained.

Multiplicity Repression Effect in Various C_2 Mutants

The multiplicity repression effect observed in the $m_3C_2h_{21}$ mutant may be the characteristic of the particular mutant, as in case of L phage, a phage closely related to P22 (2). A group of mutants having a defect in the right-hand side of gene II of L phage (equivalent to gene C_2 of P22) exhibit the multiplicity repression effect. Therefore, the infective centers formed following infection of *S. typhimurium* with a number of C_2 mutants and the burst sizes of these mutants were determined (Table IV). All the infections were carried out at a m.o.i. of 20. It is clear that all the C_2 mutants have extremely low burst size. Since the C_2 mutants chosen map over a wide range of the C_2 region, the multiplicity repression is not exerted by any particular C_2 region, as reported for L phage (2).

Table IV. Multiplicity Repression Effect
in Various C_2 Mutants[a]

Mutant	Infective centers (PFU/ml)	Burst size
$+C_1h_{21}$	2.3×10^8	325
$m_3C_2h_{21}$	2.0×10^8	10
$m_3C_2^5h_{21}$	2.4×10^8	19
$m_3C_2^6h_{21}$	1.1×10^8	11
$m_3C_2^{19}h_{21}$	1.5×10^8	19
$m_3C_2^{27}h_{21}$	1.1×10^8	12
$m_3C_2^8+$	9.7×10^7	4

[a]The procedure was essentially the same as described in Table III except that the m.o.i. was 20 in all cases.

Effect of Mutation in the m_3 Gene on the Development of Phage P22

It is rather difficult to assume that the mutation in the C_2 gene, which is responsible for the production of repressor, results in the repression of phage development. All the C_2 mutants tested had the morphology marker m_3; therefore, it was suspected that the gene m_3 may play a regulatory role in the expression of late genes of P22. To check this, various isogenic strains of P22 were isolated with respect to the m_3 marker and tested for their ability to undergo vegetative development. It is quite clear that the presence of m_3 marker is invariably associated with the multiplicity repression (Table V).

Induction of Lysozyme Following Infections with $C_1 h_{21}$ and $m_3 C_2 h_{21}$

To be sure that the m_3 gene regulates the late transcription, induction of lysozyme, a phage-specific late protein was studied. The P22 lysozyme has been

Table V. Effect of m_3 Mutation
on the Multiplication of P22[a]

Mutants	M.o.i.	Burst size
+$C_1 h_{21}$	5	183
	50	200
+$C_2 h_{21}$	5	183
	50	142
+C_1 +	5	180
	50	160
+C_2 +	5	200
	50	180
$m_3 C_1 h_{21}$	5	10
	50	1.4
$m_3 C_2 h_{21}$	5	200
	50	2.3
$m_3 C_1$ +	5	5
	50	14
$m_3 C_2$ +	5	20
	50	4

[a]The procedure was essentially the same as described in Table III.

purified from P22-infected cells, and its properties have been studied in detail in our laboratory (26). This late protein, lysozyme, was very conveniently used as a marker to follow the expression of late genes of the phage. Time courses of lysozyme induction following infections with $C_1 h_{21}$ and $m_3 C_2 h_{21}$ are shown in Fig. 8. As expected, lysozyme induction is delayed in $m_3 C_2 h_{21}$ infection, and the amount of lysozyme produced is much less than in $C_1 h_{21}$ infection.

Kinetics of Intermediate-I Formation Following Infection with $C_1 h_{21}$ and $m_3 C_2 h_{21}$

In order to be certain that the regulatory role of m_3 is in connection with late transcription only, some early gene expression had to be studied as well. Unfortunately, however, with the P22 system there is no convenient method available to follow the early gene expression. As mentioned already, the membrane complex (intermediate I), which is undoubtedly a complex between phage DNA and host cell component, plays a central role in phage DNA replication. Parental DNA starts appearing in the complex from 5 min onward. For this association, the product of gene 25 must be synthesized early in infection (19). Therefore, the kinetics of association of parental DNA to the intermediate I has been used as a measure of early transcription of P22. The two strains $C_1 h_{21}$ and $m_3 C_2 h_{21}$ behave in the same way so far as the initial kinetics of association of the parental DNA to the intermediate I is concerned (Fig. 9). In both cases, association starts from 5 min and reaches a maximum around 15 min. Appar-

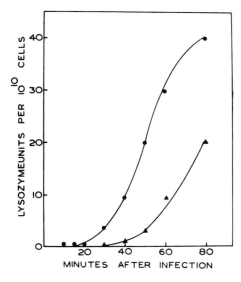

Fig. 8. Induction of lysozyme in Salmonella typhimurium following infection with $C_1 h_{21}$ and $m_3 C_2 h_{21}$ mutants of phage P22. The m.o.i. was 10. Assay of lysozyme was as described by Rao and Burma (26). The total activity (activity in the cell-free extracts plus that in the medium) was plotted. ●, $C_1 h_{21}$ infected; ▲, $m_3 C_2 h_{21}$ infected.

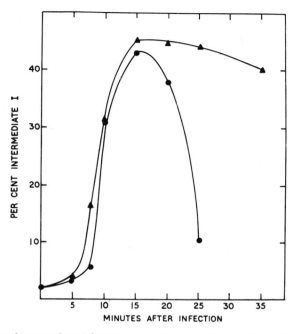

Fig. 9. Kinetics of intermediate-I formation in $C_1 h_{21}$ - *and* $m_3 C_2 h_{21}$ *-infected Salmonella typhimurium.* The m.o.i. in each case was 20. The intermediate-I formation was measured as described by Levine *et al.* (20). •, $C_1 h_{21}$ infected; ▲, $m_3 C_2 h_{21}$ infected.

ently, the invading $m_3 C_2 h_{21}$ DNA associates with the membrane complex at a normal rate and the early transcription is not affected. Although $C_1 h_{21}$ DNA is released readily from the complex, as reported earlier (20), an entirely different situation is observed in $m_3 C_2 h_{21}$ infection. In the latter case, DNA remains associated with the complex and very little is released even after another 20 min. Release of parental DNA requires expression of late genes (19). The failure to release parental DNA in $m_3 C_2 h_{21}$ infection may be connected with the repression of late transcription.

CONCLUSION

It is clear from the above presentation that complex regulatory processes are operative in the development of the temperate phage P22 in its host *S. typhimurium.* Some of these processes, occurring at the level of transcription, have been discussed above. One of the most interesting pre-early events following infection is the transient depression in macromolecular synthesis, which is due to the temporary block of the active transport processes across the membrane of the host. This is regulated by the expression of one or more pre-early genes of P22. The *sie* gene, which maps close to the second immunity region of P22, plays the most important role in this connection. Although the mechanism of interference with active transport is not understood at present, furtherance of knowledge in this area may add a new member to the list of the regulatory mechanisms known to be operative at the level of replication, transcription, and translation. The importance of the membrane of the host in the vegetative multiplication of phage has been amply justified from earlier studies as well as the present one. Even though the purpose of transcription of all the genes of P22 at the site of the membrane is not understood yet, its involvement in the replication process as well as the release of the newly synthesized DNA from the replication complex may be visualized. The regulation of late transcription of P22 is also reflected at the site of formation of replication complex. Both active transport and release of parental phage DNA from the replication complex are blocked when the expression of the late genes is repressed. Further study of these phenomena may lead to the understanding of some of the genetic regulatory mechanisms. The role of the m_3 gene, which has so far been treated as only a morphology marker, in the negative regulation of late gene expression is most intriguing. The complex relationship between the m_3 gene and the late genes needs further exploration.

ACKNOWLEDGMENTS

P.S.K. and S.T. are Junior Research Fellows of the Council of Scientific and Industrial Research, New Delhi.

The financial assistance received from the Council of Scientific and Industrial Research and the Indian Council of Medical Research is gratefully acknowledged. Sincerest thanks are due to Professor Myron Levine, Department of Human Genetics, University of Michigan, Ann Arbor, Michigan, U.S.A., for helpful suggestions and a supply of some of the mutants of phage P22. The experiments described in Figs. 6 and 7 and Table II were carried out in his laboratory, by one of the authors (M. C.). Thanks are also due to Macmillan Journals Limited for permission to reproduce Figs. 2 and 3, from the Chakravorty and Bhattacharya (11).

REFERENCES

1. M. Bezdek and J. Soska. Evidence for an early regulatory function in phage P22. *Mol. Gen. Genet.* **108:** 243-248 (1970).
2. M. Bezdek, J. Soska, and P. Amati. Properties of P22 and a related *Salmonella typhimurium* phage. (III.) Studies on clear plaque mutants of phage L. *Virology* **40:**505-513 (1970).

3. D. Botstein. Synthesis and maturation of phage P22 DNA. I. Identification of inter-mediates. *J. Mol. Biol.* **34**:621-641. (1968).

4. D. Botstein and M. Levine. Synthesis and maturation of phage P22 DNA. II. Properties of temperature sensitive phage mutants defective in DNA metabolism. *J. Mol. Biol.* **34**:643-654 (1968).

5. D. Botstein and M. Levine. Intermediates in the synthesis of phage P22 DNA. *Cold Spring Harbor Symp. Quant. Biol.* **33**:659-667 (1968).

6. J. S. K. Boyd. Observations on the relationship of symbiotic and lytic bacteriophage. *J. Pathol. Bacteriol.* **63**:445-457 (1951).

7. H. Bremmer and M. W. Konrad. A complex of enzymatically synthesized RNA and templated DNA. *Proc. Natl. Acad. Sci. (USA)* **51**:801-808 (1964).

8. M. J. Bronson and M. Levine. Virulent mutants of P22. I. Isolation and genetic analysis. *J. Virol.* **7**:559-568 (1971).

9. R. Byrne, L. G. Levine, H. A. Bladen, and M. W. Nirenberg. The *in vitro* formation of a DNA ribosome complex. *Proc. Natl. Acad. Sci. (USA)* **52**: 140-148 (1964).

10. M. Chakravorty. Induction and repression of L-arabinose isomerase in bacteriophage infected *Salmonella typhimurium. J. Virol.* **5**:541-547 (1970).

11. M. Chakravorty and A. K. Bhattacharya. Role of *sie* gene in the transient depression of macromolecular synthesis in phage P22 infected *Salmonella typhimurium. Nature New Biol.* **234**:145-147 (1971).

12. L. W. Cohen and M. Levine. Detection of proteins synthesized during the establishment of lysogeny with phage P22. *Virology* **28**:208-213 (1966).

13. M. Gough. Second locus of bacteriophage P22 necessary for maintenance of lysogeny. *J. Virol.* **2**:992-998 (1968).

14. M. Gough and M. Levine. Circularity of the phage P22 linkage map. *Genetics* **58**:161-169 (1968).

15. D. Gillespie and S. Spiegelman. A quantitative assay for DNA-RNA hybrids with DNA immobilized on a membrane. *J. Mol. Biol.* **12**:829-842 (1965).

16. R. A. Kolstad and H. H. Prell. An amber map of *Salmonella* phage P22. *Mol. Gen. Genet.* **104**: 339-350 (1969).

17. M. Levine. Mutations in the temperate phage P22 and lysogeny in *Salmonella. Virology* **3**: 22-41 (1957).

18. M. Levine. Effect of mitomycin C in interactions between temperate phages and bacteria. *Virology* **13**:493-499 (1961).

19. M. Levine. Replication and lysogeny with phage P22 in *Salmonella typhimurium. Curr. Top. Microbiol. Immunol.* **58**:135-156 (1972).

20. M. Levine, M. Chakravorty, and M. J. Bronson. Control of the replication complex of bacteriophage P22. *J. Virol.* **6**:400-405 (1970).

21. M. Levine and R. Curtiss. Genetic fine structure of the *C* region and the linkage map of phage P22. *Genetics* **46**:1573-1580 (1961).

22. M. Levine and C. Schott. Mutation of phage P22 affecting bacteriophage DNA synthesis and lysogenization. *J. Mol. Biol.* **62**:53-64 (1971).

23. M. Levine and H. O. Smith. Sequential gene action in the establishment of lysogeny. *Science* **146**:1581-1582 (1964).

24. A. Lwoff. Lysogeny. *Bacteriol. Rev.* **17**:269-337 (1953).

25. R. N. Rao. Bacteriophage P22 controlled exclusion in *Salmonella typhimurium. J. Mol. Biol.* **35**:607-622 (1968).

26. G. R. K. Rao and D. P. Burma. Purification and properties of phage P22-induced lysozyme. *J. Biol. Chem.* **246**:6474-6479 (1971).

27. G. R. K. Rao, M. Chakravorty, and D. P. Burma. Transient depression in the active transport across the membrane of *Salmonella typhimurium* after infection with bacteriophage P22. *Virology* **49**:811-814 (1972).

28. H. O. Smith. Defective phage formation by lysogens of integration deficient phage P22 mutants. *Virology* **34**:203-223 (1968).

29. H. O. Smith and M. Levine. The synthesis of phage and host DNA in establishment of lysogeny. *Virology* **25**:585-590 (1965).

30. H. O. Smith and M. Levine. A phage P22 gene controlling integration of prophage. *Virology* **31**:207-216 (1967).

31. M. M. Susskind, A. Wright, and D. Botstein. Superinfection exclusion by P22 prophage in lysogens of *Salmonella typhimurium*. II. Genetic evidence for two exclusion systems. *Virology* **45**:638-652 (1971).

32. N. D. Zinder. Lysogenisation and superinfection immunity in *Salmonella*. *Virology* **5**:291-326 (1958).

DISCUSSION

Question (Mandal): Is there any information about whether RNA polymerase of the host also transcribes the P22 genes or whether some altered RNA polymerase preferentially transcribes the P22 genes?

Answer: So far, there is no report regarding the induction of P22-specific RNA polymerase or alteration of host polymerase following P22 infection.

5

New Small Proteins Associated with DNA-Dependent RNA Polymerase of *Escherichia coli* After Infection with T4 Phage

Audrey Stevens and R. Diane Crowder

Biology Division
Oak Ridge National Laboratory
Oak Ridge, Tennessee, U.S.A.

T4 phage infection of *Escherichia coli* involves several changes in the transcription process that are very interesting with respect to control mechanisms. Almost coincident with infection, transcription of *E. coli* DNA ceases (1-4) and formation of early species of T4 messenger RNA (mRNA) begins. Shortly after T4 DNA replication starts (6–7 min after infection), a second part of the T4 DNA molecule is transcribed, producing late T4 mRNA. The early-to-late change has been studied in some detail by several investigators (5-8). Late T4 mRNA synthesis is dependent on DNA replication (9-11) or a DNA structure prepared for replication (12). This change from early to late transcription also involves a switchover in transcription from the *l* to the *r* strand of the T4 DNA (13).

We became interested in the T4 transcription process when studies suggested that the transcriptional changes might result from a modification of the DNA-dependent RNA polymerase of *E. coli*. Bautz and Dunn (14) first reported the loss of the σ subunit from the purified RNA polymerase as an early event after T4 phage infection. Seifert *et al.* (15) reported that the α subunit is altered early (2–5 min after infection at 37°C) in the infection process, and Goff and Weber (16) showed that the modification of α involves the addition of a phosphorylated compound to the α subunit. Changes in the polymerase have also been found later in the infection process. Using a mutant of *E. coli* with a temperature-sensitive RNA polymerase, Khesin (17) showed that one of the large subunits, probably β', is altered. In addition, Travers (18) showed a change in the electrophoretic properties of β', and Schachner and Zillig (19) have reported that the β, β', and a subunits all undergo amino acid changes as detected by analyses of tryptic peptides. We have found, from labeling studies after T4 phage infection, that new small proteins are bound to the polymerase starting at about 6 min after infection (20). Whether or not the new small proteins are responsible for some of the just-mentioned late changes in a, β, and β' is not yet known. All of the polymerase changes occur after infection with T4 early (Do) amber mutants.

We originally undertook labeling of proteins with amino acids to study the fate of the polymerase subunits following T4 phage infection. Figure 1 shows the end products of two labeling experiments, i.e., two different types of gel analyses of labeled purified enzyme from T4 phage infected cells. In the experiment shown in Fig. 1A, *E. coli* B cells were labeled before infection with [^{3}H]leucine and after infection with a mixture of ^{14}C-labeled amino acids. After the labeling period, normal carrier cells were added and RNA polymerase was purified as described previously (20). Normal carrier cells were used because of ease of purification. The enzyme was denatured with sodium dodecylsulfate (SDS), and the labeled subunits were examined on 11% polyacrylamide-SDS gels, run as described by Weber and Osborn (21). The results of the ^{3}H labeling (solid line) show that the main polymerase subunits—β, β', σ, and a—all are

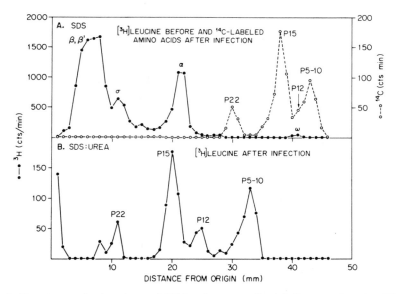

Fig. 1. Two types of gel analyses of RNA polymerase after labeling experiments with T4 amN82 phage. The experiments were carried out as described previously (20).

labeled. During infection, there is no measurable loss of ^{3}H; i.e., the main subunits have the same specific activity at 25 min after T4 phage infection as before infection. The dashed line shows the distribution of the postinfection ^{14}C on the gel. Three main ^{14}C bands are found. Figure 1B shows an analysis of a labeled enzyme on SDS-urea gels run as described by Swank and Munkres (22) and designed to separate proteins of low molecular weight. The only label used was [^{3}H]leucine after T4 infection. Four bands of small labeled proteins are found. The new small proteins are designated on the basis of their molecular weights, determined by gel analysis (20), as P22, with a mol wt of 22,000, and, accordingly, P15, mol wt 15,000; P12, mol wt 12,000; and P5 or 10, mol wt 5000 or 10,000 (depending on the gel used for analysis).

All the labeling experiments showed that there was little incorporation of label following T4 phage infection into any of the main host polymerase subunits. A small incorporation would be expected because the infection process is not 100% efficient. Table I shows a calculation of the total amount of label in the main subunits as compared to that in the new small ones after a postinfection ^{14}C amino acid labeling experiment. The total amount in the four main subunits was about 10% of that in P15. No main subunit was labeled more than another, and all were labeled after infection with different T4 phage mutants.

By pulse labels at different times after infection, it was found that P5-10 is synthesized first, starting at about 5 min after infection at 30°C (20). P22, P15, and P12 are synthesized shortly thereafter and labeled at high rates in the 8- to 11-min postinfection interval. At 20 min, some incorporation of label into P22, P15, and P12 was found, with that into P22 being highest. The kinetics of synthesis of the new small subunits suggest that they might be involved in the change from early to late mRNA synthesis, as inhibitors of early synthesis and/or as promoters of late synthesis. Certainly they are formed too late to be involved in the change from host mRNA to early T4 mRNA synthesis.

Because of the possible involvement of the new small proteins in late mRNA synthesis, T4 phage mutants in genes 55 and 33 were used in labeling experi-

Table I. Comparison of the ^{14}C Content of the Main Polymerase Subunits with That of the New Polypeptides Following a Postinfection Label with ^{14}C-Labeled Amino Acids

Subunits	^{14}C (cpm)
β, β' σ, α	60
P22	150
P15	600
P12 + P5-10	500

ments. Gene-55 and -33 mutants were first described by Bolle *et al.* (11). T4 mutants in these two genes are unique in that, upon infection, DNA replication takes place but no late mRNA is synthesized. They are called "maturation-defective" (MD) mutants. Temperature-sensitive gene-55 mutants have been studied by Pulitzer (23) and Pulitzer and Geiduschek (24). From their studies, they concluded that the gene-55 product is formed 5 min or more after infection, that it is continuously required for late T4 mRNA formation, and that it probably acts at the level of transcription. The results of checking the subunit content of the polymerase after infection with different gene-55 mutants and one gene-33 mutant are shown in Table II. Some Do mutants are shown for comparison. The experiments were done by labeling the polymerase with ^{14}C-labeled amino acids or [^{3}H]leucine after infection and determining the label in each new small subunit after gel separation, as shown in Fig. 1. After infection with Do amber mutants, the polymerase has the same content of new subunits as

Table II. Polypeptide Content of RNA Polymerase from *Escherichia coli* Infected with Different T4 Phage Mutants

Phage	Gene	Host	Percent of postinfection label			
			P22	P15	P12	P5-10
T4D^+		B	11	43	46^a	
Do						
*am*N82	44	B	11	47	42	
*am*N55-B14	42, 46	B	10	45	13	33
*am*N55-A456	42, 47	B	10	45	45	
MD						
*am*BL292	55	B	< 1	46	54	
		CR63	5	45	50	
*am*552	55	B	< 1	46	54	
		CR63 (30°C)	2	53	15	30
*ts*553	55	B (30°C)	< 2^b	41	57	
*ts*A81	55	B (30°C)	< 2^b	46	52	
*am*N134	33	B	18	54	<1	28
MD-Do						
*am*BL292-N122	55, 42	B	< 1	46	54	

^{a}When the value is shown between colums, the preparations were examined on 11% SDS gels, which do not separate P12 and P5-10, as shown in Fig. 1A.

^{b}[^{3}H]Leucine was used as the label, and the limit of detection was about 2%. Details on the labeling techniques have been described (20). All the MD mutants were gifts of Dr. E. P. Geiduschek; the Do double mutants, of Dr. John S. Wiberg; and the MD-Do double mutant, of Dr. Kay Fields.

Table III. Subunit Content of Enz$^+$ and Enz 55$^-$

Subunit	Glycerol gradient		Phosphocellulose		DNA-cellulose	
	Enz$^+$	Enz 55$^-$	Enz$^+$	Enz 55$^-$	Enz$^+$	Enz 55^{-a}
β	1	1	1	1	1	1
β'	1	1	1	1	1	1
a	2	2	2	2	2	2
σ	0.2–0.25	0.12–0.2	< 0.05	< 0.05	0.05	0.15
ω	0.5–1	0.5–1	0.5–1	0.5–1	0.5–1	0.5–1
P22	0.5–0.7	0	0.3–0.7	0	0.3–0.7	0
P15	1	1	1	1	1	1
P12	0.2	0.2	0	0	0.2	0.2
P5-10	< 0.2	< 0.2	0	0	0	0

[a]Only one preparation was examined. The values are the amount of each subunit per enzyme molecule and were calculated from densitometer scans of subunit peaks on gels.

it does after T4D$^+$ infection for 20 min at 30°C. With the first gene-55 mutant, *am*BL292, infection of the nonpermissive host B does not lead to formation of P22. Using *E. coli* CR63 as the permissive host, about 40% of the usual amount of P22 was found. With another *am*55 mutant, 552, no synthesis of P22 was found on infection of *E. coli* B, and a barely detectable amount with infected CR63. Using two temperature-sensitive T4 mutants in gene 55, no significant amount of P22 was found on the polymerase even when the infection was carried out at 30°C. One gene-33 amber mutant, N134, gave polymerase deficient in P12.

The absence of the P22 subunit from the polymerase after infection with T4 gene-55 mutants and the kinetics of its synthesis suggest that it may be the gene-55 product. Other interpretations are possible but more difficult to correlate with the properties of the gene-55 product as analyzed *in vivo* (23,24).

We have examined two enzymes isolated after T4 infection in some detail. One designated Enz$^+$ was isolated from *E. coli* B infected for 25 min at 30°C with a T4 double amber mutant (*am*N55-*am*A456) in genes 42 and 47. As analyzed in the labeling experiment of Table II, it contains all the four new small proteins. The second enzyme is called Enz 55$^-$ and was isolated from *E. coli* B infected for 25 min at 30°C with a T4 double amber mutant (*am*N122-*am*BL292) in genes 42 and 55. The gene-55 mutation caused the polymerase made after infection to be deficient in the P22 subunit.

First, the subunit content of the enzymes and some of the properties of the subunits were examined. The enzymes were purified by a protamine sulfate step, a DEAE-cellulose step, and two glycerol-gradient centrifugation steps. The

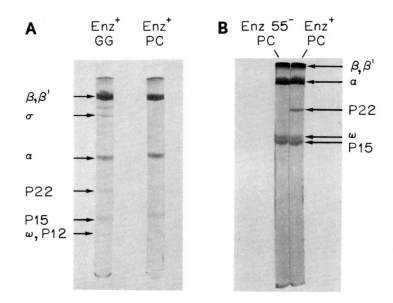

Fig. 2. Polyacrylamide gels showing the subunits of Enz⁺ and Enz 55⁻. Twenty micrograms
of each enzyme preparation were run. In A, 11% acrylamide gels, as described by Weber and
Osborn (21), were used. In B, 10% acrylamide gels, as described by Swank and Munkres
(22), were used.

glycerol-gradient purified enzymes were also examined after phosphocellulose
column chromatography, and enzymes of the protamine sulfate stage after
chromatography on DNA-cellulose columns. Table III shows the subunit content
of Enz⁺ and Enz 55⁻ purified in these different ways. The σ content was low on
both in comparison to normal enzyme (which contains about 0.6 equivalent of
σ) isolated in the same manner. The σ content of Enz⁺ was slightly higher than
that of Enz 55⁻, usually by a factor of about 1.5. Enz⁺ contained 0.5–0.7
equivalent of P22, while Enz 55⁻ had none. One P15 per enzyme molecule was
found on both Enz⁺ and Enz 55⁻. The amount of P12 was always low, about 0.2
equivalent per enzyme. P5-10 was also very low, if detectable at all, and further
studies of it are reported below.

On phosphocellulose chromatography of the glycerol-gradient purified enzymes, σ, P12, and the small amount of P5-10 were lost. The amount of P22 was
sometimes reduced on Enz⁺, maximally by about 50%. On DNA-cellulose chromatography of the more impure protamine fractions, P5-10 was lost. Sigma was
reduced in amount on Enz⁺. Whether the difference in σ content between Enz⁺
and Enz 55⁻ after DNA-cellulose chromatography is significant is not known.

Use of different purification techniques showed that P15 and P22 remain bound to the enzyme through most purification procedures.

Figure 2 shows photos of SDS gels of the enzymes. Fig. 2A shows 11% SDS gels of Enz[+], the glycerol-gradient purified (GG) enzyme and the phosphocellulose purified (PC) enzyme. The glycerol-gradient enzymes contain two main contaminating bands. One is removed by phosphocellulose chromatography, the other is not. Figure 2B shows SDS-urea gels of Enz[+] and Enz 55[-] after phosphocellulose chromatography. The enzymes are very pure in the small subunit range.

The very low amounts of P5-10 found on the purified infected enzymes led us to reexamine our labeling experiments and the use of normal vs. infected cells as carriers for enzyme isolation (20). We found that much less P5-10 is found when infected cells are used as carrier in a labeling experiment similar to that of Fig. 1A. Results of gel analyses of two labeling experiments are shown in Fig. 3.

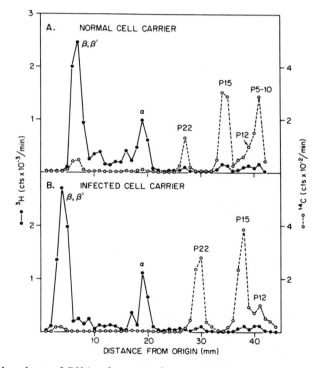

Fig. 3. Gel analyses of RNA polymerase after two labeling experiments with T4 amN82 phage and with normal (A) and infected (B) cells as carrier material for enzyme isolation. The labeling experiments were carried out as described previously (20). In A, 3 g of normal *E. coli* B was added to the labeled cells before enzyme isolation. In B, 3 g of *am*N82 phage infected cells was used. The gels used were as in Fig. 1A.

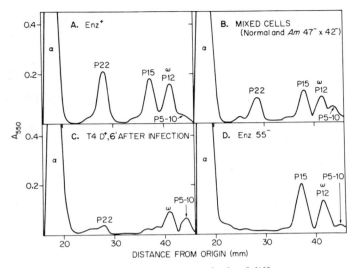

Fig. 4. Densitometer scans of the lower portions of gels of different enzyme preparations.
The gels used were as in Fig. 1A.

In A, normal cells were used as carrier for enzyme isolation; in B, infected cells. The results suggest that P5-10 is more tightly bound to normal enzyme or to enzyme not containing the other small subunits. We explored the P5-10 binding further in two ways. First, we looked at enzyme isolated 6 min after infection with wild-type T4 phage; from the kinetic studies, we knew that some P5-10, but little of the other subunits, should have been formed by 6 min. Second, we isolated enzyme from a 1:1 mixture of normal cells and infected cells. The results of gel analyses of these enzymes are shown in Fig. 4. Densitometer scans of 11% SDS gels are shown from the region of the a subunit through the region of the small subunits. Figure 4A shows Enz$^+$ and Fig. 4D Enz 55$^-$; Fig. 4B shows the enzyme isolated from the 1:1 mixture of normal and infected cells, and that more P5-10 is found than on A or D. Figure 4C shows the content of small subunits on the 6-min enzyme. Only P5-10 of those formed after infection is present in high concentration. The results support the idea that the protein P5-10 does bind to polymerase, but binds better to enzyme lacking the other small subunit modifications.

How tightly are the small subunits bound? We have looked for release of free P22, P15, and ω on gradient centrifugation of Enz$^+$ in the presence of low concentrations of urea and very low concentrations of the ionic detergent Sarkosyl. (P12 was not examined in these experiments.) In the presence of 1 M urea, no subunit was lost—not even ω, which is removed by 1 M urea from normal enzyme (25). When the enzyme was centrifuged in a 2 M urea gradient, some breakdown of the enzyme occurred. Omega was completely released, and about one-half of P22 and of α were also released. No free P15 was found. Figure 5 summarizes the results of a gradient centrifugation in the presence of 3 *M* urea. Gel analyses of enzyme fractions are shown as follows: in A, the enzyme is shown before centrifugation; in B, the β, β′ peak from the gradient is shown; and in C, the top of the gradient is shown. Figure 5C shows that one finds free ω, free P22, and free α. No free P15 is found. Rather, it is still bound to the β or β′ subunit, as demonstrated by its presence in the peak of Fig. 5B.

As shown in Fig. 6, centrifugation of the enzyme in 0.01% Sarkosyl-containing gradients leads to removal of all the ω and P22 from the enzyme, but no P15.

By chromatography of Enz$^+$ on a DEAE-cellulose column in the presence of 7 *M* urea, we have looked at the basicity of the small subunits relative to the other polymerase subunits. We were particularly interested in whether P15, P22, and P12 were small basic proteins like the small proteins described by Ghosh and Echols (26) and by Cukier-Kahn *et al.* (27). Figure 7 shows the elution of the subunits of Enz$^+$ from a DEAE-cellulose column run in the presence of 7 *M* urea. β′ and ω, both known to be relatively basic proteins (28), and P15 (which may

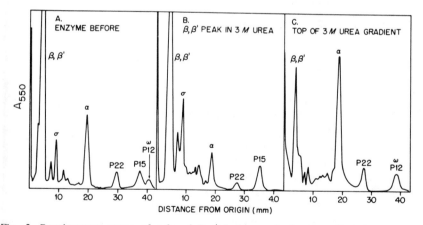

Fig. 5. Densitometer scans of gels of Enz$^+$ before and after centrifugation in a 3 M urea-containing gradient. Eighty micrograms of Enz$^+$, labeled with [^{3}H]leucine and containing 3000 cpm, was purified through glycerol-gradient centrifugation and dialyzed for 6 hr against the following buffer solution: 5% glycerol, 0.15 *M* KCl, 10 m*M* tris buffer, (*p*H 7.8), 0.1 m*M* EDTA, 0.1 m*M* dithiothreitol, and 3 *M* urea. The dialyzed enzyme solution was then layered on a 12.5–30% glycerol gradient (4.6 ml) in the same buffer. Centrifugation was for 14 hr at 34,000 rpm (Spinco L centrifuge, SW39 head). Twenty-nine fractions were collected from the bottom of the tube and analyzed for ^{3}H label to locate the fractions containing β and β′ (fractions 23 and 24, Fig. 5B). Fractions 27, 28, and 29 were examined for free subunits (Fig. 5C). Gels used were as in Fig. 1A.

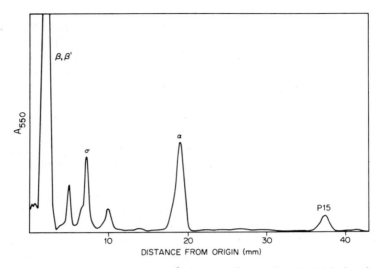

Fig. 6. Densitometer scan of a gel of Enz⁺ after centrifugation in a 0.01% Sarkosyl-containing gradient. Enz^+ (50 µg) was dialyzed for 3 hr against the following solution: 5% glycerol, 0.1 M KCl, 20 mM tris buffer (pH 8.0), 0.1 mM dithiothreitol, 0.1 mM EDTA, and 0.01% Sarkosyl. The solution was then layered on a 10–30% sucrose gradient (4.6 ml) in the same buffer and centrifuged for 14 hr at 32,000 rpm (Spinco L, SW39 head). Fractions from the gradient were assayed for enzyme activity and the peak fractions combined for gel analysis as in Fig. 1A.

also be basic, or still bound to β') do not stick to the column in the loading buffer. P22 is the first small protein to elute from the column with the gradient solution, β and α are all in the main protein peak, and P12 is the last small protein to elute from the column. The results show that P12 is probably a relatively acidic protein and that P22 is not as basic as ω. About one-half of the σ band was found in the main protein peak, and the remainder was eluted using 0.5 M KCl after the gradient was finished.

Table IV shows the specific activities of four glycerol-gradient purified enzymes—Enz⁺, Enz 55⁻, and enzyme isolated 6 min after infection with wild-type T4 phage (see Fig. 4C), and normal enzyme. There is no significant difference in the activities of the purified enzymes with calf thymus DNA as a template. The ratio of calf thymus DNA activity to that of T4 DNA activity with the first three enzymes at low salt is similar to that reported for infected enzyme by others (14,15,18)—about 5. The three enzymes are about one-half to one-third as good as normal enzyme at low salt on T4 DNA, which is about the activity one might expect on the basis of their lower σ content. At 0.2 M salt, the activities of both Enz⁺ and Enz 55⁻ on T4 DNA are 50–60% inhibited. The calf thymus DNA activity is not inhibited, so the ratio of calf thymus DNA activity to T4 DNA activity increases. The 6-min enzyme is not inhibited by salt but rather is

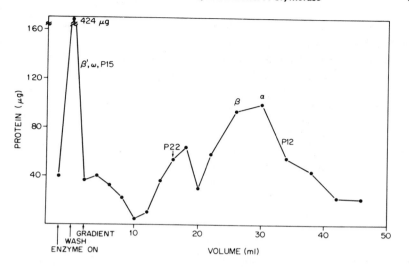

Fig. 7. Chromatography of Enz⁺ on DEAE-cellulose in the presence of 7 M urea. Glycerol-gradient purified Enz⁺, 1.5 mg in 2 ml, was dialyzed for 4 hr against the following buffer solution: 20% glycerol, 10 mM tris buffer (pH 8.0), 10 mM MgCl$_2$, 10 mM KCl, 0.1 mM EDTA, 20 mM β-mercaptoethanol, and 7 M urea. It was then applied to a 1- by 2-cm DE-23 column equilibrated with the same buffer. The column was washed with 2 ml of the same buffer and then eluted with 50 ml of a linear gradient system from 0.01 to 0.15 M KCl in the same buffer solution. Two-milliliter fractions were collected and analyzed for protein following trichloroacetic acid precipitation. Each fraction was also examined by SDS gel electrophoresis for polymerase subunit content. The notation of subunit content shows the fraction in which the subunit was highest in amount.

Table IV. Specific Activities[a] of Different Enzyme Preparations

Enzyme (GG)	Calf thymus DNA (0.05 M KCl)	Calf thymus/T4 (0.05 M KCl)	Calf thymus/T4 (0.20 M KCl)
Enz⁺	350-700	5–7	10
Enz 55⁻	350-600	4–7	10
Enz (6 min)[b]	600	6	4
Normal	350-700	2	1

[a]Specific activity = nmoles of [^{14}C]ATP incorporated into RNA in 10 min at 37°C/mg protein.

[b]Only one preparation was examined.

stimulated as is normal enzyme. The phosphocellulose-purified enzymes respond to salt in the same manner as the glycerol-gradient purified enzymes. The salt sensitivity occurs at the initiation step and in all properties is suggestive of an altered stability of the enzyme-DNA initiation complex. Further studies of the salt sensitivity will be presented elsewhere.

The RNA products made with mature T4 DNA, and either glycerol-gradient purified Enz[+] or Enz 55[-], have been examined for their content of late T4 mRNA as measured by the competitive hybridization assay of Bolle *et al.* (8), and for antimessenger content by annealing of the labeled RNA products with both 5-min and 20-min *in vivo* T4 RNA (29). Some of the results are shown in Table V. Three preparations of each enzyme were examined. Upon examination, little if any DNase activity with T4 DNA was found in preparation 1 of either enzyme. The σ contents of the enzymes are shown—those of Enz[+] being slightly higher. Enz[+] is similar to normal core enzyme (30) in that the RNA produced is high in antimessenger content. Enz 55[-] makes less symmetrical RNA in spite of a lower σ content. When Enz[+] contains about twice the amount of the σ subunit as Enz 55[-], the enzymes are rather equivalent in early T4 mRNA and antimessenger production. The results suggest that the σ activity of Enz[+] is altered, but a more detailed analysis is not yet complete.

The results show that Enz[+] and Enz 55[-] differ from normal enzyme and enzyme isolated 6 min after infection (and containing only small amounts of P15, P22, and P12) in having a salt-sensitive reaction with T4 DNA. The salt effect may be related to an alteration of the enzyme, changing the stability of the enzyme–DNA initiation complex. Modification of the conformation of the

Table V. Analyses of Labeled RNA Products Made with T4 DNA and Enz[+] or Enz 55[-] by RNA-DNA and RNA-RNA Annealing Studies[a]

Enzyme	GG preparation	σ content/ enzyme molecule	Late T4 mRNA (%)	Antimessenger (%)
Enz[+]	1	0.20	25	38
	2	0.25	15	22
	3	b	20	35
Enz 55[-]	1	0.15	7	10
	2	0.13	10	15
	3	b	8	12

[a][14C]RNA products were prepared using reaction mixtures containing the following components: [14C]ATP, 0.25 mM (30,000 cpm/nmol); UTP, CTP, and GTP each 0.25 mM; tris buffer (pH 7.8), 20 mM; MgCl$_2$, 10 mM; mercaptoethanol, 10 mM; T4 DNA, 22 μg; and Enz[+] or Enz 55[-], 8 μg. After incubation for 15 min at 37°C, the labeled RNA products were isolated as described by Bolle *et al.* (8). The percent of late T4 mRNA in the labeled RNA products was determined by a competitive hybridization technique using 5- and 20-min *in vivo* T4 RNA as described by Bolle *et al.* (8). The percent of antimessenger was determined as the percent RNase resistance of the labeled RNA products after annealing with 20-min *in vivo* T4 RNA as described by Brody *et al.* (29). Annealing with 5-min *in vivo* T4 RNA gave values about 25% lower. The percent of late T4 mRNA was not corrected for antimessenger content.

[b]Not determined.

enzyme could be part or all of the function of the new small proteins, resulting in an inhibition of early T4 mRNA formation, which is so σ dependent (30), and in a stimulation of the capacity of the enzyme to recognize late T4 mRNA initiation sites. Obviously, the subunits have to be isolated and their activities studied directly.

ACKNOWLEDGMENT

This research was sponsored by the U.S. Atomic Energy Commission under contract with the Union Carbide Corporation.

REFERENCES

1. S. S. Cohen. *J. Biol. Chem.* **174**:281 (1948).
2. L. Astrachan and E. Volkin. *Biochim. Biophys. Acta* **29**:536 (1958).
3. W. D. Hayward and M. H. Green. *Proc. Natl. Acad. Sci. (USA)* **54**:1675 (1965).
4. M. Nomura, C. Witten, N. Mantei, and H. Echols. *J. Mol. Biol.* **17**:273 (1966).
5. T. Kano-Sueoka and S. Spiegelman. *Proc. Natl. Acad. Sci. (USA)* **48**:1942 (1962).
6. B. D. Hall, A. P. Nygaard, and M. H. Green. *J. Mol. Biol.* **9**:143 (1964).
7. R. B. Khesin, M. F. Shemyakin, Z. M. Gorlenko, S. L. Bogdanova, and T. P. Afanaseva. *Biokhimya* **27**:1092 (1962).
8. A. Bolle, R. H. Epstein, W. Salser, and E. P. Geiduschek. *J. Mol. Biol.* **31**:325 (1968).
9. J. S. Wiberg, M. A. Dirksen, R. H. Epstein, S. E. Luria, and J. M. Buchanan. *Proc. Natl. Acad. Sci. (USA)* **48**:293 (1962).
10. Y. N. Zograff, N. Yu, V. G. Nickiforov, and M. F. Shemyakin. *Mol. Biol.* **1**:94 (1962).
11. A. Bolle, R. H. Epstein, W. Salser, and E. P. Geiduschek. *J. Mol. Biol.* **33**:339 (1968).
12. A. Cascino, E. P. Geiduschek, R. L. Cafferata, and R. Haselkorn. *J. Mol. Biol.* **61**:357 (1971).
13. A. Guha, W. Szybalski, W. Salser, A. Bolle, E. P. Geiduschek, and J. F. Pulitzer. *J. Mol. Biol.* **59**:329 (1971).
14. E. K. F. Bautz and J. J. Dunn. *Biochem. Biophys. Res. Commun.* **34**:230 (1969).
15. W. Seifert, P. Qasba, G. Walter, P. Palm, M. Schachner, and W. Zillig. *Europ. J. Biochem.* **9**:319 (1969).
16. C. G. Goff and K. Weber. *Cold Spring Harbor Symp. Quant. Biol.* **35**:101 (1970).
17. R. B. Khesin. In L. Silvestri (ed.), *Lepetit Colloquium on RNA Polymerase and Transcription,* North-Holland, Amsterdam (1970), p. 167.
18. A. Travers. *Cold Spring Harbor Symp. Quant. Biol.* **35**:241 (1970).
19. M. Schachner and W. Zillig. *Europ. J. Biochem.* **22**:531 (1971).
20. A. Stevens. *Proc. Natl. Acad. Sci. (USA)* **69**:603 (1972).
21. K. Weber and M. Osborn. *J. Biol. Chem.* **244**:4406 (1969).
22. R. T. Swank and K. D. Munkres. *Anal. Biochem.* **39**:462 (1971).
23. J. F. Pulitzer. *J. Mol. Biol.* **49**:473 (1970).
24. J. F. Pulitzer and E. P. Geiduscheck. *J. Mol. Biol.* **49**:489 (1970).
25. D. Berg, K. Barrett, and M. Chamberlin. In L. Grossman and K. Moldave (eds.), *Methods in Enzymology,* Vol. 21D, Academic Press, New York (1971), p. 506.
26. S. Ghosh and H. Echols. *Proc. Natl. Acad. Sci. (USA)* **69**:3660 (1972).
27. R. Cukier-Kahn, M. Jacquet, and F. Gros. *Proc. Natl. Acad. Sci. (USA)* **69**:3643 (1972).

28. R. R. Burgess. *J. Biol. Chem.* **244**:6168 (1969).
29. E. N. Brody, H. Diggelmann, and E. P. Geiduschek. *Biochemistry* **9**:1289 (1970).
30. E. K. F. Bautz, F. A. Bautz, and J. J. Dunn. *Nature* **223**:1022 (1969).

DISCUSSION

Question (Mandal): What is your explanation of the fractional molar ratio of the smaller subunits per mole of enzyme?

Answer: There is one P15 per enzyme molecule. That the others are not found in stoichiometric amount could be explained in several ways, but of course we don't know yet. They may be lost on purification, or they may be catalytic in action, or they may not all occur on the same enzyme molecule.

Question (Murthy): Of the four small proteins that you observe, is it possible that one of the proteins functions as a termination factor for terminating the synthesis of host RNA?

Answer: The small proteins are formed after host mRNA synthesis is terminated.

Question (Biswas): Can you explain in what way the lower molecular weight subunits are necessary for RNA polymerase activity? Is there any possibility that these subunits are the products of a number of proteases? Perhaps in the mutants a particular protease is defective and therefore a particular subunit band is absent. Do these smaller subunits have any nuclease activity?

Answer: Unfortunately, the studies at present do not show a unique activity of any of the new small subunits. Since we presume they are required for late T4 mRNA synthesis, it may require a good *in vitro* late RNA synthesizing system to demonstrate their activity. They could be the products of proteases or they could be some sort of proteases or transpeptidases, altering the main polymerase subunits. Enz$^+$ has little or no DNase activity. RNase activity has not been measured.

6

The Stringent Response—21 Years On

Andrew Travers
Division of Cell Biology
MRC Laboratory of Molecular Biology
Cambridge, England

During normal growth, bacteria synthesize no more ribosomes than can be engaged with high efficiency in protein synthesis (1). The molecular mechanism maintaining this fine balance is clearly of crucial importance in determining the growth characteristics of the cell. The first inkling that the synthesis of an essential component of the ribosome, the ribosomal RNA, might be directly coupled to protein synthesis was provided in 1952 by Sands and Roberts (2). They observed that when a particular bacterial strain was deprived of a required amino acid, not only did protein synthesis stop but also the net synthesis of RNA was substantially reduced. This phenomenon, subsequently christened the "stringent response," has recently been the subject of several excellent reviews (1,3,4). In this chapter, I argue that the stringent response is an extreme manifestation of the normal processes of the gross control of RNA synthesis in the bacterial cell. I further suggest that a major mode of effecting the selective coupling of stable RNA species to protein synthesis is mediated by EF-TuTs, a protein synthesis elongation factor, and ppGpp, a metabolic product of the ribosome (5).

CONTROL OF RNA ACCUMULATION

The accumulation of stable RNA species in bacteria is regulated in accordance with the physiological state of the cell. During balanced growth, the rate of accumulation of stable RNA is approximately proportional to the square of the growth rate (1,6,7). Thus the commonly observed fivefold variations in growth rate can encompass at least a twentyfold change in the net rate of stable RNA synthesis.

The stringent response is a more extreme example of the regulation of RNA accumulation and is defined genetically by the *rel* or *RC* locus (8). When *rel*⁺ strains of *Escherichia coli* are functionally deprived of an amino acid, the rate of RNA accumulation is rapidly reduced at least fiftyfold (9). Nor are the physiological effects of the stringent response restricted to RNA synthesis. The synthesis of nucleotides, glycolytic esters, and lipids is inhibited (10-14), the uptake of certain exogenous metabolites is blocked (10,14,15), and the rate of protein breakdown increases (16). None of these phenomena is exhibited when strains carrying the recessive (17) *rel*⁻ allele are starved for an amino acid. Such strains are said to possess relaxed control of RNA synthesis.

A rapid turnoff of RNA synthesis can be evoked in circumstances other than amino acid starvation. In such cases, the response is independent of the allelic state of the *rel* gene. One example is a temperature-sensitive aldolase mutant that ceases net RNA synthesis on being shifted to the restrictive temperature (18).

A fundamental characteristic of the changes in the rate of RNA accumulation so far described is that they are both rapid and reversible. Thus when the required amino acid is restored to a culture of starved stringent bacteria, net synthesis of RNA resumes within 40 sec (19).

CONTROL OF RNA ACCUMULATION—SYNTHESIS OR DEGRADATION?

The stability of different RNA species in the bacterial cell is extremely varied. After incorporation into the structure of the ribosome, rRNA can remain intact for several bacterial generations, yet under similar conditions *trp* operon mRNA is being degraded before its synthesis is terminated (20). Thus a measurement of the incorporation of a radioactive RNA precursor into RNA *in vivo* must inevitably reflect the balance between synthesis and degradation, and thus the longer the period of incorporation the greater will be the contribution of the more stable RNA species to the measurement. Variation in the rate of RNA accumulation could be a consequence of either a change in the rate of RNA synthesis or a change in the stability of particular RNA species. The complications of degradation can be minimized, but not excluded, by measuring RNA synthesis in as short a time period as possible. Using such a method, Lazzarini and Dahlberg (21) and Gallant and Margarson (22) concluded that amino acid starvation of stringent *E. coli* or *Bacillus subtilis* reduces the instantaneous rate of total RNA synthesis by about 70%. This result argues that the regulation of RNA accumulation is largely a consequence of control of synthesis. However, Donini (9) has challenged this view, suggesting that the principal control is at the level of degradation. This conclusion depends on the observation that the rate of nascent RNA synthesis in starved stringent cells at $42.5°C$ is 65–150% of the rate in unstarved cells at $29°C$. Since both growth rate and RNA accumulation increase with temperature (23), such a comparison could minimize or even obliterate an actual inhibition of the rate of synthesis.

In principle, RNA synthesis could be controlled by restricting the initiation and/or the elongation of RNA molecules. A control of initiation would alter the actual number of RNA polymerase molecules actively transcribing DNA. By the simple expedient of extracting the *E. coli* genome intact from normally growing and starved stringent cells, Stomato and Pettijohn (19) showed that the number of RNA polymerase molecules transcribing the rRNA genes was at least twelve-fold lower in starved cells. Thus most evidence points to the rate of RNA synthesis as the prime determinant of the rate of RNA accumulation. Such a conclusion by no means excludes the possibility that normally stable RNA species are degraded during stringency. Indeed, the results of Donini (9) imply that such degradation does occur, although only to a limited extent. Similarly, Nierlich (24) has suggested that degradation of nascent rRNA and tRNA may immediately follow a carbon source downshift.

COORDINATE OR NONCOORDINATE CONTROL?

Is the control of RNA synthesis during normal growth and during the stringent response coordinate or noncoordinate? In other words, is the synthesis of all RNA species equally affected, or is the synthesis of a particular class of RNA species selectively regulated? During balanced growth, the proportion of stable RNA (i.e., rRNA plus tRNA) in the transcript decreases as the growth rate falls (7). At slow growth rates (μ = approximately 0.5 doublings/hr), stable RNA comprises 20% of the *E. coli* transcript; at the fastest growth rates (μ = 2.5), this proportion rises to 65–70% (7). Clearly, in this instance, control is noncoordinate.

In contrast, the problem of coordinacy during the stringent response is far from resolution. It is beyond dispute that the synthesis of stable RNA is virtually completely shut off through the operation of amino acid control. Thus the extent to which mRNA synthesis is similarly restricted should determine the degree of coordinacy. If the synthesis of all mRNA were not curtailed during starvation, the RNA synthesized under these conditions should be relatively enriched in mRNA species and conversely depleted of stable RNA species. Furthermore, the reduction in the overall rate of instantaneous RNA synthesis should reflect only the restriction of stable RNA synthesis. In fact, Lazzarini and Dahlberg (21) noted that in *E. coli* the total instantaneous rate is reduced by 70% on amino acid starvation, although the formation of stable RNA represents only 40% of the normal total. In *B. subtilis,* where stable RNA synthesis comprises only 16% of the normal instantaneous rate, starvation likewise reduces this rate by about 70% (22). In these examples, therefore, there is evidence for the inhibition of RNA species other than rRNA or tRNA. This conclusion is emphasized by the characterization of up to 30% of the total nascent RNA in starved *E. coli* as rRNA or tRNA (9,25,26). Studies on the stringent control of selected mRNA species suggest that the synthesis of functional messengers for both *E. coli* ornithine transcarbamoylase (27) and *B. subtilis* flagellar proteins may be inhibited by as much as 75% during stringency. In contrast, other experiments indicate that the synthesis of *lac* mRNA (29), *trp* mRNA (30), T4 mRNA (31), and φ80 mRNA (32) proceeds at a rate close to normal during amino acid starvation.

The experimental evidence clearly implies that the response of mRNA synthesis to stringency is heterogeneous: one class of mRNA species is not under stringent control, while another class is restricted in a similar manner to stable RNA synthesis. This second class could be comprised of the messengers for those proteins whose production is geared to the growth rate of the cell. An obvious example would be the messengers for ribosomal proteins (33). Messengers not under stringent control could code for the bacterial "luxury" proteins, which would not normally be required for growth in rich media. Thus we can eliminate models invoking coordinate control of RNA synthesis. Nevertheless, the observed pattern of noncoordinate control probably does not reflect the classical dichotomy between mRNA and stable RNA but instead may represent a functional distinction between those RNA species that are required for growth independent of the circumstances of the cell and those that are only occasionally needed.

ppGpp, AN EFFECTOR FOR STRINGENT CONTROL

The rapidity of the *in vivo* response of stable RNA synthesis to amino acid starvation or to its relief suggests that control may be effected by a low molecular weight compound. Furthermore, the dominance of the *rel*$^+$ allele is consistent with the existence of a functional inhibitor of RNA synthesis. A very early and apparently invariant manifestation of *rel*$^+$ gene function during amino acid starvation is the accumulation of guanosine-5'-diphosphate-3'- (or 2'-) diphosphate, ppGpp (34-36). The accumulation of ppGpp after amino acid starvation is very rapid in cells bearing *rel*$^+$ but not *rel*$^-$ alleles, the *in vivo* concentration of the nucleotide attaining and usually exceeding the levels of GTP (pppG) within 2 min (27,35). Conversely, on amino acid resupplementation, ppGpp rapidly disappears (35). Comparison of the rate of RNA synthesis (R) and the intracellular ppGpp levels under conditions of partial amino acid starvation reveals a linear relationship between $1/R$ and ppGpp concentration (23) compatible with the hypothesis that ppGpp acts as a noncompetitive inhibitor of stable RNA synthesis with a K_i of 0.1–0.2 mM.

The correlation between ppGpp and RNA synthesis is also maintained during balanced growth when both rel^+ and rel^- strains contain low levels of ppGpp whose concentration is inversely related to both the RNA content and growth rate of the cells (37,38). ppGpp also accumulates to high levels when bacterial cells, either rel^+ or rel^-, are strongly stressed by starvation for an energy source, nitrogen, or sulfur (39) or by osmotic shock in hypertonic sodium chloride (40). In all these cases, RNA synthesis is concomitantly severely restricted. Thus the *in vivo* behavior of ppGpp fulfills the criteria required for a low molecular weight inhibitor of RNA synthesis.

In addition to ppGpp, a second guanine nucleotide, pppGpp, accumulates in rel^+ strains during the stringent response (34-36). In *E. coli*, the levels of pppGpp are generally low compared to those of ppGpp (35). Moreover, certain *E. coli* strains exist that, although accumulating ppGpp, fail to accumulate pppGpp on amino acid starvation. Such strains maintain stringent control of RNA synthesis. Nevertheless, in *B. subtilis*, the level of pppGpp exceeds that of ppGpp (22).

SYNTHESIS OF ppGpp

A prerequisite for the efficient operation of a regulatory low molecular weight effector is a precise and rapidly responding control of its intracellular concentration. Such a control must thus regulate either or both of the processes concerned with the biosynthesis and degradation of the effector.

During stringency, ppGpp rapidly accumulates as a consequence of amino acid starvation. A critical step in this response is the failure to aminoacylate a transfer RNA species (41), suggesting that a process intimately linked with protein synthesis may determine the level of ppGpp. This conclusion is supported by the observation that the presence of mRNA in cells is absolutely required for ppGpp accumulation (42). Moreover, treatment of amino acid starved rel^+ cells with antibiotics, which inhibit ribosomes actively engaged in protein synthesis, results in the rapid decay of the accumulated ppGpp with a consequent resumption of RNA synthesis (35,43). Such antibiotics include chloramphenicol (35), erythromycin, tetracycline, and fusidic acid (43). Significantly, streptomycin, whose target is believed to be free ribosomes (44), does not induce ppGpp decay (43). In addition to its effect on ppGpp levels during stringency, chloramphenicol also causes the disappearance of ppGpp accumulated in both rel^+ and rel^- strains as a consequence of energy starvation (43).

Thus the *in vivo* accumulation of ppGpp during stringency requires an uncharged tRNA, mRNA, ribosomes, and an active *rel* gene product. These requirements are met by a reconstituted *in vitro* system for ppGpp synthesis (5,45). In such a system, GDP (ppG) acts as a precursor for ppGpp and pppG acts as a precursor for pppGpp (5). The 3'- (or 2'-) pyrophosphates arise from the donation of the β and γ phosphates of ATP (5). The *in vitro* synthesis of ppGpp is blocked by fusidic acid (5) and tetracycline (45) but, in contrast with *in vivo* accumulation, is unaffected by either chloramphenicol or erythromycin (45). Net ppGpp synthesis thus appears to be elicited by the codon-dependent binding of uncharged tRNA to the aminoacyl site of the ribosome (45). Subsequent translocation may (5) or may not (45) be necessary. Thus the *rel* gene product could function as a sensor for the uncharged state of tRNA and trigger the net synthesis of ppGpp by either itself or another protein. This process would be compatible with the original concept of ppGpp synthesis by an idling reaction of the ribosome (34) and leaves open the possibility that ppGpp and pppGpp may be synthesized as normal transient intermediates in protein synthesis.

The mechanism of ppGpp accumulation independent of *rel* gene function is unknown. It remains to be established whether this accumulation is a consequence of the ribosomal synthetic mechanism responding to a different signal or of a completely different synthetic pathway. Another unsolved puzzle is the mode of breakdown of ppGpp in the cell.

STRINGENT CONTROL *IN VITRO*

A major consequence of stringency is the selective curtailment of a specific class of RNA synthesis. Therefore, if ppGpp is the effector for stringent control, its target should be a component of the transcription machinery. There are two general mechanisms for regulating the synthesis of specific RNA species. Either the activity of a promoter can be regulated by a DNA binding protein such as a repressor, or the initiation specificity of RNA polymerase can be altered (46,47). The regulation of the synthesis of both stable RNA species and certain mRNA species during stringency suggests that the operative control system has a broad specificity spectrum. Such a characteristic is typical of regulation of polymerase initiation specificity. In contrast, regulatory proteins that bind to DNA normally have a highly specific effect limited to the control of a very few RNA species.

One mechanism proposed for the general control of RNA synthesis in *E. coli* suggests that the initiation specificity of RNA polymerase holoenzyme is regulated by interaction of the polymerase with auxiliary specificity factors, the ψ factors (46,48,49). By stabilizing a particular initiation conformation of RNA polymerase, each ψ factor allows efficient initiation of RNA synthesis only from a specified set of promoters (50). This model is derived from studies on the *in vitro* transcription of rRNA from *E. coli* and *B. subtilis* DNA (48-55). A critical determinant of the character of rRNA synthesis by holoenzyme is the conformation of the DNA template (55). When sheared *E. coli* DNA (56) is used as template, two forms of the rRNA promoter can be distinguished; below $35°C$, the promoter is closed, above $36°C$ it is open (55). The conversion between these conformational states is effected by a cooperative transition. The ability of

RNA polymerase to utilize these different structural forms of the rRNA promoter is strongly KCl dependent. Thus whereas transcription from the closed promoter is tenfold higher at 0.01 M KCl than at 0.1 M KCl, the rate of rRNA synthesis from the open promoter is relatively insensitive to changes in KCl concentration. However, rRNA synthesis by holoenzyme alone from either form of the promoter is not selectively inhibited by physiological concentrations of ppGpp (50), implying that an additional component is required for regulation. rRNA transcription from the closed promoter is selectively enhanced by the ψ_r factor (50), now equated with the protein synthesis elongation factor EF-TuTs (57). This preferential stimulation is inhibited by ppGpp, the proportion of rRNA in the transcript falling from about 15% in the absence of ppGpp to about 2% at 0.5 mM ppGpp (50). The K_i for this selective inhibition of rRNA synthesis by ppGpp is about 0.1–0.2 mM and thus is similar to that observed *in vivo*. In contrast to its stimulatory effect on synthesis from the closed promoter, EF-TuTs substantially inhibits rRNA synthesis from the open promoter at 0.01 M KCl, yet has little effect at 0.1 M KCl. Nor does ppGpp reduce the proportion of rRNA in the transcript under these conditions. Thus, *in vitro,* the closed rRNA promoter and EF-TuTs are prerequisite for selective control by ppGpp.

The response of rRNA synthesis to changes in polymerase specificity is not unique. tRNA^{Tyr} synthesis is preferentially inhibited by ppGpp under similar conditions to those required for the control of rRNA synthesis (50). The activities of T4 DNA and poly(dA-dT) as templates resemble the open rRNA promoter, while that of poly(dG)̄poly(dC) is similar to the closed rRNA promoter (50,60).

A simple model that accounts for these observations proposes that RNA polymerase holoenzyme can exist in two conformational states, $(E\sigma)_m$ and $(E\sigma)_s$, formerly termed $(E\sigma)_A$ and $(E\sigma)_G$, respectively (50,58,59). In this model, $(E\sigma)_m$ initiates RNA synthesis efficiently at certain mRNA promoters, as exemplified by T4 promoters, and at open rRNA promoters, while $(E\sigma)_s$ initiates efficiently at closed rRNA and tRNA promoters. A corollary to this pattern of template specificity is that $(E\sigma)_s$ should initiate RNA chains with pppG much more efficiently than $(E\sigma)_m$ (59). Similarly, $(E\sigma)_m$ should utilize pppA as the preferred initiating triphosphate. These polymerase forms are assumed to be in equilibrium such that at high KCl concentrations $(E\sigma)_m$ is strongly favored, while at low KCl concentrations neither form is favored. The role of EF-TuTs is to stabilize the $(E\sigma)_s$ conformation. Consequently, in the presence of EF-TuTs, neither form is favored at high KCl, while at low KCl $(E\sigma)_s$ is the dominant form. Thus in the extreme situations where one form of the polymerase is limited, synthesis of the corresponding RNA is markedly restricted. ppGpp binds to EF-TuTs (57), consequently inhibiting transcription factor activity.

Two independent lines of evidence also indicate that RNA polymerase can exist in different conformational states with differing initiation specificities.

First, a mutant RNA polymerase, $ts103$ (61), in comparison with the parent enzyme, synthesizes RNA more efficiently from the closed promoter and much less efficiently from the open promoter (62). $ts103$ polymerase thus behaves as though the equilibrium between $(E\sigma)_m$ and $(E\sigma)_s$ were shifted in favor of $(E\sigma)_s$ as a consequence of the mutation. *In vivo,* the $ts103$ mutant fails to restrict rRNA synthesis to the same extent as its parent bacterial strain; that is, it exhibits a relaxed phenotype as a consequence of mutation in RNA polymerase (Jacobson and Gillespie, personal communication). *In vitro,* this situation is mimicked by the comparative rates of rRNA synthesis by mutant and parent holoenzymes from only the closed rRNA promoter.

A second type of evidence is the finding that RNA polymerase in crude extracts of *B. subtilis* (63) and *E. coli* (60,64) is heterogeneous. In *E. coli,* three polymerase activities can be distinguished, sedimenting at 16S, 21S, and 27S, respectively. None of these activities behaves either physically or functionally like the purified holoenzyme. The initiation specificities of the 16S and 21S polymerase activities are characteristic of stabilized $(E\sigma)_s$ and $(E\sigma)_m$ conformations, respectively (60), a view supported by the cosedimentation of EF-TuTs with the 16S form. The nature of the 27S species is more problematical since it initiates efficiently at both T4 promoters and closed rRNA promoters (60). This heterogeneity of polymerase function suggests that in crude extracts, and perhaps *in vivo,* nontranscribing RNA polymerase does not exist as the free holoenzyme but rather in a complex association with other proteins.

Both the 16S and 27S polymerases, but not the 21S polymerase, are strongly inhibited by ppG and ppGpp (60). Thus only those polymerase activities that synthesize rRNA from the closed promoter are sensitive to ppGpp, and consequently the effect of ppGpp on a mixture of these crude polymerases is the selective restriction of the synthesis of certain classes of RNA molecules.

Is the physical and functional heterogeneity of crude RNA polymerase of biological significance? The strongest argument that the heterogeneity does reflect the internal state of the cell is that under two very different circumstances where rRNA synthesis is preferentially turned off *in vivo,* those polymerase activities that synthesize rRNA *in vitro* are no longer detectable. Thus in extracts of both stationary-phase cells and T4-infected cells (64), only the 21S activity can be observed. The disappearance of the 16S and 27S activities can be mimicked *in vitro* by isolating the polymerases in the presence of 1 mM ppG (60). This selective loss of polymerase activity is a consequence of the direct inhibition of the crude polymerases and not of their dissociation into holoenzyme and auxiliary factor.

The protein synthesis factor EF-TuTs is also required for another mode of RNA synthesis, the replication of RNA phages (57). Clear analogies exist between this role of EF-TuTs and its involvement in transcription. In both cases, EF-TuTs interacts directly with other polypeptides to form either the phage replicase (65,66) or a complex with polymerase holoenzyme. In neither case does EF-TuTs appear to bind independently to the template. Further, both in transcription (50) and in phage replication (67,68) EF-TuTs stimulates the synthesis of RNA molecules initiated with pppG. It has been suggested that EF-TuTs functions in phage replication by recognizing a structure resembling tRNA in the phage RNA molecule, and thus the functions of EF-TuTs in protein synthesis and in phage replication would be analogous (57). However, EF-TuTs is also required for replicase function with poly(C) templates, whose only resemblance to tRNA is the dicytidylate sequence adjacent to the 3'-terminal nucleotide. Consequently, it appears more reasonable to parallel EF-TuTs function in transcription and replication.

MOLECULAR MECHANISMS FOR STRINGENT CONTROL *IN VIVO*

The characteristics of the stringent control of RNA synthesis *in vivo* are closely paralleled *in vitro* by the sensitivity to ppGpp of EF-TuTs-dependent RNA synthesis from the closed rRNA promoter. There is little evidence relating to the normal state of the rRNA promoter *in vivo*. Nevertheless, it is particularly striking that the supercoiled form of the *E. coli* genome (69,70) appears to restrain the rRNA promoter so that it remains in the closed configuration at temperatures where on sheared DNA the configuration would normally be open (54,55). Again, this evidence points to the closed form of the promoter as the operative *in vivo* configuration. Moreover, DNA must also bind polyamines and/or basic proteins *in vivo*. Conceivably, such interactions could also determine the conformational state of promoters. Consistent with this view is the observation that rRNA synthesis can be "relaxed" *in vivo* by exogenous spermidine (71). Regardless of the exact mechanism of action of polyamines, it is clear in principle that if the rRNA promoters could be converted to an open form *in vivo* then rRNA synthesis would no longer be under stringent control.

By what mechanism is the pattern of RNA polymerase specificity determined? One possibility is that the initiation specificity of a given RNA polymerase molecule is fixed immediately after it has terminated the synthesis of an RNA chain. On termination, the polymerase is released from the template, presumably in the form of core polymerase. The core then binds σ factor to reconstitute holoenzyme. I have argued that holoenzyme can exist in two, or perhaps more, initiation conformations that are in rapid equilibrium with each other, and that each of these conformations is specific for a certain class of promoters. An initiation conformation would be stabilized when a holoenzyme in that conformation formed a complex with the appropriate auxiliary factor. Such complexes, which would correspond to the polymerase activities observed in crude extracts, would be stable. Consistent with this model is the observation that the mutant phenotype of the *ts*103 polymerase, in which the equilibrium position between conformations may be altered, is apparent only when the enzyme is pure. The crude *ts*103 polymerase activity behaves in a similar manner to the parent enzyme (61).

In this model, the pattern of the initiation of RNA synthesis in bacteria could be controlled by regulating either the activity of the polymerase-factor complexes or the association of polymerase with a factor. Direct inhibition by a low molecular weight effector, such as ppGpp, would create a pool of inactivated RNA polymerase molecules which could thus be kept in reserve by the cell until the inhibition is lifted. The existence of such a pool of nontranscribing polymerases has in fact been inferred by Pato and von Meyenburg (7) on the basis of the very rapid increase in RNA synthesis following a carbon-source upshift.

Control of association of factor and polymerase could be operative under conditions where a very high proportion of polymerase molecules are engaged in the synthesis of a particular class of RNA species. Such a situation would occur at high growth rates, when stable RNA synthesis accounts for up to 70% of the instantaneous rate of synthesis (7). Under these conditions, constitutive transcription from the *trp* operon is sharply depressed (72). Fiil *et al.* (23) have pointed out that the variation of ppGpp concentration as a function of growth rate is much too small to suffice as the sole controlling element for the wide range of stable RNA synthesis rates that are observed. Consequently, they have suggested that the concentration of the polymerase factor controlling rRNA synthesis should vary in proportion to the growth rate. EF-TuTs fits this model exactly, since its concentration is proportional to the amount of ribosomes (73) and thus to the growth rate (33). A similar correlation of RNA polymerase production with growth rate would ensure maximal rates of RNA synthesis.

A simplified scheme of the central role that EF-TuTs may play in cellular macromolecular synthesis is shown in Fig. 1. Free EF-TuTs is generated by synthesis and recycling from the ribosome. Its specific activity, either free or in association with RNA polymerase, is determined principally by the concentration of ppGpp, whose synthesis in turn is triggered by the absence of EF-Tu-dependent binding of an aminoacyl-tRNA to the ribosome. However, since EF-TuTs also binds pppG, albeit 100 times less tightly than ppGpp (57), its activity should depend on the ppGpp/pppG ratio, although this is unlikely to be apparent from normal *in vivo* studies because of the large difference in the binding constants of the two nucleotides. In this context, it is pertinent to ask why the intracellular concentration of ppGpp should be so high. Its concentration can exceed that of another regulatory nucleotide, cyclic AMP, by 100- to 10,000-fold. Such a high concentration suggests either that the target of ppGpp is very abundant or that the regulatory role of ppGpp may involve some competition with another guanine nucleotide. An interesting feature of the

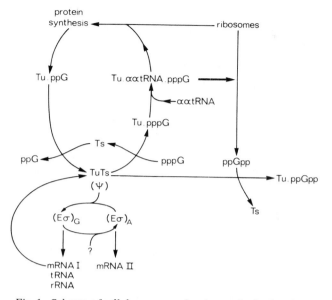

Fig. 1. Scheme of cellular macromolecular synthesis, showing possible central role of EF-TuTs.

scheme in Fig. 1 is that if the EF-TuTs messenger should be under stringent control the synthesis of EF-TuTs would be autocatalytic.

The major characteristics of the selective control of RNA synthesis during normal growth are thus compatible with the regulation of a set of RNA species, including the stable RNA species by EF-TuTs and ppGpp. There is no positive evidence for an alternative model of control of stable RNA synthesis invoking a repressor binding to DNA (52,74). During the stringent response, the concentration of ppGpp is much higher than during balanced growth. While the same control on polymerase specificity probably operates, a less selective inhibition of all polymerase molecules by ppGpp (75) could account for at least part of the decrease in total RNA synthesis (76) and thus could obscure specific control. Finally, a *caveat:* The flexibility of natural control systems is such that the possibility remains open that ppGpp control is not the only means of regulating bacterial RNA synthesis selectively. Conceivably, other low molecular weight compounds could also influence the activity of any of the crude polymerases.

REFERENCES

1. O. Maaløe. Twenty-eighth Symposium of Society for Developmental Biology: Communication in Development, University of Colorado (1969).

2. M. K. Sands and R. B. Roberts. *J. Bacteriol.* **55**:505 (1952).
3. G. Edlin and P. Broda. *Bacteriol. Rev.* **32**:206 (1968).
4. A. Ryan and E. Borek. *Progr. Nucleic Acid Res.* **11**:212 (1971).
5. W. A. Haseltine, R. Block, W. Gilbert, and K. Weber. *Nature* **238**:381 (1972).
6. A. L. Koch. *J. Theoret. Biol.* **28**:303 (1969).
7. M. L. Pato and K. von Meyenburg. *Cold Spring Harbor Symp. Quant. Biol.* **35**:497 (1970).
8. G. S. Stent and S. Brenner. *Proc. Natl. Acad. Sci. (USA)* **47**:2005 (1961).
9. P. Donini. *J. Mol. Biol.* **72**:553 (1972).
10. J. Gallant and M. Cashel. *J. Mol. Biol.* **24**:225 (1967).
11. M. Cashel and J. Gallant. *J. Mol. Biol.* **25**:545 (1967).
12. J. Irr and J. Gallant. *J. Biol. Chem.* **244**:2233 (1969).
13. Y. Sokawa, E. Nakao, and Y. Kaziro. *Biochem. Biophys. Res. Commun.* **33**:108 (1969).
14. D. P. Nierlich. *Proc. Natl. Acad. Sci. (USA)* **60**:1345 (1968).
15. Y. Sokawa and Y. Kaziro. *Biochem. Biophys. Res. Commun.* **34**:99 (1969).
16. A. J. Sussman and C. Gilvarg. *J. Biol. Chem.* **244**:6304 (1969).
17. N. Fiil. *J. Mol. Biol.* **45**:195 (1969).
18. A. Bock and F. C. Neidhardt. *J. Bacteriol.* **92**:470 (1966).
19. T. D. Stomato and D. E. Pettijohn. *Nature New Biol.* **234**:99 (1971).
20. R. D. Mosteller, J. K. Rose, and C. Yanofsky. *Cold Spring Harbor Symp. Quant. Biol.* **35**:461 (1970).
21. R. A. Lazzarini and A. E. Dahlberg. *J. Biol. Chem.* **246**:420 (1971).
22. J. Gallant and G. Margason. *J. Biol. Chem.* **247**:2289 (1972).
23. N. P. Fiil, K. von Meyenburg, and J. Friesen. *J. Mol. Biol.* **71**:769 (1972).
24. D. P. Nierlich. *J. Mol. Biol.* **72**:765 (1972).
25. J. D. Friesen. *J. Mol. Biol.* **20**:559 (1966).
26. J. D. Stubbs and B. D. Hall. *J. Mol. Biol.* **37**:303 (1968).
27. J. Gallant, B. Hall, H. Erlich, and T. Laffler. *Cold Spring Harbor Symp. Quant. Biol.* **35**:397 (1970).
28. K. Dimitt, S. Bradford, and M. Simon. *J. Bacteriol.* **95**:801 (1968).
29. D. W. Morris and N. O. Kjeldgaard. *J. Mol. Biol.* **31**:145 (1968).
30. G. Edlin, G. S. Stent, R. F. Baker, and C. Yanofsky. *J. Mol. Biol.* **37**:257 (1968).
31. L. Legault-Demare, A. Malhie, and F. Gros. *Europ. J. Biochem.* **8**:482 (1969).
32. P. Primakoff and P. Berg. *Cold Spring Harbor Symp. Quant. Biol.* **35**:391 (1970).
33. R. F. Schleif. *J. Mol. Biol.* **27**:41 (1967).
34. M. Cashel and J. Gallant. *Nature* **221**:838 (1969).
35. M. Cashel. *J. Biol. Chem.* **244**:3133 (1969).
36. M. Cashel and B. Kalbacher. *J. Biol. Chem.* **245**:2309 (1970).
37. R. A. Lazzarini, M. Cashel, and J. Gallant. *J. Biol. Chem.* **246**:4381 (1971).
38. R. B. Harshman and H. Yamazaki. *Biochemistry* **10**:3980 (1971).
39. G. Edlin and P. Donini. *J. Biol. Chem.* **246**:4371 (1971).
40. R. B. Harshman and H. Yamazaki. *Biochemistry* **11**:615 (1972).
41. F. C. Neidhardt. *Bacteriol. Rev.* **30**:701 (1966).
42. E. Lund and N. O. Kjeldgaard. *FEBS Letters* **26**:306 (1972).
43. E. Lund and N. O. Kjeldgaard. *Europ. J. Biochem.* **28**:316 (1972).
44. D. Schlessinger, C. Gurgo, L. Luzzatto, and D. Apirion. *Cold Spring Harbor Symp. Quant. Biol.* **34**:231 (1969).
45. F. S. Pedersen, E. Lund, and N. O. Kjeldgaard. *Nature New Biology* **243**:13 (1973).
46. A. A. Travers. *Nature New Biol.* **229**:69 (1971).
47. E. K. F. Bautz. *Progr. Nucleic Acid Res.* **12**:129 (1972).

48. A. A. Travers, R. I. Kamen, and R. F. Schleif. *Nature* **228**:748 (1970).
49. A. A. Travers, R. I. Kamen, and M. Cashel. *Cold Spring Harbor Symp. Quant. Biol.* **35**:415 (1970).
50. A. A. Travers. *Nature* **224**:15 (1973).
51. C. Hussey, J. Pero, R. G. Shorenstein, and R. Losick. *Proc. Natl. Acad. Sci. (USA)* **69**:407 (1972).
52. W. A. Haseltine. *Nature* **235**:329 (1972).
53. D. E. Pettijohn, K. Clarkson, C. R. Kossman, and O. G. Stonington. *J. Mol. Biol.* **52**:381 (1970).
54. D. E. Pettijohn. *Nature New Biol.* **235**:204 (1972).
55. A. A. Travers, D. L. Baillie, and S. Pedersen. *Nature New Biology* **243**:161 (1973).
56. J. Marmur. *J. Mol. Biol.* **3**:208 (1961).
57. T. Blumenthal, T. A. Landers, and K. Weber. *Proc. Natl. Acad. Sci. (USA)* **69**:1313 (1972).
58. A. A. Travers. *New Scientist* **53**:324 (1972).
59. A. A. Travers. *Proceedings of 11th Latin American Symposium: Protein Synthesis and Nucleic Acids* (1972), p. 43.
60. A. A. Travers and R. Buckland. *Nature New Biology* **243**:257 (1973).
61. A. Jacobson and D. Gillespie. *Cold Spring Harbor Symp. Quant. Biol.* **35**:85 (1970).
62. A. A. Travers. Manuscript in preparation (1973).
63. J. J. Pene. *Nature* **223**:705 (1969).
64. L. Snyder. *Nature New Biology* **243**:131 (1973).
65. R. I. Kamen. *Nature* **228**:527 (1970).
66. M. Kondo, R. Gallerani, and C. Weissmann. *Nature* **228**:525 (1970).
67. R. Roblin. *J. Mol. Biol.* **31**:51 (1968).
68. M. Watanabe and J. T. August. *Proc. Natl. Acad. Sci. (USA)* **59**:513 (1968).
69. O. G. Stonington and D. E. Pettijohn. *Proc. Natl. Acad. Sci. (USA)* **68**:6 (1971).
70. A. Worcel and E. Burgi. *J. Mol. Biol.* **71**:127 (1972).
71. A. Raina, M. Jansen, and S. S. Cohen. *J. Bacteriol.* **94**:1684 (1967).
72. J. K. Rose and C. Yanofsky. *J. Mol. Biol.* **69**:103 (1972).
73. J. Gordon. *Biochemistry* **9**:912 (1970).
74. R. Losick. *Ann. Rev. Biochem.* **41**:409 (1972).
75. M. Cashel. *Cold Spring Harbor Symp. Quant. Biol.* **35**:407 (1970).
76. R. M. Winslow and R. A. Lazzarini. *J. Biol. Chem.* **244**:3387 (1970).

DISCUSSION

Question (Shubrahmanyam): In *B. subtilis,* there are relaxed mutants which accumulate ppGpp but rRNA synthesis is not shut off. How do you explain this on the basis of your hypothesis?

Answer: rRNA synthesis would depend on the conformation of the DNA as well as on the ppGpp level.

Question (Shubrahmanyam): After the cells are starved for an amino acid and the required amino acid is added back, rRNA synthesis continues even though there is already accumulated ppGpp?

Answer: ppGpp is degraded very fast after restoration of the required amino acid.

Question (Singh): It seems like you are putting a lot of emphasis on the initiation of rRNA transcription. In a nutritionally deficient condition, assuring that the necessary synthesis of messages and hence that protein synthesis continues uninhibited, then one would expect an accumulation of free ribosomal proteins in a cell. We find, on the contrary, that the amount of free protein goes down in proportion to the amount of mature ribosomes in a cell.

Answer: It is quite probable that the synthesis of r protein mRNA is controlled in a similar manner to rRNA synthesis (33).

Question (Wickner): Have you purified the 16S RNA polymerase?
Answer: No.

Question (Wickner): When you mix purified RNA polymerase with TuTs, can you observe any cosedimentation in a glycerol gradient?
Answer: I have tried this and have failed.

Question (Rutter): Have you tested whether the effects are on initiation or on other phases of synthesis?
Answer: Psi factor must be present prior to the formation of the rifampicin-resistant complex between DNA and RNA polymerase in order to change the quality of the transcript.

Question (Rutter): Is the RNA synthesis symmetrical or asymmetrical?
Answer: The synthesis of at least tRNA is asymmetrical.

Question (Bautz): According to your last scheme, if protein synthesis is very active TuTs should become limiting and rRNA synthesis should go down. Is there enough TuTs?
Answer: There is a substantial excess of TuTs over RNA polymerase in the bacterial cell.

Question (Brahmachary): I would like to mention, from an interdisciplinary point of view, that some of your results might be of interest to embryologists. It is known, for example, that in many species of embryos rRNA begins to be synthesized markedly only as late as the gastrula stage. Also, some Japanese workers claim to have detected inhibitors of rRNA synthesis in amphibian embryos. Some of your results might be useful for embryologists to investigate.

Answer: This will be an interesting problem.

7

Elucidation of RNA Initiation (DNA Promoter?) Sequences in T4 DNA Transcription Using *Escherichia coli* RNA Polymerase and Dinucleoside Monophosphates

Salil K. Niyogi and David J. Hoffman

Biology Division
Oak Ridge National Laboratory
and
University of Tennessee — Oak Ridge Graduate School of Biomedical Sciences
Oak Ridge, Tennessee, U.S.A.

The RNA polymerase reaction can be divided into four main steps: (a) binding to DNA, (b) chain initiation, (c) chain propagation, and (d) chain termination. Steps (a) and (b) seem to be intimately related to each other.

The σ subunit of bacterial RNA polymerase (1-3) is required for accurate and asymmetrical initiation of RNA synthesis on certain phage DNA templates (4-7). The stimulatory effect of σ depends on both the base composition and the secondary structure of the template, as well as the ribonucleoside triphosphate concentration, as shown by studies with well-defined templates (8). These studies also showed that a similar type of stimulation is exerted on chain initiation by oligoribonucleotides complementary to the templates. Earlier studies indicated that chain initiation is the rate-limiting step and can be bypassed only by *complementary* oligoribonucleotides (with a free 3′-OH group), which act as chain initiators (9). Gros *et al.* (10) observed small stimulations by certain oligoribonucleotides at normal substrate concentration with *Escherichia coli* DNA as a template. Similarly, Downey *et al.* (11), using 0.2 *M* KCl, reported stimulation by certain dinucleoside monophosphates at extremely low substrate levels with T4 DNA and holoenzyme or T5 DNA in the absence and presence of σ.

Our present studies with T4 DNA show that the type of dinucleoside monophosphates stimulating the reaction is influenced by the ratio of σ to core enzyme; a low ratio favors guanosine starts, whereas adenosine starts are predominant at higher values. With holoenzyme, A-U, C-A, G-U, and U-A are the most effective and stimulate the synthesis of T4 "early" RNA, suggesting that these may act at T4 "early" initiation regions. Studies with combinations of dinucleoside monophosphates and incorporations of ^{3}H-labeled stimulatory dinucleoside monophosphates suggest that these compounds may recognize part of a continuous sequence in T4 DNA. On the basis of these studies, a *speculative* model for T4 "early" RNA initiation (DNA promoter?) sequences is proposed.

RESULTS

Effect of 0.2 *M* KCl on Dinucleoside Monophosphate Stimulation

At low (30 μM and lower) ribonucleoside triphosphate concentration, 0.2 *M* KCl strongly inhibits RNA synthesis (12). At 10 μM NTP concentration, RNA synthesis is inhibited by 90%; under these conditions, a variety of dinucleoside monophosphates produce seemingly high stimulations relative to the KCl-inhibited control value. The highest stimulation was by U-A (about thirteen-fold), agreeing with the tenfold stimulation reported by Downey *et al.* (11) under similar conditions. C-A, A-U, G-U, U-G, and A-G stimulated 7.5-, 6.5-, 4.5-, 3.0-, and 2.5-fold, respectively. In the absence of KCl, more modest, yet consistent, stimulations are obtained relative to the tenfold higher control value; A-U, C-A, U-A, and G-U produced 4.1-, 3.9-, 3.5-, and 2.9-fold stimulations, respectively.

Because of the inhibitory effect of KCl at low NTP concentrations, subsequent experiments were done in the absence of KCl.

Effect of σ-Factor Concentration on Dinucleoside Monophosphate Stimulation.

With core enzyme alone, there were small stimulations by G-G and G-A (Table I), indicating a preference for 5'-G initiations. With 10 μg of core enzyme plus 1 μg of σ factor, U-A, G-G, G-U, G-A, and G-C stimulated over threefold, showing a predominance of 5'-G initiations. When σ was increased to 5 μg along with 10 μg of core enzyme, U-A, C-A, A-U, G-U, and U-G stimulated quite well, suggesting a transition toward adenosine starts. With 5 μg of σ plus 5 μg of core enzyme, C-A, U-A, A-U, and G-U showed maximal stimulations and resembled

Table I. Effect of Dinucleoside Monophosphates on RNA Synthesis[a]

Dinucleoside monophosphate added[b]	[14C]UMP incorporated (pmoles)	Stimulation (-fold)	Dinucleoside monophosphate added	[14C]UMP incorporated (pmoles)	Stimulation (-fold)
20 μg core RNA polymerase			10 μg core RNA polymerase, 1 μg σ		
None	6	–	None	6	–
G-G	16	2.7	U-A	46	7.6
G-A	13	2.1	G-G	42	7.0
			G-U	39	6.5
			G-A	26	4.3
			G-C	22	3.7
10 μg core RNA polymerase, 5 μg σ			5 μg core RNA polymerase, 5 μg σ		
None	21	–	None	15	–
U-A	84	4.0	C-A	72	4.8
C-A	74	3.5	A-U	69	4.6
A-U	65	3.1	U-A	68	4.5
G-U	53	2.5	G-U	47	3.1
U-G	47	2.3			

[a]Reaction conditions were as described in *Materials and Methods* of ref. 17 for measuring the overall rate of RNA synthesis. Dinucleoside monophosphates (where added) were 0.21 mM with respect to phosphate.
[b]The remaining dinucleoside monophosphates, not shown in this table, stimulated less than twofold, if at all.

the situation with holoenzyme in the absence of KCl. These results agree with previous ones showing that σ factor favors initiation by ATP rather than by GTP (8,12).

Dinucleoside Monophosphates as Initiators—Incorporation Data

In order to show conclusively that stimulatory dinucleoside monophosphates act as chain initiators, ^{3}H-labeled A-U and G-U were prepared with high specific activities and tested for incorporation into the RNA product. As shown in Fig. 1, the incorporation of [^{3}H]A-U increased with its concentration, whereas that of [γ-^{32}P]ATP correspondingly decreased. Thus it seems clear that A-U is replacing ATP as an initiator during RNA synthesis. Other evidences confirm that A-U is incorporated at the 5' terminus of the RNA chain and not internally. It is evident from Fig. 1 that, under proper conditions, all the RNA starts can be made unique, namely, with A-U. Similar studies with [^{3}H]G-U and [γ-^{32}P]GTP suggest that G-U can effectively replace GTP as an initiator during RNA synthesis.

Dinucleoside Monophosphates Competing with ATP and GTP in Chain Initiation: Complexities of Recognizing Adjacent Sequences

If the stimulatory dinucleoside phosphates are indeed acting as chain initiators, one would expect a reduction of $[\gamma\text{-}^{32}P]$ ATP incorporation in the case of ATP initiation and of $[\gamma\text{-}^{32}P]$ GTP incorporation in the event of GTP initiation. It is known that RNA polymerase can initiate new RNA chains with phage DNA templates almost exclusively with either ATP or GTP (13,14). At the maximum stimulatory concentration of C-A and A-U (as judged by $[^{14}C]$ UMP incorporation), $[\gamma\text{-}^{32}P]$ ATP incorporation was very effectively reduced (Fig. 2), whereas that of $[\gamma\text{-}^{32}P]$ GTP remained essentially constant, thereby suggesting that A-U and C-A are selectively acting at an ATP-initiation site. In the case of U-A, there was a significant decrease (to a value of 30%) in ATP initiation even at low concentrations of U-A; however, at higher concentrations, GTP initiation was reduced to about 50% of control. G-U had a greater effect on GTP initiation than on ATP initiation. Similarly, A-G and U-G, which stimulated moderately, had a greater effect on GTP initiation (not shown). In the case of G-C, which had little effect on holoenzyme-directed synthesis, there was no appreciable effect on either ATP or GTP initiation. Thus A-U, U-A, and C-A appear to have a greater effect on ATP initiation than on GTP initiation, whereas with G-U, A-G, and U-G the reverse is true. The fact that some dinucleoside phosphates affect

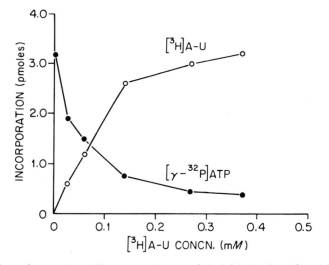

Fig. 1. Effect of increasing A-U concentration on chain initiation by either A-U or ATP. Reaction conditions were the same as those described in *Materials and Methods* of ref. 17 for measuring the rate of initiation of RNA synthesis. Ten micrograms of holo RNA polymerase was used for each reaction mixture.

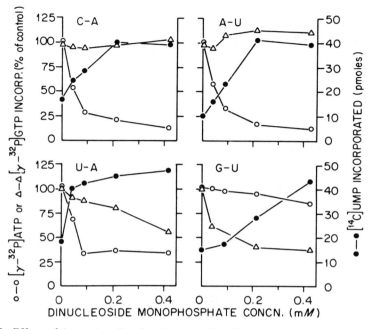

Fig. 2. *Effect of increasing dinucleoside monophosphate concentration on [¹⁴C] UMP, [γ-³²P] ATP, and [γ-³²P] GTP incorporations.* Reaction conditions were the same as those described in *Materials and Methods* of ref. 17 for measuring the overall rate of RNA synthesis ([¹⁴C] UMP incorporation) and for measuring the rate of initiation of RNA synthesis ([γ-³²P] ATP and [γ-³²P] GTP incorporation). Five micrograms of core enzyme and 5 μg of σ factor were used for each reaction mixture.

chain initiations by both ATP and GTP, although to different degrees, suggests that these dinucleoside phosphates may recognize adjoining DNA dinucleotide sequences. This is further suggested by other experiments, as described below.

Effects of Combinations of Dinucleoside Monophosphates

In order to further explore the idea that the stimulatory dinucleoside phosphates may recognize continuous DNA dinucleotide sequences, A-U, C-A, G-U, and U-A were examined in all combinations of two to see whether there were additive effects. The rationale behind these experiments is that the degree of additivity of stimulation may be inversely proportional to the proximity of the DNA dinucleotide regions. With A-U, C-A, and U-A, the net effect with any combination of two was not additive. Results with A-U and U-A are shown in Fig. 3. However, a combination of G-U with A-U (Fig. 3) or U-A (Fig. 4) or C-A (not shown) produced additive effects. On the other hand, a combination of G-U

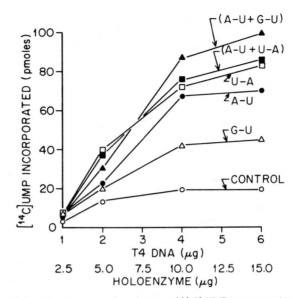

Fig. 3. *Effects of dinucleoside monophosphate on [¹⁴C] UMP incorporation with increasing concentrations of T4 DNA and holoenzyme.* Reaction conditions were the same as described in *Materials and Methods* of ref. 17 for measuring the overall rate of RNA synthesis. Each dinucleoside monophosphate concentration was 0.21 m*M* with respect to phosphate.

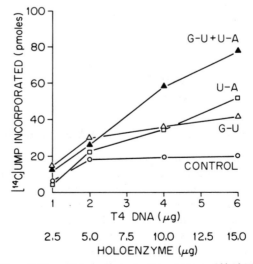

Fig. 4. *Effect of either G-U or U-A or their combination on [¹⁴C] UMP incorporation.* Reaction conditions were as described in Fig. 3.

with other G-containing dinucleoside phosphates, such as A-G and U-G, produced no additive effect. These results suggest the possibility that C-A, A-U, and U-A may recognize one continuous DNA sequence, whereas A-G, G-U, and U-G may recognize another such sequence in T4 DNA.

Competition Between Dinucleoside Monophosphates in Chain Initiation

As a further examination of the possibility that the stimulatory dinucleoside phosphates may recognize continuous DNA dinucleotide sequences, the incorporation of [³H] A-U was examined with increasing concentrations of cold C-A or U-A. As seen in Fig. 5, either U-A or C-A very effectively reduced [³H] A-U incorporation. On the other hand, compounds such as G-C (nonstimulating), G-U, A-G, and U-G (the latter three possibly representing G starts) had little effect on [³H] A-U incorporation. These results suggest that C-A, A-U, and U-A initiate the synthesis of an RNA chain(s) by recognizing adjacent DNA dinucleotide sequences that may be part of an ATP-initiation region. Similarly, from preliminary studies (Table II), [³H] G-U incorporation is effectively reduced by U-G or A-G, whereas C-A, A-U, and U-A have little effect. This suggests that A-G, G-U, and U-G recognize another set of adjoining DNA dinucleotide sequences comprising part of the GTP-initiation region in T4 DNA.

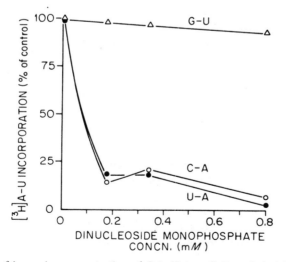

Fig. 5. *Effect of increasing concentration of C-A, U-A, or G-U on chain initiation by A-U.* Reaction conditions were similar to those described in *Materials and Methods* of ref. 17 for measuring the rate of initiation of RNA synthesis. The [³H] A-U was 0.10 mM with respect to phosphate. Ten micrograms of holo RNA polymerase was used for each reaction mixture.

Table II. Effect of Dinucleoside Monophosphates on [^{3}H] G-U Incorporation

Addition[a]	[^{3}H] G-U incorporated (pmoles)[b]
None	1.2
A-U	1.1
U-A	1.4
A-G	0.2
U-G	0.2

[a]Concentration of additions was 0.05 mM with
respect to phosphate.
[b][^{3}H] G-U concentration was 0.025 mM with respect to phosphate.

Dinucleoside Monophosphates: Recognition of T4 "Early" Promotor Regions by Competition-Hybridization Studies

It is well established that holo RNA polymerase transcribes only "early" T4 DNA genes (15). The results shown in Fig. 6 indicate that the RNAs produced with holoenzyme and dinucleoside phosphate (C-A, A-U, U-A, or G-U) stimulation indeed fall in this category. The 5-min "early" unlabeled T4 RNA competes very well with all RNAs. Adding 20-min "late" unlabeled T4 RNA had little additional competitive effect. These results suggest that these dinucleoside monophosphates act on T4 DNA regions recognized by RNA polymerase containing σ, namely, T4 "early" initiation regions. The results also support our conclusion that the stimulatory dinucleoside monophosphates initiate the synthesis of RNA chains by recognizing closely associated DNA dinucleotide sequences.

CONCLUSIONS

The ratio of σ factor to core RNA polymerase is important in determining which dinucleoside monophosphate will stimulate T4 DNA directed RNA synthesis; low ratios favor stimulation by G-containing ones, whereas A-containing ones are active at higher ratios (Table I). This agrees with previous observations (8,12) that σ factor selectively stimulates ATP over GTP initiations. These dinucleoside phosphates are acting as initiators, as suggested by their competition with [γ-^{32}P] ATP and [γ-^{32}P] GTP and confirmed by incorporation data using [^{3}H] A-U and [^{3}H] G-U.

Various results suggest that the stimulatory dinucleoside phosphates may recognize complementary DNA sequences in close proximity to one another.

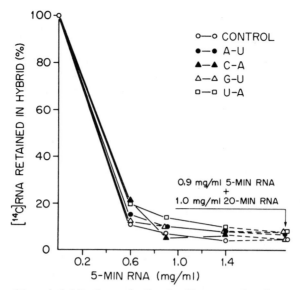

Fig. 6. Competition hybridization of dinucleoside monophosphate stimulated T4 [^{14}C] RNA against 5- and 20-min unlabeled T4 RNA. Reaction conditions were as described in *Materials and Methods* of ref. 17.

First, different combinations of C-A, A-U, and U-A exhibit little additivity in stimulatory effect. Combinations of G-U, A-G, and U-G display a similar phenomenon. The competition in chain initiation between [^3H] A-U and unlabeled C-A and U-A (Fig. 5) and that between [^3H] G-U and unlabeled A-G and U-G (Table II) support the above. In addition, competition-hybridization experiments demonstrate that the stimulatory dinucleoside phosphates act on T4 DNA sequences recognized by RNA polymerase containing σ, namely, T4 "early" initiation regions. The facts that higher concentrations of U-A cause some inhibition of GTP initiation as well as of ATP initiation and that G-U in excess has similar effects on ATP initiation besides that of GTP further suggest a complex relation in which these compounds may recognize complementary dinucleotide sequences in a continuous region(s) in T4 DNA. It should be pointed out that these conclusions are based on previous studies (8,9,16) showing that RNA synthesis is stimulated only by oligoribonucleotides *complementary* to the template. Confirmation of the purity and sequences of the dinucleoside monophosphates (17) supports the specificity of the stimulatory effects. A possible, although speculative, T4 RNA initiation (DNA promoter?) sequence that is compatible with our results is given below:

$$\text{DNA} \cdots 3' \cdots \text{G-T-A-T-}(N)_n\text{-A-T-C-A-C} \cdots 5'$$
$$\text{RNA} \cdots 5' \cdots \text{C-A-U-A-}(N)_n\text{-U-A-G-U-G} \cdots 3'$$

C-A is placed at the 5′ end of the RNA since no compounds of the type N-C were stimulatory. C-A would stimulate by initiating a start that would normally occur with A-U [since A-U is the most common starting sequence with T4 DNA as template (5)]. In a similar manner, U-A could substitute for A-U. This reasoning is supported by the competition by C-A and U-A during A-U initiation. Of the compounds of the type N-G, both A-G and U-G were somewhat stimulatory; these could stimulate by substituting for a normal G-U initiation. Indeed, A-G and U-G compete with G-U for RNA initiation. We have tested compounds such as A-A-A, A-A-C, A-A-G, A-A-U, A-U-U, A-U-G, A-U-A, and U-A-G. Of these only A-U-A and U-A-G showed significant stimulation, in agreement with our proposed model. The DNA region complementary to C-A-U-A could represent a sequence for ATP initiations, whereas that for A-G-U-G may represent one for GTP initiations. The fact that some dinucleoside monophosphates affect both ATP and GTP starts, although to different degrees, suggests that the distance between these two regions in the model may comprise a small number of nucleotides.

Studies from our laboratory (unpublished) have shown that RNA polymerase − bound "promoter" regions in T4 DNA have a high $(A+T)/(G+C)$ ratio and are about 54–60 nucleotides long. If all nucleotides are involved, one could postulate a multiple sequence of the above model. Our proposed model has features characteristic of a poly(dA-dT) structure, which is known to be preferred by RNA polymerase (18,19). A high (A+T) region should possess a low T_m and could have a partially "melted" structure that might serve as a target or recognition region for RNA polymerase on an otherwise duplex molecule. There may be about 10–12 σ-recognized promoter regions per T4 genome (20). For strand selection, the base sequences adjacent to the poly(dA-dT) region on the "proper" strand in our model must have some specificity determinants that enable σ-containing RNA polymerase to select and transcribe that particular strand. A conclusive proof of our tentative model will have to await a direct sequence analysis of T4 "early" RNA initiation (promoter?) regions. The present studies suggest the possibility of using dinucleoside monophosphates to probe RNA initiation (DNA promoter?) sequences *in vitro*. Our studies suggest the interesting possibility of using oligoribonucleotides to initiate the synthesis of specific RNAs with unique starts on various DNA templates. Such RNAs should be useful for other studies, such as sequence determinations and specific protein synthesis *in vitro*. With regard to mapping promoter sites, it should be pointed out that although dinucleoside monophosphates initiate T4 DNA directed "early" RNA synthesis, it has yet to be established whether these initiation sites are identical to the promoter regions. There is compelling evidence from the studies of Blattner *et al.* (21,22) that, in the case of λ DNA, the promoter region is not transcribed. We prefer to call the sites recognized by dinucleoside monophosphates "RNA initiation regions."

ACKNOWLEDGMENTS

D. J. H. is a Postdoctoral Investigator supported by a Research in Aging Training Grant; PHS Grant No. HD 00296 from the NICHD. Oak Ridge National Laboratory is operated by Union Carbide Corporation for the U.S. Atomic Energy Commission.

REFERENCES

1. R. R. Burgess, A. A. Travers, J. J. Dunn, and E. K. F. Bautz. *Nature* **221**:43-46 (1969).
2. J. S. Krakow, K. Daley, and M. Karstadt. *Proc. Natl. Acad. Sci. (USA)* **62**:432-437. (1969).
3. D. Berg, K. Barrett, and M. Chamberlin. In L. Grossman and K. Moldave (eds.), *Methods in Enzymology*, Vol. 21D, Academic Press, New York, p. 506 (1971).
4. A. A. Travers and R. R. Burgess. *Nature* **222**:537-540 (1969).
5. E. Mauro, L. Snyder, P. Parino, A. Lamberti, A. Coppo, and G. P. Tocchini-Valentini. *Nature* **222**:533-537 (1969).
6. E. K. F. Bautz, F. A. Bautz, and J. J. Dunn. *Nature* **223**:1022-1024 (1969).
7. M. Sugiura, T. Okamoto, and M. Takanami. *Nature* **225**:598-600 (1970).
8. S. K. Niyogi. *J. Mol. Biol.* **64**:609-618 (1972).
9. S. K. Niyogi and A. Stevens. *J. Biol. Chem.* **240**:2593-2598 (1965).
10. F. Gros, J. Dubert, A. Tissieres, S. Burgeois, M. Michelson, R. Soffer, and L. Legault. *Cold Spring Harbor Symp. Quant. Biol.* **28**:299-313 (1963).
11. K. M. Downey, B. S. Jurmark, and A. G. So. *Biochemistry* **10**:4970-4975 (1971).
12. D. J. Hoffman and S. K. Niyogi. *Biochim. Biophys. Acta* **299**:588-595 (1973).
13. U. Maitra and J. Hurwitz. *Proc. Natl. Acad. Sci. (USA)* **54**:815-822 (1965).
14. H. Bremer, M. W. Konrad, K. Gaines, and G. S. Stent. *J. Mol. Biol.* **13**:540-553 (1965).
15. E. N. Brody and E. P. Geiduschek. *Biochemistry* **9**:1300-1309 (1970).
16. K. M. Downey and A. G. So. *Biochemistry* **9**:2520 (1970).
17. D. J. Hoffman and S. K. Niyogi. *Proc. Natl. Acad. Sci. (USA)* **70**:574-578 (1973).
18. O. W. Jones and P. Berg. *J. Mol. Biol.* **22**:199-209 (1966).
19. K. Shishido and Y. Ikeda. *Biochem. Biophys. Res. Commun.* **44**:1420-1428 (1971).
20. E. K. F. Bautz, F. A. Bautz, and E. Beck. *Mol. Gen. Genet.* **118**:199-207 (1972).
21. F. R. Blattner and J. E. Dahlberg. *Nature New Biol.* **237**:227-232 (1972).
22. F. R. Blattner, J. E. Dahlberg, J. K. Boeitinger, M. Fiandt, and W. Szybalski. *Nature New Biol.* **237**:232-236 (1972).
23. S. K. Niyogi and C. A. Thomas, Jr. *J. Biol. Chem.* **234**:1220 (1968).

DISCUSSION

Question (Burma): What happens when you use pApU, that is, a dinucleotide which starts with 5'-phosphate? Will it affect the initiation?

Answer: Based on our earlier studies, a compound such as pApU should act as an initiator because it still has a free 3'-hydroxyl end. ApUp would not be expected to stimulate, and it does not. Because of the higher stability of complexes formed by 5'-phosphate-containing oligonucleotides with complementary polynucleotides (23), one might expect pApU to be more efficient than ApU in acting as a chain initiator.

Question (Mehrotra): What happens with a short pulse of a mixture of these dinucleoside monophosphates, to find out the preference the RNA polymerase has in the initiation?

Answer: The experiment has not been done with all 16 compounds together. It is an interesting suggestion and should be tested. However, they have been tested in many combination of twos, threes, and fours to test additivity in stimulation; the RNA polymerase seems to prefer the most stimulatory compound in cases where there is no additivity.

Question (Rutter): The apparent specificity of initiation you get is most interesting (competition by early T4 messages) since one would predict from random binding of nucleotides artificial initiation at many sites. One explanation is that there is a specific conformation of the DNA itself, perhaps a node formed by intrachain hydrogen bonds. I know that this is not stable by itself, but the interaction with the polymerase may stabilize such a node, and the dinucleotide could then operate at that site. Your tentative model for initiation site region might take into account this possibility.

Answer: Both of your points are quite plausible. We have also envisioned that the high (A+T) content of the initiation region may have a partially melted structure at $37°C$, thereby providing a region that the polymerase can "see" on an otherwise duplex DNA molecule. It is known from our studies with well-defined templates and complementary oligonucleotide initiators that the polymerase can indeed stabilize complexes that would not otherwise occur.

Question (Sambrook): Two alternative models for the structure of the promoter site are under discussion: (a) Rutter (last question) and (b) Niyogi. It seems to me that (a) cannot be correct because hairpin structures of this sort are much less stable than the linear duplex, as a consequence of loss of stacking energy. Thus it seems unlikely that polymerase would be able to find such structures to use for initiation *in vitro. In vitro,* of course, hairpin structure could exist because of superhelical twists in DNA or because of protein which stabilizes the unstacked bases in the hairpin. Model (b) may be correct, but then it becomes difficult to explain the action of dinucleoside monophosphates. For if the base composition of the promoter site renders it so unstable that it is partially denatured *in vitro,* I do not see how binding of a dinucleotide to the denatured region could occur.

Answer: I believe that the polymerase itself can help the binding of a dinucleotide to the denatured region. It may be pointed out that even a nucleoside triphosphate can presumably bind to a complementary DNA nucleotide in the presence of the enzyme. This stabilizing effect of the enzyme may play a key role in promoter site selection by specific dinucleoside monophosphates.

Question (Szybalski): We are planning to see the effects of various di- and trinucleotides on the priming of *in vitro* λ RNA synthesis, since in this system there are only four starts, and we know the exact sequences of all four RNA starts. Do you believe that the effects of the di- and trinucleotide primers will be just as predicted from the five terminal sequences (see ref. 21)?

Answer: I believe and certainly hope so.

8

Stringent Coupling Between Transcription, Translation, and Degradation of Messenger RNA in an Inducible Enzyme System: A Theoretical Analysis

U. N. Singh

Molecular Biology Group
Tata Institute of Fundamental Research
Bombay, India

Many of the studies on the mechanism of expression of genetic information in recent years have centered around various "factors" or functional elements needed to ensure a minimal level of fidelity in the transcription and translation of a messenger RNA. Instability of mRNA—one of the major postulates of Jacob and Monod (6) implicated in the regulation of induced β-galactosidase synthesis and now amply supported by direct experimental evidence—may have profound influence on the fidelity of translation in a whole cell. This aspect, of course, is not immediately obvious in the studies on isolated systems. A question of fundamental significance, which refers to a still higher level of organization in the cellular hierarchy, is, how are these *unit processes*—transcription, translation, and degradation of mRNA implicated in the regulation of protein synthesis—coordinated in a cell? In 1966, Stent (14) proposed a very provocative hypothesis in this direction and envisioned translational movement of ribosomes to have an obligatory role to play in an orderly transcription of mRNA. These concepts are still in a very fluid state and are being widely debated in the literature. Inducible enzyme systems, which so richly contributed to the development of some of our most basic ideas on the expression of genetic information, also provide a versatile experimental model for an investigation of many of these questions. In recent years, the precision achieved in the DNA·RNA hybridization technique by the use of transducing phage containing various segments of host genome has given fresh impetus to such studies. An optimal exploitation of these developments needed a strong formal base for the induced enzyme synthesis. A number of workers (2-5,7,8,10,15) made attempts in this direction in the past. The relevance of many of these theoretical investigations to the real system, however, remained obscure in the absence of a rational basis for the instability of mRNA. A model of protein synthesis described elsewhere (11,12) gave adequate considerations to these limitations and has thus greatly rectified the situation. A unique feature of this model is that it enables us to define unstable mRNA in a way that is operationally meaningful from an experimentalist's point of view, i.e., quantitation of mRNA based on DNA·RNA hybridization. In this chapter, I examine various aspects of the kinetics of enzyme induction under a variety of experimentally realizable constraints. An extended version of these analyses has appeared elsewhere (13).

THEORETICAL FORMULATION

Basic Postulates and Definitions

The analysis of the inducible enzyme system presented here is based essentially on a model of protein synthesis described earlier (11). The basic postulates of the model may be summarized as follows: (a) Transcription, translation, and degradation of mRNA proceed in a $5'$- to $3'$-end direction. (b) The three processes are stringently coupled. (c) The decay of mRNA is attributed to two distinct processes, (i) a stochastic process implying a random inactivation of initiation sites, and (ii) a deterministic process that defines the processive (stepwise and sequential) degradation of mRNA coupled with the translational movement of ribosomes. In essence, the dynamics of protein synthesis on polyribosomes with initiation sites successively exposed to the degradative enzyme, either free or a part of ribosomes, constitutes a special case of the so-called Markov chain. The details of mathematical formulation and its varied consequences have been discussed in our earlier communications (11,12).

We consider a simple model operon comprising a single cistron with the operator region O as shown in Fig. 1A. Following our original convention, we define the length of an mRNA or of a DNA template in units of δ, the average distance between adjacent ribosomes on the mRNA. The unit of time τ is defined as the time required by a ribosome to traverse a distance δ. It is obvious that in a stringently coupled system τ also represents the time required by an RNA polymerase to traverse the same distance δ on the DNA template. The average distance T between adjacent polymerases in Fig. 1A is related to the transcription frequency.

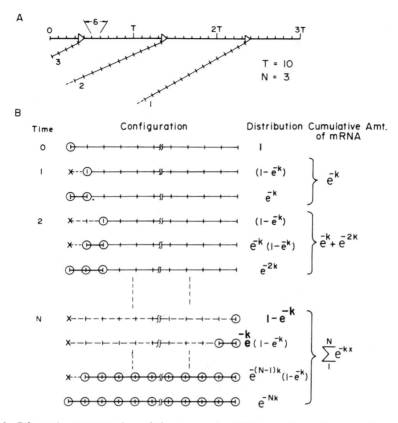

Fig. 1. Schematic representation of the states of mRNA in a stringently coupled system.
A: A "transcription-translational complex" with three RNA polymerases acting simultaneously on a DNA template. Ribosomes on the growing RNA chains are not shown for the sake of clarity. δ refers to the distance between adjacent ribosomes and is considered as a unit of length. T is the distance between adjacent polymerases expressed in units of δ. Note that T also represents the time interval, expressed in units of τ, between successive initiations of transcription. B: Schematic description of the method used in calculating cumulative amount (number of unit lengths, δ) of an mRNA present in a cell following its initiation at 0 time. The thin lines indicate segments still to be synthesized, the thick lines the segment detectable by DNA·RNA hybridization, and the dashed lines the degraded parts of mRNA. In a stringently coupled system, RNA polymerase is supposed to be moving immediately ahead of the first ribosome.

Cumulative Amounts of mRNA as Determined by DNA·RNA Hybridization

We have emphasized earlier (11,12) that a considerable amount of unstable mRNA in a cell may exist in nascent and partially degraded states that nevertheless, in association with polyribosomes, constitute a major fraction of the protein-synthesizing machinery. This has led to serious conceptual difficulties in the characterization and quantitation of mRNA. The only analytical method available at present that provides most explicit estimates of the total amount of unstable mRNA existing in a cell is that based on DNA·RNA hybridization. The postulation of a functional relationship between the amounts of mRNA obtained from such measurements and the observed rate of protein synthesis, however, has been little more than presumptive. Indeed, a major objective in the analyses presented here is to develop a formal base for such a relationship.

It is apparent that the amount of mRNA, defined as the total number of unit lengths δ in our model system, is compatible with the quantitation of mRNA in a cell by DNA·RNA hybridization, assuming of course that hybridization conditions favor the formation of stable hybrids with all mRNA fragments $\geq \delta$. Before coming to a complex situation represented by Fig. 1A, we consider a simpler case of the synthesis of mRNA by one RNA polymerase. Figure 1B represents essentially a "transcription-translational complex" (9) in a stringently coupled system and shows configurations of polyribosomes at different times following initiation of transcription. For convenience, we further consider the mRNA existing in two distinct states: (a) nascent mRNA associated with the "transcription-translational complex" as shown in Fig. 1A and (b) completed mRNA chains present in free polyribosomes. In the distribution values shown in column 3 of Fig. 1B, k represents the first-order rate constant for the inactivation of initiation site. The expressions for the cumulative amount of mRNA, $M(t)$, at any time t, where $t \leq N$ is defined as the total number of unit lengths δ, may be written as

$$M_i(t) = M(t) = \frac{e^{-k}(1-e^{-kt})}{1-e^{-k}} \tag{1}$$

The subscript i here refers to nascent mRNA chains, and 0 time refers to the time of attachment of the first ribosome. Note that for $t > N$, mRNA will exist in association with free polyribosomes, and

$$M_c(t) = M(t) = \frac{e^{-k}(e^{kN}-1)e^{-kt}}{1-e^{-k}} \tag{2}$$

where the subscript c refers to completed mRNA chains.

Enzyme Synthesis

Continuous Induction

The method outlined in the previous section can be readily extended to a more complex and realistic situation in which a DNA template is transcribed simultaneously by more than one RNA polymerase, as depicted schematically in

Fig. 1A. In a model inducible enzyme system, we consider the time of initiation of transcription by the first polymerase molecule following addition of inducer as the 0 time. Without getting into algebraic details, the expressions for the amounts of mRNA in nascent $M_i(t)$ and completed $M_c(t)$ states at any time t may be summarized as follows:

For $t \leqslant N$, where N is the transcription time,

$$M_i(t) = M(t) = \frac{te^{-k}}{T(1-e^{-k})} - \frac{e^{-2k}(1-e^{-kt})}{T(1-e^{-k})^2} \tag{3}$$

For all values of $t > N$, it is apparent that the amount $M_i(t)$ of mRNA in nascent state will be equal to $M_i(N)$ and will remain constant. The amount $M_c(t)$ of mRNA in free polyribosomes for $t = N + \sigma$, where $\sigma = 1, 2, 3, \ldots$, can be written as

$$M_c(t) = \frac{e^{-2k}(e^{kN}-1)(e^{k\sigma}-1)e^{-kt}}{T(1-e^{-k})^2} \tag{4}$$

The expression for the total amount $M(t)$ of mRNA for $t > N$ can be readily derived from the above equations and shown to be

$$M(t) = \frac{Ne^{-k}}{T(1-e^{-k})} - \frac{e^{-2k}(e^{kN}-1)e^{-kt}}{T(1-e^{-k})^2} \tag{5}$$

In considering the synthesis of the corresponding complete protein, i.e., induced enzyme, we note that, in view of the finite time required for the transcription or translation of an mRNA, there will be a minimal time difference between the appearance of mRNA (as measured by DNA·RNA hybridization) and the enzyme, which will correspond to the transcription (or translation) time of the mRNA concerned. Assuming 0 time in this case as the time at which the first enzyme molecule appears, the cumulative amount $E(t)$ of enzyme at any time t during continuous induction is given by

$$E(t) = \frac{t}{T(1-e^{-k})} - \frac{e^{-2k}(1-e^{-kt})}{T(1-e^{-k})^2} \tag{6}$$

Pulse Induction

Another extensively studied experimental variation of induced enzyme synthesis is often referred to as "pulse induction." We consider a model system in which initiations of transcription are allowed for a finite period η where $\eta < N$. Further initiations are prevented either by removing inducer or by using an appropriate inhibitor such as rifampicin. Expressions for the amount of mRNA in this case are summarized below.

It is apparent that for $t < \eta$, $M(t)$ is again given by equation (3): When $\eta < t \leqslant N$, we have

$$M_i(t) = M(t) = \frac{\eta e^{-k}}{T(1-e^{-k})} - \frac{e^{-2k}(e^{k\eta}-1)e^{-kt}}{T(1-e^{-k})^2} \tag{7}$$

For $t > N$, let $t = N + \sigma$, where $\sigma = 1, 2, 3, \ldots, \eta$. $M_i(t)$ and $M_c(t)$ are then given by

$$M_i(t) = \frac{(\eta-\sigma)e^{-k}}{T(1-e^{-k})} - \frac{e^{-2k}(e^{k(\eta-\sigma)}-1)e^{-kN}}{T(1-e^{-k})^2} \tag{8}$$

and

$$M_c(t) = \frac{e^{-2k}(e^{kN}-1)(e^{k\sigma}-1)e^{-kt}}{T(1-e^{-k})^2} \tag{9}$$

From equations (8) and (9), we have

$$M(t) = \frac{(\eta-\sigma)e^{-k}}{T(1-e^{-k})} - \frac{e^{-2k}[e^{k\eta}-1-e^{kN}(e^{k\sigma}-1)]e^{-kt}}{T(1-e^{-k})^2} \tag{10}$$

It is seen from equation (8) that, as σ approaches the limiting value η, $M_i(t) = 0$ and all the messenger RNA chains for $t > (N + \eta)$ will be associated with free polyribosomes as given by equation (9). It is further apparent that the amount of mRNA for $t > (N + \eta)$ will decay in a strictly exponential fashion. This conclusion, I believe, is not so trivial and is of considerable significance from an experimental point of view. While the model does provide a formal justification for the observed exponential decay of rapidly labeled RNA as measured either by DNA·RNA hybridization or by trichloroacetic acid precipitation, it also lays down an important condition often not fully appreciated by experimental workers. It requires that DNA·RNA hybridization conditions employed should lead to the formation of stable hybrids in quantitative amounts with all mRNA fragments of size greater than a certain minimal size; it can be shown to be immaterial what this minimal size is. In this connection, if I may venture to say so, some pretreatment of cellular extracts in order to break the larger polyribosomes into smaller fragments before extracting RNA may lead to an improvement in the quantitation of mRNA by hybridization with DNA.

BEHAVIOR OF A MODEL SYSTEM

In this section, I propose to examine briefly the behavior of a model system on the basis of the expressions derived in the previous section. Figure 2 shows theoretical curves calculated for $N = 30$ and $k = 0.1$ time^{-1} in units of σ and τ, respectively. The order of magnitude of the value for k here corresponds to an estimate based on the observed translational rate and half-life of mRNA in

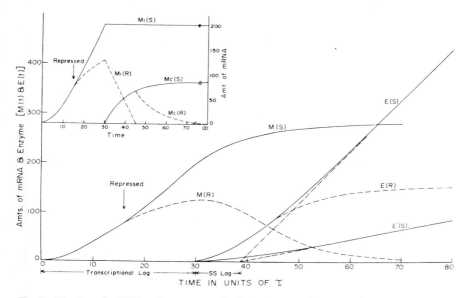

Fig. 2. Kinetics of mRNA and enzyme synthesis during asynchronous induction. The curves were calculated for a model system; the length of mRNA, $N = 30$ and $k = 0.1$, the inducer being added at 0 time. Continuous induction approaching a steady state: $M(S) = $ mRNA, $E(S) = $ enzyme. $E'(S)$ refers to enzyme synthesis for transcription frequency one-fifth that in $E(S)$. $M(R)$ and $E(R)$ represent mRNA and enzyme synthesis, respectively, in pulse-induction type experiments; the vertical arrow indicates removal of inducer. The inset describes the behavior of mRNA in nascent and completed (in free polyribosomes) states during continuous (solid curves) and pulse induction (dashed curves). Subscripts i and c refer to nascent and free mRNA, respectively.

Escherichia coli. Curves $M(S)$ and $E(S)$ refer to the cumulative amounts of mRNA and enzyme, respectively, during continuous induction for $T = 1$. Note that while mRNA begins to appear immediately after derepression, the enzyme appears only after a finite lag that corresponds to the transcription time of mRNA.

The intercept on the time axis by an extrapolation of the linear synthetic rate in the steady state as shown by the dashed line, often considered as the lag period, has been the subject of considerable controversy in the literature (1). It is interesting to note that curve $E(S)$ calculated for $T = 5$, i.e., the transcription frequency being one-fifth of that assumed for the curve $E(S)$, also has the same intercept. This implies that the lag period is independent of transcription frequency, or of induction level as experimentally demonstrated by Branscomb and Stuart (1). To be more explicit, we must emphasize here that the lag period as observed in enzyme induction should be considered as being composed of two physiologically distinct components: (a) "transcriptional (or translational)" lag and (b) "steady-state" lag, as shown in Fig. 2. It can be easily shown that the steady-state lag, *LS*, is given by $e^{-2k}/(1-e^{-k})$ in units of τ. For $k \ll 1$, we can further show that $LS \simeq t_{1/2}/\ln 2$. Thus, assuming the half-life of mRNA to be 1–2 min, the model predicts a steady-state lag period of 1½–3 min. This is not far from an estimate derived from the data reported by Branscomb and Stuart (1).

The dashed curves $M(R)$ and $E(R)$ in Fig. 2 refer to the behavior of mRNA and enzyme, respectively, during pulse induction. The inset in Fig. 2 describes changes in the relative amounts of mRNA in nascent and completed states during continuous and pulse induction.

In considering the role of mRNA as a template in protein synthesis, it is generally assumed that the rate of protein synthesis is directly proportional to the amount of mRNA. However, if a protein is measured by its biological activity, as in the case of enzymes, and the amount of mRNA by DNA·RNA hybridization, such a formalism breaks down or is applicable only under certain conditions. In view of the considerable interest in recent years in the functional *vs.* physical decay of mRNA, this deviation from linearity as indicated in Fig. 2

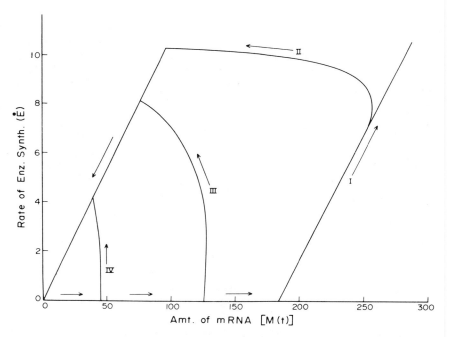

Fig. 3. Phase diagram describing the relationship between the rate of enzyme synthesis and the amount of mRNA as determined by DNA·RNA hybridization. Straight line I refers to continuous induction. Curves II, III, and IV were calculated for varying durations (40, 15, and 5 in units of τ, respectively) of pulse induction.

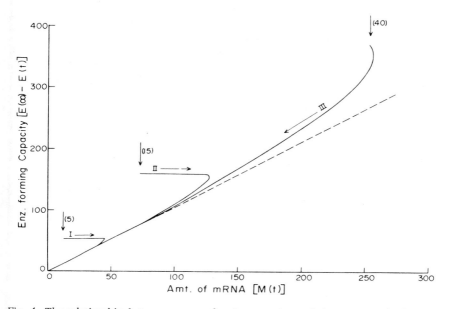

Fig. 4. The relationship between enzyme-forming capacity and the amount of mRNA as estimated by DNA·RNA hybridization. The numbers in brackets represent durations of pulse induction.

needs a more precise formulation. The phase diagram shown in Fig. 3, in which we have plotted rate of enzyme synthesis *vs.* amount of mRNA for both continuous and pulse induction, clearly emphasizes the nonlinear relationship. An important point that is apparent from this plot is that the slope of the ascending part of the straight line during continuous induction is the same as that of the descending linear part of the curves for pulse induction. This feature, indeed, may provide a useful guideline for an investigation of the stringency in the coupling between transcription, translation, and degradation of mRNA.

Another parameter derived from the studies on pulse induction, which has been widely used to define the dynamic properties of the template involved in the enzyme synthesis, is the so-called enzyme-forming capacity. In the present notation, this is simply $[E(\infty) - E(t)]$, where t now refers to η, the duration of pulse induction. It is instructive to know the relationship between this hypo-thetical entity and the amount of mRNA as determined directly by DNA·RNA hybridization. This is shown in Fig. 4, in which $[E(\infty) - E(t)]$ for varying durations of pulse induction is plotted against the amount of mRNA present at the time of its termination. The analysis emphasizes that the enzyme-forming capacity should vary linearly with amounts of mRNA only over a limited range and that the nature and extent of deviation from linearity depend on the duration of pulse induction.

I have tried to develop in this presentation a theoretical base for the synthesis of induced enzyme within the framework of our present notion about transcription, translation, and degradation of mRNA. The only *a priori* postulate I have advanced here is that the inactivation of an initiation site at the 5′ end of mRNA is a stochastic process and that it is immaterial whether the 5′ end belongs to an incomplete or a complete chain. It is true that the inferences derived from these analyses apply strictly to a system in which transcription, translation, and degradation of mRNA are stringently coupled. To dispel any misgivings, and this fear is not entirely unfounded, I must reiterate that this is only a model system. At this stage, I do not pretend to postulate how stringent this coupling is. In fact, the usefulness of this model lies in its role as a suitable reference system for experimental investigations directed to some of these very questions related to the mechanism of coordination between the three processes implicated in the regulation of protein synthesis.

As a concluding remark, which is very much relevant to the approach used in these investigations, I recall a statement of Sir Arthur Eddington in *Pathways in Science*—". . . it is also a good rule not to put overmuch confidence in the observational results that are put forward until they have been confirmed by theory."

REFERENCES

1. E. W. Branscomb and R. N. Stuart. *Biochem. Biophys. Res. Commun.* **32**:731 (1968).
2. B. C. Goodwin. In G. Weber (ed.), *Advances in Enzyme Regulation,* Vol. 3, Pergamon Press, Oxford (1965), p. 425.
3. R. Gordon. *J. Theoret. Biol.* **22**:515 (1969).
4. M. D. Garrick. *J. Theoret. Biol.* **17**:19 (1967).
5. F. Heinmets. *Quantitative Cellular Biology,* Marcel Dekker, Inc., New York (1970).
6. F. Jacob and J. Monod. *J. Mol. Biol.* **3**:318 (1961).
7. C. T. MacDonald and J. H. Gibbs. *Biopolymers* **7**:707 (1969).
8. J. Maniloff. *J. Theoret. Biol.* **23**:441 (1969).
9. O. L. Miller, Jr., B. R. Beatty, B. A. Hamkalo, and C. A. Thomas, Jr. *Cold Spring Harbor Symp. Quant. Biol.* **35**:505 (1970).
10. R. D. Parker and T. L. Lincoln. *J. Theoret. Biol.* **15**:218 (1967).
11. U. N. Singh. *J. Theoret. Biol.* **25**:444 (1969).
12. U. N. Singh and R. S. Cupta. *J. Theoret. Biol.* **30**:603 (1971).
13. U. N. Singh. *J. Theoret. Biol.,* **40**:553 (1973).
14. G. S. Stent. *Proc. Roy. Soc. B* **164**:181 (1966).
15. J. M. Zimmerman and R. Simha. *J. Theoret. Biol.* **13**:106 (1966).

DISCUSSION

Question (Burma): Your model depends heavily on the existence of 5'-exonuclease, which has not yet been found. Suppose there is endonuclease involved, then how will you modify your model? If a combination of an endonuclease and a 3'-exonuclease is involved, then what will be the situation?

Answer: Although it is true that no 5'-exonuclease has been isolated, the nature of degradative products of mRNA during translation does indicate the existence of such an enzymic activity. It is conceivable that the enzyme functions only in association with ribosomes (like many of the proteins of the ribosome which do not exhibit any biochemical activity in isolation). As regards the behavior of a model based on an endonuclease or 3'-exonuclease, or a combination of both, I am afraid I have not found the notion sufficiently provocative to get into, either conceptually or on the strength of experimental evidence.

Question (Szybalski): In the case of the leftward λ mRNA, we know the mechanism of mRNA degradation. First, there is an endonucleolytic cleavage to ½ and ¼ mRNA molecules. Second, they are cleaved to 4-5S size, especially the promoter-proximal fragment. Finally, the 4-5S fragments are degraded exonucleolytically in the 3'→5' direction. Some fragments are more resistant to this final degradation than others. How does this experimental fact relate to your theoretical scheme?

Answer: I think one should be cautious in extrapolating the inferences derived from observations on viral mRNA, the functions of which may be under an entirely different set of constraints geared to viral multiplication. It is conceivable that in this case translation and degradation are temporally separated, and in such a situation I do not visualize any conceptual difficulty in the degradation of mRNA either by an endonuclease or by a 3'-exonuclease. However, experimental evidences for unstable mRNA implicated in the synthesis of induced enzymes do not indicate such a temporal separation. I only wish to emphasize that in the latter case a model evisaging 5'→3' degradation demands the minimum number of assumptions.

9

Gene-Specific Changes in Induced Enzyme Synthesis in *Escherichia coli* Infected with Phage pX174

Amit Ghosh and Ramendra K. Poddar

Biophysics Laboratory
Saha Institute of Nuclear Physics
Calcutta, India

A few simple experiments involving measurement of induced enzyme synthesis in *Escherichia coli* cells infected with single-stranded DNA phage ϕX174 which indirectly suggest a peculiar type of *in vivo* control of transcription of the genes of the infected cells are described in this chapter. The intracellular replication of this phage, which contains only eight genes and about 5500 nucleotides in its DNA, may be summed up as follows (1). Upon entry into the cell, the single-stranded circular DNA ("plus" strand) of the virus is quickly converted to a double-stranded circular DNA, called "replicative form" or RF, as a result of synthesis of the complementary strand ("minus" strand) mediated by the host enzymes. This parental RF becomes associated with a site on the bacterial membrane; it then replicates semiconservatively and symmetrically, releasing a number of daughter RF molecules into the cytoplasm in such a manner that the input viral "plus" strand always remains associated with the site, exchanging partners at each replication. RF replication, for which both host and viral functions are necessary, is initiated about 2-3 min after infection (37°C) and continues until about 12 min, when it practically comes to a halt. At this time, an asymmetrical replication of the daughter RF molecules sets in at a very rapid rate. Phage capsid proteins, which have already been made in the cell, are essential for this switchover to asymmetrical DNA replication. During this stage, only the "minus" strand of the RF molecule serves as template for synthesis of a new complementary "plus" strand, expelling thereby the old "plus" strand, which is immediately encapsulated by the capsid proteins to produce a mature phage.

In spite of some uncertainties about details, the above scheme is generally considered to be correct. Our knowledge regarding what happens to the infected cell itself is, however, much less precise. If one measures the total DNA, RNA, and protein synthesis, one detects hardly any difference between an infected and a healthy cell (2,3). However, at about the time, i.e., 12-15 min after infection, when symmetrical replication of RF ceases and asymmetrical replication of viral "plus" strand ensues, the host DNA synthesis also ceases (4,5). As regards RNA synthesis, if pulse-labeled RNA is first allowed to degrade and then turn into stable 16S and 23S RNA, this rate seems to be considerably slowed down in the infected cell (6). Regarding synthesis of host-specific proteins, it has been found that a ϕX-infected *E. coli* cell, although its genome is not replicating, retains the ability to synthesize β-galactosidase (7). This phenomenon has not, however, been thoroughly investigated. We believe that a detailed quantitative study of this phenomenon may reveal some interesting features of control of transcription and/or translation of the nonreplicating genome of ϕ X-infected *E. coli* cells. Some preliminary results of such a study are presented herein, based on measurement of synthesis of three inducible enzymes specified by three more-or-less equispaced genes on the genetic map of *E. coli*. The first one is the *lac* gene at the 2 o'clock position, responsible for the formation of β-galactosidase in response to its specific inducer, isopropylthiogalactoside. The second one is the *dsd* gene at the 6 o'clock position, which codes for the enzyme D-serine deaminase. This enzyme is formed when D-serine is added to the culture medium. The third gene is the *ind* located at the 9 o'clock site, which triggers the synthesis of tryptophanase when induced with tryptophan.

MATERIALS AND METHODS

All the strains were obtained from Dr. R. L. Sinsheimer, California Institute of Technology, U.S.A.

Bacterial Strains

Bacterial strains used were *E. coli* C, normal host of ϕX174 *wt*; *E. coli* 15 *t*3 $\overline{\text{TAU}}$, a temperature-sensitive mutant which supports ϕX174 growth at 30°C but not at 40°C and requires thymine, arginine, and uracil for growth; and *E. coli* HF 4714, an amber suppressor strain used for plating ϕX174 *am*3.

Phage

The phage used was ϕX174 *am*3, a lysis-defective mutant of ϕX174..

Medium

Tris-glycerol medium contained 12 g tris, 35 mg KCl, 1 g NH$_4$Cl, 0.2 g MgCl$_2$J6H2O, 2.7 mg FeCl$_3$J6H2O, 58 mg NaCl, 0.4 g KH$_2$PO4, 0.3 g Na$_2$SO$_4$, 25% glycerol (10 ml) per 1000 ml of distilled water, the *p*H being adjusted to 7.5 with 6 *N* HCl.

Induced Enzyme Studies

Inducer used for β-galactosidase was isopropylthiogalactoside, 1 mg/10 ml of culture medium; for tryptophanase, DL-tryptophan, 1 mg/ml culture medium; for D-serine deaminase, DL-serine, 300 μg/ml culture medium.

E. coli cells were allowed to grow to a log phase concentration of 3 X 10^8 cells/ml. These were then divided into two parts, one part being used as control, the other for infection. Fifteen minutes after infection, the specific inducers mentioned above were added. One-milliliter aliquots were withdrawn at specified intervals and collected over 0.5 ml toluene at ice

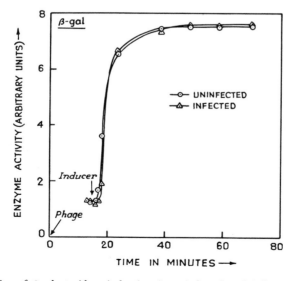

Fig. 1. Kinetics of β-galactosidase induction in uninfected and infected cells. To one-half of a culture of *E. coli* C growing in tris-glycerol medium ϕX174 *am*3 was added at m.o.i. = 5 at 0 min. Isopropylthiogalactoside was added 15 min later.

temperature. The tubes were shaken vigorously. After the sampling was complete, the enzymes were assayed following the methods of Pardee and Prestidge (8,9) as modified by Pollard and Davis (10). Optical densities were measured in a Zeiss PMQ II spectrophotometer.

RESULTS AND DISCUSSION

Studies on the *lac* Gene

Figure 1 shows the formation of induced β-galactosidase in infected cells. It is seen that the *lac* gene was transcribed and translated normally and that apparently there was no effect due to φX. However, a closer look reveals something interesting. Figure 2 shows that the growth kinetics of un-infected and infected cells are different. The increase in OD $_{440}$ of the unin-

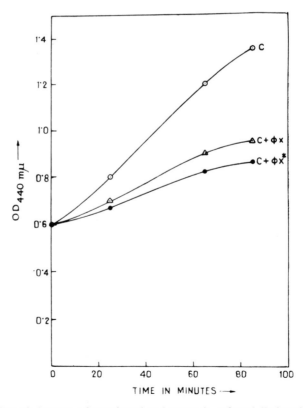

Fig. 2. Growth kinetics of uninfected and variously infected Escherichia coli C.

fected culture is due to an increase in bacterial number, while that of the infected culture is due to an increase in the total protein of the infected cells. If we assume one DNA molecule per cell, the total number of the DNA molecules in the control culture at 70-80 min is almost double that of the infected culture, and therefore we should expect the level of induction to be greater in the uninfected culture commensurate with the number of bacterial genomes. The apparent equality of induction thus hides the fact that a greater amount of β-galactosidase is synthesized in the infected cells.

Studies on the *ind* and *dsd* Genes

Next we examined the induction of the enzyme tryptophanase. In the infected cells, there is a marked reduction (75-80%) in the amount of tryptophanase formed (Fig. 3). This reduction is more than what can be ac-

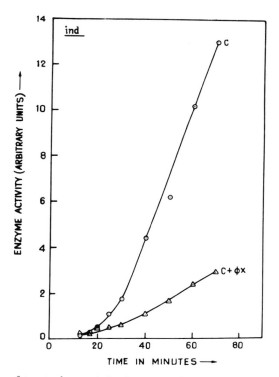

Fig. 3. Kinetics of tryptophanase induction in uninfected and infected Escherichia coli C. Experimental details as in Fig. 1. Inducer was DL-tryptophan.

counted for by the reduced growth of infected cells. A similar repression is also observed in the case of induction of D-serine deaminase from the *dsd* locus (Fig. 4). Thus these results lead to conclusions that are the opposite of those from the *lac* gene study; i.e., ϕX infection causes a reduction of the synthesis of tryptophanase and D-serine deaminase.

To check if any phage-specified function is responsible for the observed changes in enzyme induction, we measured the synthesis of induced tryptophanase in *E. coli* infected with ϕX174, heavily UV-irradiated to a survival of $10^{-5}\%$. We observed that the synthesis of the enzyme is still repressed, but to a slightly lesser extent compared to the cells infected with nonirradiated phage (Fig. 5). To gain some further insight into this aspect of the problem, we next used a temperature-sensitive mutant of *E. coli*, *E. coli t3* $\overline{\text{TAU}}$, which supports normal growth of ϕX at 30°C but blocks the formation of parental RF at 40°C and hence ϕX-specified products. When such a strain was used for infection and for induction of D-serine deaminase at 40°C, again an intermediate type of repression was observed (Fig. 6). These experiments thus indicate that ϕX-specific products are at least partially in-

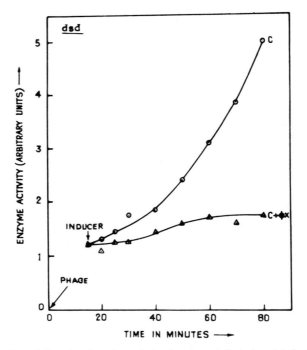

Fig. 4. Kinetics of D-serine deaminase induction in uninfected and infected Escherichia coli C. Experimental procedure as in Fig. 1. Inducer was DL-serine.

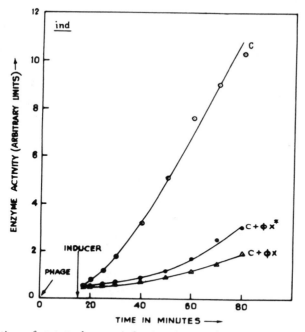

Fig. 5. Kinetics of tryptophanase induction in uninfected and variously infected Escherichia coli C. Log phase (3 × 10⁸ cells/min). The culture was divided into three parts; one part was used as the control, a second part was infected with φX *am*3 (m.o.i. = 5), and the third part was infected with UV-irradiated (to a survival level of 10⁻⁵%) φX *am*3.

volved in the observed changes in the pattern of induced enzyme synthesis in the infected cells.

It has been proposed that the rate of decay of enzyme-forming capacity after inducer removal is a reflection of the stability of enzyme-specific mRNA. The decay rate of enzyme-forming capacity in both infected and uninfected cells, induced for tryptophanase for 6 min, was determined. It was found that although the final level of enzyme attained in infected cells is less than that in uninfected cells (Fig. 7), the decay rate is the same in both cases (Fig. 8). This result indicates that, most probably, once enzyme-specific mRNAs are formed, they are translated at the same rate in both infected and uninfected cells, only there are fewer such mRNAs in the former.

To summarize, we may state that φX infection in *E. coli* cells leads to an increase in induction of β-galactosidase but a decrease in induction of tryptophanase and D-serine deaminase. Some φX-specific function is partially involved in this peculiar type of control phenomenon, which is exerted at

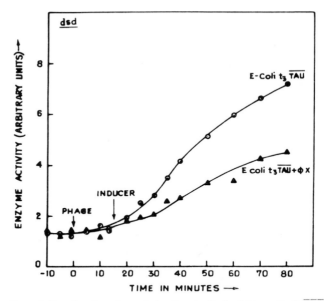

Fig. 6. Kinetics of D-serine deaminase induction in Escherichia coli t3 TAU uninfected and infected with ϕX174 am3 at 40°C. Experimental details as in Fig. 4.

the level of transcription. At present, we are unable to offer a fully satisfactory explanation for our results. It has been suggested, in a different context, that viruses may bring about changes in fibroblasts by lowering the level of intracellular cyclic AMP (11). We cannot, however, invoke any such scheme since, if the viral infection caused such a lowering, we should have observed repression in the case of β-galactosidase, also (12). On the other hand, if the virus somehow increased the intracellular concentration of cyclic AMP, we should have observed stimulation, not repression, of the tryptophanase synthesis (13). The contrary observation obtained in the case of two different systems thus clearly rules out the involvement of cyclic AMP. If alteration in membrane permeability were the major cause for the observed changes, one must assume that ϕX infection causes a very highly differentiated modification in the transport of the inducers used in these experiments; i.e., infection must have facilitated entry of a galactoside, such as isopropylthiogalactoside, while retarding the entry of amino acids, such as tryptophan and D-serine. Such a possibility, although it cannot be completely ruled out without further experimentation, does not seem to be very likely. One possibility that appears attractive to us is that the *lac* and the other two genes, *dsd* and *ind*, are not transcribed from the same strand of the *E. coli* DNA and that some phage-specified factor in conjunction with host RNA polymerase makes the latter transcribe one particular strand more

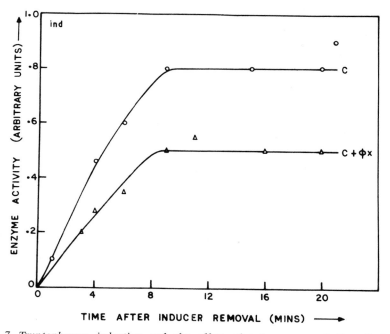

Fig. 7. Tryptophanase induction and the effect of inducer removal. E. coli C was grown in tris-glycerol medium. One-half of the medium was infected with ϕX174 *am*3 (m.o.i. = 5). DL-Tryptophan was added 7 min after infection. Inducer was removed from both uninfected and ϕX *am*3 infected culture at 6 min by filtration and resuspended 3 min later in inducer-free medium.

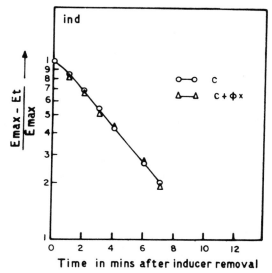

Fig. 8. Decay of tryptophanase synthesis as a function of time following inducer removal in uninfected and ϕX am3 infected cultures. Experimental details as in Fig. 8. The points represent $(E_{max}-E_t)/E_{max}$ at any given time t (from Fig. 8). E_{max} is the final level of enzyme activity reached after inducer removal.

efficiently than the complementary strand of the nonreplicating *E. coli* DNA. It is relevant to remember here that a switchover from symmetrical to asymmetrical replication of DNA does occur in the ϕX-infected *E. coli,* as described at the beginning of this chapter.

REFERENCES

1. R. L. Sinsheimer, R. Knippers and T. Komano. *Cold Spring Harbor Symp. Quant. Biol.* 33:443 (1968).
2. R. R. Rueckert and W. Zillig. *J. Mol. Biol.* 5:1 (1962).
3. S. R. Pal Chaudhury and R. K. Poddar. *Biochim. Biophys. Acta* 103:693 (1965).
4. B. Lindqvist and R. L. Sinsheimer. *J. Mol. Biol.* 28:87 (1967).
5. E. Tessman. *J. Mol. Biol.* 17:218 (1966).
6. S. R. Pal Chaudhury and R. K. Poddar. *J. Mol. Biol.* 32:505 (1968).
7. M. Hayashi, M. N. Hayashi, and S. Spiegelman. *Proc. Natl. Acad. Sci. (USA)* 50:664 (1963).
8. A. B. Pardee and N. L. Prestidge. *J. Bacteriol.* 70:667 (1955).
9. A. B. Pardee and N. L. Prestidge. *Biochim. Biophys. Acta* 49:77 (1961).
10. E. C. Pollard and S. A. Davis. *Radiation Res.* 41:375 (1970).
11. J. Otten, J. Bader, G. S. Johnson and I. Pastan. *J. Biol. Chem.* 247:1632 (1972).
12. R. Perlman and I. Pastan. *Biochem. Biophys. Res. Commun.* 37:151 (1964).
13. I. Pastan and R. Perlman. *J. Biol. Chem.* 244:2226 (1969).

DISCUSSION

Question (Chakravorty): As a result of ϕX174 infection, there is preferential depression of tryptophanase and D-serine deaminase. Do you have any explanation for that? My feeling is that as a result of phage infection you are preferentially knocking off permease, which is reflected in your result. From our experience with P22, we know that immediately following P22 infection there is drastic depression of the active transport process across the host membrane. You might check the respective transport system.

Answer: Further experiments are obviously needed. I have explained our reservation regarding this sort of explanation.

Question (Sarkar): Could the differential response of the three enzymes to induction be due to differential sensitivity toward catabolite repression? Is it possible that phage infection may alter the level of cyclic AMP and other factors required for the expression of catabolite-repressible genes.

Answer: If there were any alteration in cyclic AMP level due to ϕX infection, both β-galactosidase and tryptophanase induction would have been affected in the same manner.

10

Initiation of Transcription by RNA Polymerases of *Escherichia coli* and Phage T3

E. K. F. Bautz, W. T. McAllister, H. Küpper, E. Beck, and F. A. Bautz

Institut für Molekulare Genetik
Universität Heidelberg
Heidelberg, West Germany

Any enzyme able to initiate RNA synthesis at specific sites along the DNA template must undergo a series of reactions that can be summarized as follows:

Association:

    a. Enzyme + DNA $\rightleftharpoons$ enzyme·DNA

    b. Enzyme·DNA $\underset{15°C}{\overset{20°C}{\rightleftharpoons}}$ Enzyme*·DNA

Initiation:

    c. Enzyme*·DNA + $(NTP)_1$ + $(NTP)_2$ $\rightleftharpoons$ enzyme*·DNA·$(NTP)_1$·$(NTP)_2$

    d. Enzyme*·DNA·$(NTP)_1$·$(NTP)_2$ $\rightleftharpoons$ enzyme*·DNA·$(NTP)_1$–$(NMP)_2$ + PP_i

Polymerization:

    e. Translocation of enzyme on DNA template

    f. Enzyme*·DNA·$(NTP)_1$–$(NMP)_2$ + $(NTP)_3$ $\rightleftharpoons$ enzyme*·DNA·$(NTP)_1$–$(NMP)_2$–$(NMP)_3$ + PP_i

The initial binding of the enzyme to promoter sites must be rather complicated, as it involves the seeking out of specific initiation signals encoded in the DNA sequence. However, once bound and in the proper configuration, the enzyme is able to start synthesis immediately upon addition of nucleoside triphosphates. Thus polymerase molecules bound at promoter sites are resistant to rifampicin if the drug is added simultaneously with substrate, whereas those enzymes not occupying a site where they may start immediately are rapidly inactivated by the drug (1,2). This resistance to rifampicin is found only if the enzyme contains the σ factor, which suggests that the function of σ is to promote the formation of a binary complex between DNA and RNA polymerase at sites from which RNA chains can be started.

Further studies summarized here have led us to conclude that the σ factor affects the stability of these DNA·RNA polymerase complexes in such a way that only holoenzyme is able to discriminate between promoter and nonpromoter sites on native DNA templates.

The later steps in initiation of RNA synthesis, including the formation of the first few phosphodiester linkages, have been studied with the RNA polymerase of bacteriophage T3. This enzyme, because of its simpler structure and more stringent specificity, yields kinetic data that are more easily interpreted than those obtained with the *Escherichia coli* RNA polymerase.

SELECTIVE BINDING OF HOLOENZYME TO PROMOTERS

The half-life of enzymes bound to promoter sites is rather long, and the binding is so tight that polymers such as polyinosinic acid [poly(I)] which have a stronger affinity for polymerase than native DNA templates, are unable to

Table I. Protection of ^{32}P-Labeled DNA by
Escherichia coli RNA Polymerase[a]

	Percent of input DNA resistant to DNase
Holoenzyme - poly(I)	1.8
Holoenzyme + poly(I)	0.4
Core enzyme - poly(I)	1.2
Core enzyme + poly(I)	0.04

[a]T7 [^{32}P]DNA (7 μg) was incubated with 2 μg holo or core polymerase for 30 min at 24°C in 1 ml binding buffer (9). Then, where indicated, 40 μg poly(I) was added and incubation was continued for 1 hr. DNase (2 × 40 μg) was added in two 10-min intervals at 37°C, and after another 10 min the complexes were filtered through Millipore filters at 37°C according to Jones and Berg (9). The filters were washed with 20 ml of binding buffer prewarmed to 37°C, dried, and counted in a liquid scintillation system.

remove the promoter-bound enzyme molecules from the template (3). This finding suggested that it should be possible to remove those enzyme molecules not specifically bound to a few strong binding sites by competition with another strongly binding polymer such as poly(I). Subsequent digestion of the unprotected regions of the template with DNase would then permit the isolation of sequences of DNA corresponding to strong binding sites. We have performed such experiments with T7 DNA and have found that, in the absence of any competing polymer, very large amounts of the DNA template are protected, but that following competition with poly(I) only 0.4% of the total genome is protected (Table I). Practically no DNA escapes degradation if core enzyme is bound and then competed by poly(I), which indicates that the tight binding to promoter sites requires σ factor. On degradation to apurinic acid, the material gives an oligo(pyrimidine nucleotide) pattern which is quite unique, indicating that the protected sequences are not random but occur at only a few sites. We estimate that there are only two or three such tight binding sites on the bacteriophage T7 genome and that the protected regions themselves are 35-40 base pairs long (4).

We have summarized the conclusions of these studies in Fig. 1. Whereas holoenzyme has a low affinity for regions of DNA that do not contain initiation signals (promoter sites), the association of holoenzyme with promoter sites results in a tightly bound complex. Core enzyme, on the other hand, appears not to discriminate between the two types of sequences but has an intermediate affinity. Core enzyme binds to promoter sites much less strongly than the holoenzyme but shows a somewhat higher affinity for

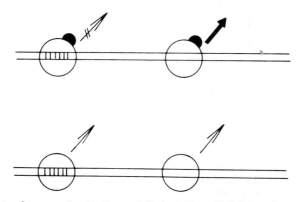

Fig. 1. *Effect of σ on the binding of Escherichia coli RNA polymerase to DNA.* Holoenzyme containing the σ subunit binds very tightly to promoter regions (crosshatched areas) of double-stranded DNA, but has a low affinity for nonpromoter regions. Core enzyme, on the other hand, exhibits an intermediate affinity for both promoter and nonpromoter regions.

nonpromoter regions than the holoenzyme. This behavior of the two forms of RNA polymerase offers an explanation for the σ cycle (5) in that, following initiation, loss of the σ factor would facilitate binding of the enzyme to nonpromoter regions of the DNA.

INITIATION OF RNA CHAINS BY T3 RNA POLYMERASE

The data above give some information about the binding of RNA polymerase, but do not indicate much about the further steps in the initiation reaction, which involve the addition of the first and second nucleoside triphosphates. For this purpose, the RNA polymerase made after bacteriophage T3 infection is a good subject of study, as it appears to have a high degree of template specificity. After infection, the early region of the T3 phage

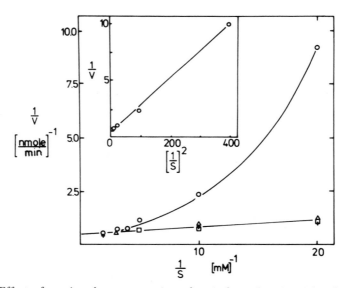

Fig. 2. *Effect of varying the concentration of a single nucleoside triphosphate on the rate of nucleotide incorporation by the T3 RNA polymerase.* Reaction mixtures contained, in 0.25 ml, 0.04 M tris-Cl (pH 7.9), 0.01 M MgCl$_2$, 0.05 M KCl, 0.01 M 2-mercaptoethanol, 0.1 mM Na$_3$EDTA, 12 μg T3 DNA, 0.5 mg/ml bovine serum albumin, and three of the four nucleoside triphosphates at a concentration of 0.4 mM. The was initiated by the addition of enzyme (to a final concentration of 5 μg/ml), and after 5 min at 37°C the reactions were terminated by the addition of 2 ml of 5% trichloroacetic acid. Terminated reactions were filtered through Whatman GF/A filters, which were washed with 20 ml of 5% acid, dried, and counted in a toluene-based liquid scintillation system. The initial rate of synthesis (V) has been calculated as nmoles [^{3}H]UMP incorporated/min. The variable substrates were GTP (○), CTP (□), ATP (△), and UTP (+).

genome is transcribed by the RNA polymerase of the host. This region comprises about 20% of the total genome and is demarcated by a strong termination signal past which the *E. coli* polymerase cannot read. The late region (the other 80% of the genome) is transcribed by the protein product of gene 1. This enzyme is less complicated in structure than the host enzyme and consists of only one polypeptide chain having a molecular weight of 110,000 (6).

To determine the dependence of enzyme activity on the concentration of the nucleoside triphosphates, which serve as substrates, one can vary the concentration of one triphosphate and keep that of the other three at a high level. The results of such experiments can be graphically displayed in a Lineweaver-Burk plot in which the inverse of the initial velocity $(1/V)$ of the reaction is plotted against the inverse concentration $(1/S)$ of the variable substrate. While varying the concentration of either ATP, CTP, or UTP resulted in a straight line, changing the concentration of GTP gave a curvilinear plot that became linear when plotted as $1/V$ vs. $1/S^2$ (Fig. 2). This suggests that the simultaneous addition of two GTP moieties is required at some stage during the synthesis reaction. Studies on the exchange of pyrophosphate, which measures the reverse reaction of synthesis, support the contention that it is initiation with the sequence pppGpG which causes this unusual dependence of enzyme activity on the concentration of GTP; i.e.,

Table II. Exchange of $[^{32}P]$Pyrophosphate with Nucleoside Triphosphates by Bacteriophage T3 and T7 RNA Polymerases

Nucleoside triphosphates present:	DNA template:	Enzyme: T3 T3	T7	T7 T3	T7
2 × GTP		0.59^a	0.03	0.24	0.24
GTP + ATP		0.45	0.31	0.22	0.18
GTP + CTP		0.61	0.06	0.27	0.20
GTP + UTP		0.55	0.07	0.36	0.30
ATP + UTP		0.01	0.01	–	–
2 × ATP		–	–	0.05	0.05

[a]Assays of pyrophosphate exchange were performed in 0.25 ml containing 0.05 M tris-C1 (pH 7.9), 0.02 M MgCl$_2$, 0.05 M 2-mercaptoethanol, 0.1 mM Na$_3$EDTA, 0.5 mg bovine serum albumin, 100 nmoles of the indicated triphosphate, 250 nmoles of Na^{32}PP$_i$ having a specific activity of between 6000 and 10,000 cpm/nmole, 10 μg/ml of T3 or T7 RNA polymerase, and 60 μg/ml of template DNA. After 10 min at 37°C, the reactions were terminated and the conversion of ^{32}PP$_i$ into Norite-adsorbable nucleoside triphosphates was determined by the procedure of Krakow and Fronk (10) except that the membrane-retained Norite was counted in a liquid scintillation system.

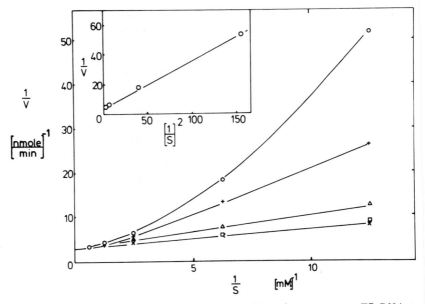

Fig. 3. *Kinetics of RNA synthesis by the T3 RNA polymerase on a T7 DNA template.* The effect of varying the concentration of either one or two nucleoside triphosphates on the rate of nucleotide incorporation was examined as described in Fig. 2. The concentration of T7 DNA in the reaction mixtures was 50 μg/ml. The variable substrates were GTP (+), ATP (□), CTP (×), GTP and ATP (○), ATP and CTP (△).

the fact that one obtains high levels of PP_i exchange in the presence of only GTP as substrate indicates that the sequence of at least the first two nucleotides is G-G (Table II). In contrast, with T7 DNA as template, almost no PP_i exchange is observed with GTP alone but only when GTP and ATP are both present, suggesting that, in this case, an adenylate residue occupies one of the first two positions at the 5′ end of the message.

Checking the dependence of enzyme activity on the concentration of each of the substrates with T7 DNA template, variation of the concentration of GTP alone did not give the type of curvilinear plot observed with T3 DNA, but a curvilinear plot was obtained if the concentrations of both GTP and ATP were varied simultaneously (Fig. 3). This corroborates the PP_i exchange data, indicating that, indeed, the T3 RNA polymerase is forced to start RNA chains with another sequence on T7 DNA than on T3 DNA. The T7 RNA polymerase, however, appears to be able to start with G-G on both T7 and T3 DNA templates (Table II).

The T3 RNA polymerase is sensitive to either the rifampicin derivative AFO/13 or heparin. Binding of enzyme to DNA does not render it resistant to heparin, and unlike *E. coli* RNA polymerase (7) the T3 enzyme remains sensitive to heparin or high salt concentrations even after the formation of the first dinucleotide, since a prior incubation with GTP alone does not render the enzyme resistant (8). If incubated with GTP and ATP, however, the enzyme becomes almost fully resistant to heparin. It was therefore of interest to determine the size of the products that accumulate under the two conditions, i.e., incubation with GTP alone or with GTP and ATP. The results are rather clear-cut (Figs. 4 and 5); incubation with GTP alone resulted in the production of almost exclusively the dinucleotide pppGpG, whereas incubation with both GTP and ATP yielded a tetranucleotide as the major product and tri- and pentanucleotides as minor components. These results indicate that most RNA chains start with the sequence pppGpGpApR (R = A or G). Quantitatively, there are many more dinucleotides produced during incubation with GTP alone than tetranucleotides when ATP is also present, indicating

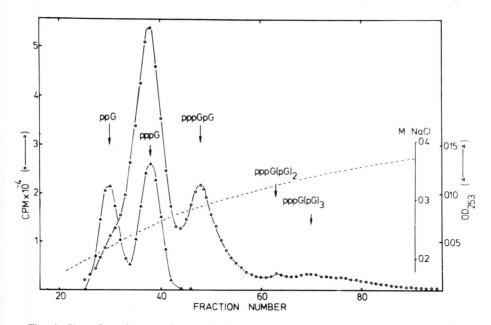

Fig. 4. Size of products made by the T3 RNA polymerase with GTP alone as a substrate. Reaction mixtures containing 150 μg/ml T3 DNA, 20 μg/ml T3 RNA polymerase, and 0.108 mM [^{3}H]GTP (specific activity = 400 c/mole) were prepared as described in Fig. 2 in a final volume of 1 ml. After incubation for 60 min at 37°C, the products of the reaction were analyzed on a column of DEAE-Sephadex in the presence of 7 M urea according to the procedure of Takanami (11). Approximately 0.1 mg each of unlabeled GDP and GTP was added to the samples before application to the column as optical density markers.

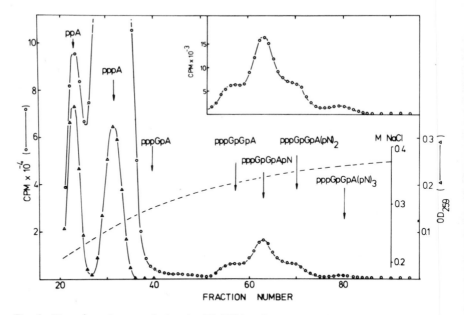

Fig. 5. Size of products made by the T3 RNA polymerase in the presence of GTP and ATP. Reaction mixtures containing 150 μg/ml T3 DNA, 20 μg/ml T3 RNA polymerase, 0.4 mM GTP, and 0.022 mM [³H]ATP (specific activity = 500 c/mole) were incubated for 60 min at 37°C. The products were then analyzed as described in Fig. 4.

that the enzyme recycles much more quickly if it can produce only dinucleotides. Thus during polymerization the T3 RNA polymerase is more tightly bound to DNA than during initiation. This accounts for the observation that complexes of enzyme·DNA and dinucleotide product are labile, while complexes containing a tetranucleotide are resistant to heparin or high salt.

REFERENCES

1. A. Sippel and G. Hartmann. *Europ. J. Biochem.* **16**:152 (1970).
2. E. K. F. Bautz and F. A. Bautz. *Nature* **226**:1219 (1970).
3. E. K. F. Bautz, F. A. Bautz, and E. Beck. *Mol. Gen. Genet.* **118**:199 (1972).
4. E. Beck. Diplomarbeit Heidelberg (1972).
5. A. A. Travers and R. R. Burgess. *Nature* **222**:537 (1969).
6. J. J. Dunn, F. A. Bautz, and E. K. F. Bautz. *Nature New Biol.* **230**:94 (1971).
7. A. G. So and K. M. Downey, *Biochemistry* **9**:4788 (1970).
8. W. T. McAllister, H. Küpper, and E. K. F. Bautz. *Europ. J. Biochem.,* **34**:489 (1973).
9. O. W. Jones and P. Berg. *J. Mol. Biol.* **22**:199 (1966).
10. J. S. Krakow and E. J. Fronk. *Proc. Natl. Acad. Sci. (USA)* **55**:1616 (1969).
11. M. Takanami, *J. Biol. Chem.* **244**:5988 (1969).

DISCUSSION

Question (Wickner): Is there any evidence, in λ or any other system, that RNA polymerase binding sites are identical with promoters defined genetically?

Answer: As you know, in λ the site specifying the 5' end of the N message does not coincide with the genetically defined leftward promoter. Whether the tight binding sites we isolate correspond to the genetically defined promotors or whether they correspond to the chain start signal or both, we don't know.

Question (Burma): How does the T3 enzyme recognize the promoter site? Is the same protein involved in recognition of the promoter as well as for chain elongation?

Answer: The answer to your first question is I don't know. To your second question, the answer is yes, as the enzyme is composed of a single polypeptide chain; therefore, it has to do both.

Question (M. Takanami): How many promoter sites have you detected by the RNA polymerase binding experiments? According to our terminal sequence analysis of the synthesized products on T3 DNA by *E. coli* RNA polymerase, we detected two unique starting sequences: pppAUG ---- and ppp GU ----.

Answer: Under the conditions given in Table I, about three. However, more recently, with a new enzyme preparation and less input of polymerase we obtain consistently less protected DNA, suggesting two binding sites, a result which seems to agree well with your two unique starting sequences.

11

Transcription of Native and Denatured DNA Preparations by Bacteriophage T3 Induced RNA Polymerase

Umadas Maitra, Prasanta R. Chakraborty, Rino A. Salvo, Henry H. Huang, Pradip Bandyopadhyay, and Probir Sarkar

Department of Developmental Biology and Cancer
Division of Biology
Albert Einstein College of Medicine
Bronx, New York, U.S.A.

It is now well established that the expression of genetic information in bacteriophages, as well as in more complex organisms, is subject to temporal control; not all genes are expressed simultaneously. Early- and late-functioning cistrons have been distinguished in λ, T-even, and other bacteriophages. In these viruses, temporal regulation of gene expression seems to occur at the transcriptional level. At a certain time after infection, mRNA synthesis, originally specific for early phage proteins, is altered to produce RNA that directs the synthesis of late phage proteins. Evidence for this control mechanism has been reviewed (1,2). The change in transcription specificity leading to the synthesis of late mRNA may be achieved either by modification of the host RNA polymerase or by *de novo* synthesis of a new RNA polymerase coded by the viral genome. The modified or the new RNA polymerase can initiate RNA synthesis corresponding to late bacteriophage genes.

Chamberlin *et al.* (3) were the first to demonstrate that bacteriophage T7 codes for the *de novo* synthesis of a new RNA polymerase in T7 phage infected *Escherichia coli*. The template specificity of the T7 RNA polymerase is striking; the only efficient template besides T7 DNA is T3 DNA and poly(dG·dC) (3,4).

Since this original discovery by Chamberlin *et al.*, reports from this laboratory (5) and that of Bautz (4) have described the isolation of a new DNA-dependent RNA polymerase in *E. coli* infected with bacteriophage T3. The phage-induced polymerase was shown to be physically and biochemically distinct from the *E. coli* RNA polymerase. The phage polymerase uses only T3 DNA as template and is inactive with native T2, T4, *E. coli*, calf thymus DNA, or poly[d(A-T)]. T7 DNA was shown to be approximately 5% as active as T3 DNA. In contrast, *E. coli* RNA polymerase is nonspecific in its DNA requirements. T3 RNA polymerase can, however, transcribe poly(dG·dC) to make poly(G) exclusively, which indicates that the polymerase may initiate chains only with GTP. A subsequent report from this lab-

Table I. Properties of T3 RNA Polymerase Compared to Those of *Escherichia coli* RNA Polymerase[a]

T3 RNA polymerase	*E. coli* RNA polymerase
1. Induced early after T3 phage infection	1. Host enzyme
2. Active with Mg^{2+} only (20 mM optimum)	2. Active with Mg^{2+} or Mn^{2+}
3. Single polypeptide chain (molecular weight 100,000 ± 5000)	3. Multiple subunits ($\sigma\beta\beta'\alpha_2$) (molecular weight 470,000)
4. Insentitive to antisera against *E. coli* RNA polymerase	4. Sensitive to *E. coli* RNA polymerase antisera
5. Active only with T3 DNA among a variety of native DNAs tested so far; 2-5% activity with native T7 DNA, as compared to T3 DNA; poly(dG · dC) highly active but not poly[d (A-T)]	5. Active with a wide variety of native DNA templates; both poly(dC · dC) homopolymer and poly[d (A-T)] highly active
6. Insensitive to rifampicin and streptolydigin	6. Inhibited by rifampicin and streptolydigin
7. Highly inhibited by salt concentrations above 0.04 M	7. Stimulated by salt concentrations above 0.15 M
8. *E. coli* RNA chain release factor ρ has no effect on the rate, yield, or size of RNA produced by T3 RNA polymerase	8. Rho factor causes inhibition of RNA synthesis without affecting the initial rate of RNA synthesis; RNA chains formed in the presence of ρ factor are smaller and more discrete in size than are those formed in its absence

[a]This information was obtained from data published previously (4-8).

oratory (6) has shown that RNA chains made by T3 RNA polymerase with native T3 DNA template are initiated exclusively with GTP and that completed RNA chains are released free of template DNA. Polymerase is also released in this process and, acting catalytically, reinitiates new RNA chains. Some of the pertinent results substantiating these conclusions are shown in Tables I-III and in Fig. 1.

Table I compares the physical and biochemical properties of T3 RNA polymerase with those of *E. coli* RNA polymerase. It is clear that T3 RNA polymerase is physically and biochemically distinct from the *E. coli* RNA polymerase.

Initiation, Release, and Reinitiation of RNA Chains by T3 RNA Polymerase

Table II summarizes the results of chain initiation obtained by the incorporation of ^{32}P from each of the four γ-^{32}P-labeled nucleoside triphosphates using T3 DNA as template. These results show that [γ-^{32}P]GTP is

Table II. Requirements for the Incorporation of γ-^{32}P-Labeled Nucleoside Triphosphates into RNA Polymerase Products[a]

Additions	[^{14}C]UMP incorporated (nmoles)	[γ-^{32}P]Nucleotide incorporated (pmoles)			
		GTP	ATP	UTP	CTP
Complete system	12.4	7.2	0.2	< 0.1	< 0.1
Omit UTP or CTP or ATP	< 0.1	< 0.1	< 0.1	< 0.1	< 0.1
Omit T3 polymerase	< 0.1	< 0.1	–	–	–
Omit T3 DNA	< 0.1	< 0.1	–	–	–
Complete + pancreatic DNase (1 μg)	< 0.1	< 0.1	–	–	–
Complete + pancreatic RNase (1 μg)	< 0.1	< 0.1	–	–	–

[a]The initiation reaction was measured by the incorporation of γ-^{32}P-labeled ribonucleoside triphosphates into an acid-insoluble RNA product. Total RNA synthesis was measured by the incorporation of ^{14}C- or ^{3}H-labeled ribonucleoside triphosphates. The conditions of the assay were as follows: each reaction mixture (0.5 ml) contained 50 mM tris-Cl buffer (pH 7.8), 20 mM MgCl$_2$, 4 mM dithiothreitol, 20 μg recrystallized bovine serum albumin, 20 nmoles (as deoxynucleotide residues) T3 DNA, and 120 nmoles (each) UTP, CTP, GTP, and ATP. γ-^{32}P-Labeled nucleoside triphosphates (3 ×10^9 cpm/μmole) were used to measure initiation; [^{14}C]- or [^{3}H]UTP (5 × 10^6 cpm/μmole) was used to measure total RNA synthesis. The polymerase reaction was initiated by the addition of 6 units of T3 RNA polymerase. After incubation at 37°C for 2 hr, the reaction was terminated and the amount of ^{32}P, ^{14}C, or ^{3}H incorporated into an acid-insoluble RNA product was determined as described previously (15). Incorporation of each of the four γ-^{32}P-labeled nucleoside triphosphates was measured in separate reaction mixtures.

the only γ-^{32}P-labeled nucleoside triphosphate incorporated into RNA chains. Furthermore, the incorporation of $[\gamma$-^{32}P]GTP into RNA displays the same requirements as those found for RNA synthesis as measured by $[^{14}$C]UMP incorporation. The site of incorporation of $[\gamma$-^{32}P]GTP into RNA by T3 RNA polymerase is at the 5' end of the RNA chains, since after alkaline hydrolysis of the labeled RNA formed with $[\gamma$-^{32}P]GTP all the ^{32}P was recovered as guanosine tetraphosphate (^{32}pppGp) (data not shown). This result shows that all RNA chains formed by T3 RNA polymerase are initiated exclusively with GTP (pppG-N----).

The rates of incorporation of $[\gamma$-^{32}P]GTP and of RNA synthesis are shown in Table III. These results can be summarized as follows: (a) Both RNA synthesis and RNA chain initiation (measured by incorporation of $[\gamma$-^{32}P]GTP) continued during the entire period of incubation. The increase in RNA synthesis with time could be quantitatively accounted for by the increase in the number of RNA chains initiated. (b) The number of RNA chains synthesized per molecule of enzyme increased progressively with time. After 4 hr of incubation, about 28 RNA chains were synthesized per molecule of polymerase. These results indicate that T3 RNA polymerase can terminate and reinitiate new RNA chains during the course of RNA synthesis. (c) The average chain length of the product during the entire course of the reaction was 5000-6000 nucleotides. This corresponds to an average molecular weight per chain of about 1.8×10^6.

Reinitiation of RNA chains by T3 polymerase represents repetitive copying of the same regions of the template DNA, as demonstrated by DNA·RNA hybridization studies (Table IV). RNA products synthesized during the first 15 min of incubation effectively prevented the hybridization to

Table III. Kinetics of RNA Synthesis and of $[\gamma$-^{32}P] GTP Incorporation[a]

Time (min)	$[\gamma$-^{32}P]GTP incorporated (pmoles)	RNA synthesis (nmoles)	Average chain length
10	2.4	15.6	6500
30	4.6	28.0	6100
60	6.7	37.6	5600
120	9.7	56.0	5700
240	12.7	72.0	5600

[a]In each reaction mixture (0.5 ml), 6 units (equivalent to 0.42 pmole) of T3 RNA polymerase was added. The other conditions of the assay were as described in the footnote to Table II. Incubation was at 37°C for the indicated time. The average chain length was calculated as the ratio of total RNA nucleotides synthesized to total initiation obtained with GTP. Total RNA nucleotides were calculated by multiplying the amount of $[^{14}$C]UMP incorporated by 3.85.

Table IV. Repetitive Copying of T3 DNA *in Vitro*[a]

Unlabeled 15-min RNA product added (μg)	Relative hybridization of 4-hr [³H] RNA product to denatured T3 DNA (%)
0	100
0.38	35
0.76	20
1.50	7

[a]Two sets of T3 RNA polymerase reaction mixtures were prepared. Reaction mixture A (total volume 5 ml) contained all four unlabeled nucleoside triphosphates with 25 units of T3 RNA polymerase and was used for the isolation of the nonradioactive RNA product at 15 min. Reaction mixture B (0.5 ml) contained UTP labeled with tritium to a final specific activity of 2×10^9 cpm/μmole and 2.5 units of T3 RNA polymerase, and was used for the isolation of the 4-hr [³H] RNA product. Reaction mixture A was incubated for 15 min and reaction mixture B was incubated for 4 hr at 37°C. RNA free of T3 DNA was subsequently isolated from each reaction mixture by DNase treatment followed by phenol extraction (16) and was used for competition-hybridization studies. The competition-hybridization mixture contained (in 0.5 ml) 1 μg of heat-denatured T3 DNA, 1×10^4 cpm of [³H] RNA product, and increasing amounts of unlabeled competing RNA (15-min product). Incubation was for 4.5 hr at 65° C. The resulting DNA · RNA hybrids were then estimated by the method of Nygaard and Hall (17). The absolute hybridization efficiency was more than 70% in the absence of unlabeled competitor RNA.

denatured T3 DNA strands of RNA products synthesized in 4 hr, indicating a competition for complementary sites on the DNA. Thus almost all of the RNA sequences present in the RNA products synthesized in 4 hr were present in products produced in 15 min. Since the extent of synthesis was increased severalfold by 4 hr (as is also shown in Table III), reinitiation and repetitive copying over the same regions of DNA occurred during RNA synthesis.

The above experiment was done under conditions in which the polymerase was the limiting component. The demonstration that under these conditions T3 polymerase can reinitiate synthesis of new RNA chains by repetitive copying of a region of the DNA also provided indirect evidence for release of polymerase from the template in termination-reinitiation reactions.

Release of RNA Chains from T3 DNA

During *in vitro* transcription of T3 DNA by T3 RNA polymerase, the completed RNA chains produced in the reaction mixture were released free of template DNA and accumulated as free RNA (Fig. 1). The amount of free RNA formed increased with time; within 5 min of incubation, almost all RNA chains already accumulated as free RNA.

The results presented above clearly demonstrate that T3 RNA polymerase can terminate and initiate new chains *in vitro*. Furthermore, the termination and reinitiation are associated with the release of both free RNA and free enzyme. Since the T3 RNA polymerase used in the present studies is electrophoretically pure and consists of a single polypeptide chain, it follows that T3 RNA polymerase alone can bring about termination and reinitiation of RNA chains without additional protein factors. Thus recognition signals on the DNA template in the form of unique nucleotide sequences and/or structural alteration(s), are responsible for the termination of RNA synthesis by T3 RNA polymerase. It is noteworthy that the addition of ρ factor to T3 RNA polymerase reaction mixtures is without effect on the rate, yield, or size of RNA produced (6-8). However, the possibility exists that a termination factor coded by T3 exists. This possibility will become a reality if

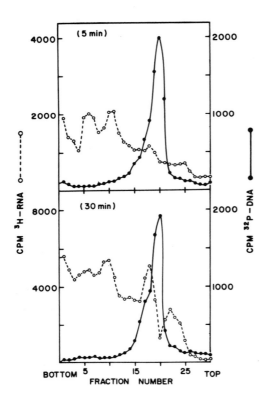

Fig. 1. Sucrose gradient analysis of T3 RNA polymerase reaction mixtures. Each reaction mixture was prepared as described in the footnote to Table II except that [^{32}P]DNA T3 was used as template and [^{3}H]-RNA was synthesized by using [^{3}H]-UTP as the labeled ribonucleoside triphosphate. At the indicated time, 0.1-ml aliquots of chilled reaction mixture were layered on chilled 5-20% linear sucrose gradients (5.0 ml) containing 50 mM tris-Cl buffer (pH 7.8), 0.1 M NH$_4$Cl, 20 mM MgCl$_2$, and 1 mM dithiothreitol. The tubes were centrifuged for 100 min at 48,000 rpm in a SW50 rotor at 5°C. The acid-insoluble radioactivity was measured in 0.15-ml fractions collected from the bottom of the tube. Radioactivity was measured in a liquid scintillation counter under conditions in which no ^{3}H was detected in the ^{32}P channel and less than 2% of ^{32}P was detected in the ^{3}H channel. ●, T3 [^{32}P]DNA; ○, [^{3}H]UMP.

the RNA products formed *in vitro* by T3 RNA polymerase are found to terminate improperly when compared with RNA formed in T3-infected cells *in vivo*.

Further Studies on the Specificity of RNA Chain Initiation by T3 RNA polymerase

Although the data are not presented in this chapter, studies carried out by us on the T3 DNA dependent PP_i exchange reaction between GTP and any one of the other three nucleoside triphosphates along with our studies on the direct determination of the nucleotide sequence at the 5′ end of RNA chains have clearly demonstrated that all RNA chains formed in the T3 RNA polymerase reaction contain the sequence $pppGp(Gp)_n Ap$----. This indicates a very high degree of specificity of initiation of RNA chains by T3 RNA polymerase from native T3 DNA templates.

COMPARISON OF *IN VIVO* AND *IN VITRO* RNA PRODUCTS

The nature of the RNA products made *in vitro* by T3 RNA polymerase and by *E. coli* RNA polymerase on T3 DNA templates was also investigated by specific DNA·RNA hybridization studies with separated strands of T3 DNA. For comparison, the hybridization patterns of "early" (0-2 min) and of "late" (8-11 min) *in vivo* [³H] RNA to T3 DNA strands were also determined. In addition, [³H] RNA isolated from cells infected with phage T3 in the presence of chloramphenicol (called "chloramphenicol" RNA) was also used in these studies. *In vivo* [³H] RNA was isolated from T3 phage infected cells pulsed with [³H] uridine for various times during the infective cycle. Although the data are not shown here, it was observed that both the *in vitro* T3 RNA polymerase product and *in vivo* RNA ("early," "late," or "chloramphenicol" RNA) hybridized exclusively with the H strand of T3 DNA. Thus *in vitro* T3 RNA polymerase copies the biologically correct strand—the strand that is copied *in vivo* at all times following T3 phage infection. With the *E. coli* RNA polymerase products, nearly 85-90% of RNA chains, as expected, hybridized with the H strand. However, approximately 10-15% of the *in vitro* E. *coli* RNA polymerase product hybridized with the L strand—the strand that is never copied *in vivo*. The reason for this small extent of copying of the "wrong" strand *in vitro* by the *E. coli* RNA polymerase is not clear.

We have used the technique of competition hybridization to determine the regions of the T3 genome transcribed *in vitro* by either T3 RNA polymerase or by *E. coli* RNA polymerase. Figure 2 shows the results of competition of *in vitro* T3 RNA polymerase product by "early," "chlorampheni-

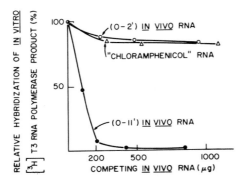

Fig. 2. Competition of in vitro T3 RNA polymerase product by in vivo RNA isolated from T3 phage infected cells. The ^{3}H-labeled T3 RNA polymerase product was synthesized from native T3 DNA template in a reaction mixture identical to that described in the footnote to Table I except that the specific radioactivity of [3H]UTP was 1×10^9 cpm/μmole and incubation was for 30 min at 37°C with 5 units of T3 RNA polymerase. The [3H]RNA product free of T3 DNA was subsequently isolated from the reaction mixture by DNase treatment, followed by phenol extraction (16), and was used for competition-hybridization studies. "Early" or "late" *in vivo* nonradioactive RNA was isolated from T3 phage infected cells as follows. *E. coli* B was grown in Casamino acid medium at 37°C as described by Gefter (18). When the cell density reached 7×10^8 cells/ml, the culture was infected with phage T3 at a multiplicity of infection of 10. For the preparation of "early" (0-2 min) RNA, infected cells were harvested after 2 min following phage infection, while for the preparation of "late" (0-11 min) RNA, cells were harvested at 11 min after infection with T3. (Under these conditions of infection, cell lysis was complete in 16 min.) Harvesting of cells was carried out by pouring the infected cells onto 0.5 vol of crushed frozen azide buffer (0.02 *M* tris-Cl, *p*H 7.4, 5 m*M* MgCl$_2$, and 0.01 *M* sodium azide), followed by centrifugation. For preparation of "chloramphenicol-early" RNA, chloramphenicol was added to a concentration of 200 μg/ml to the bacterial culture 5 min before infection with T3. Infection was then carried out for 5 min. *In vivo* RNA was isolated from infected cells by the hot-phenol extraction method of Young and Houwe (19). The H and L strands of T3 DNA were separated in CsCl gradients in the presence of poly(U,G) as described by Guha and Szybalski (20) for the separation of T4 DNA strands. Each competition-hybridization mixture (0.5 ml) contained 1 μg of H strand of T3 DNA, 10 pmoles of T3 [3H]RNA polymerase product $(1 \times 10^4$ cpm), and increasing concentrations of nonradioactive competitor *in vivo* RNA as shown in the figure. Incubation was for 5 hr at 65°C. The resulting DNA·RNA hybrids were then estimated by the method of Nygaard and Hall (17). The absolute hybridization efficiency was greater than 90% in the absence of nonradioactive competitor RNA. ●, "Late" (0-11 min) *in vivo* RNA as competitor RNA; ○, "early" (0-2 min) *in vivo* RNA as competitor; △, "chloramphenicol" *in vivo* RNA as competitor.

col," and "late" *in vivo* RNA isolated from T3 phage infected cells. The hybridization of *in vitro* [3H]RNA product made by T3 RNA polymerase to the H strand of T3 DNA can be completely prevented by *in vivo* "late" mRNA isolated 11 min after T3 phage infection (Fig. 2). Thus the *in vitro* T3 RNA polymerase product contains all the sequences present in "late" *in vivo* RNA. The experiment presented in Fig. 2 also shows that an excess of "early" (0-2 min) or "chloramphenicol" RNA can also compete with a small fraction (10-15%) of the *in vitro* T3 polymerase product for sites on the DNA. This indicates that T3 RNA polymerase *in vitro*, in addition to copying the "late" regions, may copy "early" regions of the T3 genome.

The complementary experiment, competition of "late" (8-11 min) *in*

Fig. 3. Competition of "late" in vivo [³H] RNA (upper panel) and in vitro T3 [³H] RNA polymerase product (lower panel) by in vitro RNA products made by T3 RNA polymerase and by Escherichia coli RNA polymerase. In vitro RNA product made by (a) T3 RNA polymerase, (b) E. coli RNA polymerase, and (c) E. coli RNA polymerase in the presence of saturating amounts of E. coli RNA chain release factor ρ was prepared as follows: Three separate RNA polymerase reaction mixtures, A, B, and C (5 ml each), were prepared. The molar concentrations of all components in the three reaction mixtures were the same as those described in the footnote to Table II except that all four nucleoside triphosphates were unlabeled. Reaction mixture A contained 50 units of T3 RNA polymerase, while B and C contained 100 units of E. coli RNA polymerase instead of T3 RNA polymerase. Reaction mixture C contained, in addition, 10 μg of ρ factor. After incubation at 37°C for 1 hr, unlabeled RNA product was isolated from each reaction mixture by DNase treatment,

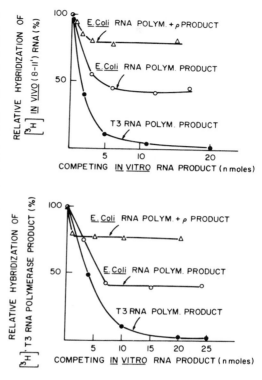

followed by phenol extraction (16), and was used as competitor RNA for competition-hybridization studies. For preparation of labeled "late" in vivo RNA, [³H]uridine was added (25 μc/ml) to infected bacterial culture at 8 min after infection with phage T3. The infection was allowed to proceed for an additional 3 min following addition of the label, and the infected cells were harvested and RNA isolated as described in the caption of Fig. 2. The synthesis and isolation of ³H-labeled T3 RNA polymerase product and the determination of hybridization were carried out as described in the caption of Fig. 2. Each competition-hybridization mixture (0.5 ml) contained the following components. Upper panel: 1 μg of H strand of T3 DNA, 0.5 μg (10⁴ cpm) of "late" in vivo (8-11 min) [³H]RNA, and increasing concentrations of nonradioactive competitor in vitro RNA products; lower panel: 1 μg of H strand of T3 DNA, 10 pmoles (10⁴ cpm) of T3 [³H]RNA polymerase product, and increasing concentrations of nonradioactive competitor in vitro RNA products. △, RNA product made by E. coli RNA polymerase in the presence of ρ factor as competitor; ○, RNA product made by E. coli RNA polymerase as competitor; ●, RNA product made by T3 RNA polymerase.

vivo [³H]RNA by unlabeled in vitro T3 RNA polymerase product, is shown in Fig. 3 (upper panel). It is clear that the unlabeled T3 RNA polymerase product can completely prevent the hybridization of "late" in vivo [³H]RNA, indicating that the in vitro T3 RNA polymerase product contains all the sequences present in "late" *in vivo* RNA. The experiment presented in Fig. 3 (upper panel) also shows that an excess of unlabeled *E. coli* RNA polymerase product made in the absence of ρ factor can prevent the hybridization of "late" *in vivo* [^{3}H] RNA to the extent of nearly 55%, while the RNA product made by *E. coli* RNA polymerase in the presence of ρ factor can only prevent the hybridization of "late" *in vivo* RNA to the extent of approximately 20%.

These experiments clearly demonstrate that T3 RNA polymerase can transcribe the entire "late" region of the T3 genome. However, in the absence of the ρ factor, *E. coli* RNA polymerase also can "read through" the early termination signal to transcribe part of the "late" region. The presence of ρ factor prevents this "read through" by *E. coli* RNA polymerase and presumably restricts the *E. coli* RNA polymerase to copying largely the "early regions."

The competition-hybridization experiments presented in the lower panel of Fig. 3 also support the above conclusion. An excess of unlabeled *in vitro E. coli* RNA polymerase product made in the absence of ρ factor can prevent the hybridization of [^{3}H] RNA product made by T3 RNA polymerase to the extent of nearly 60%, while the product made by *E. coli* RNA polymerase in the presence of ρ factor is unable to prevent such hybridization to this high extent. This indicates that nearly 60% of the RNA sequences present in the T3 RNA polymerase product are identical to those present in *E. coli* RNA polymerase product made in the absence of ρ factor. Thus, *in vitro, E. coli* RNA polymerase, in the absence of ρ factor, copies regions of the T3 DNA that are also copied by T3 RNA polymerase.

TRANSCRIPTION OF DENATURED DNA PREPARATIONS BY T3 RNA POLYMERASE

Effect of Denaturation of DNA on RNA Synthesis and [γ-^{32}P] Nucleotide Incorporation

Although T3 RNA polymerase copies only T3 DNA when native double-stranded template is used, the polymerase will copy a variety of heat-denatured or naturally occurring single-stranded DNAs (Table V). The properties of RNA synthesis primed by denatured DNA can be summarized as follows: (a) the extent of RNA synthesis with denatured DNA was markedly less than with native T3 DNA; (b) in contrast to the results obtained with native T3 DNA, reactions with denatured DNA yielded RNA chains containing both ATP and GTP termini, although more than 85% of chains were initiated with GTP. Even with denatured DNA, RNA chains were not initiated with [γ-^{32}P] UTP or -CTP (data not shown). It is also clear that under these conditions extensive reinitiation of RNA chains occurred. In experiments presented in Table V, 40-45 pmoles of RNA chains was initiated by 1.1 pmoles of T3 RNA polymerase in 30 min in some cases. The average chain length of RNA synthesized, 200-300 nucleotides, was considerably shorter than that obtained with native T3 DNA.

The rate of RNA synthesis with denatured DNA as template varied between 5 and 10% of that observed with native T3 DNA depending on the denatured DNA used in the T3 polymerase reaction. This difference does not appear to be a function of DNA concentration. The rate of RNA synthesis was maximal with 28 nmoles/ml of denatured T3 DNA or with 28 nmoles/ml of ϕX174 DNA. With native T3 DNA, the system was saturated at 14 nmoles/ml of DNA (data not shown).

Identification of Denatured DNA Directed RNA Synthesis as DNA·RNA Hybrid

In the T3 RNA polymerase system, the product formed with native T3 DNA was shown to be free RNA (6). This was true with the *E. coli* RNA polymerase as well (9,10). In contrast, products formed with *E. coli* RNA polymerase and denatured DNA are DNA·RNA hybrids and free RNA is

Table V. Effect of Denaturation of DNA on RNA Synthesis and $[\gamma\text{-}^{32}\text{P}]$ Nucleotide Incorporation by T3 RNA Polymerase[a]

DNA template	$[\gamma\text{-}^{32}\text{P}]$ Nucleotide incorporated (pmoles)		RNA synthesis (pmoles)	Approximate average chain length
	GTP	ATP		
Native T3	17.6	< 0.1	110,800	6000
Denatured T3	40.3	1.2	11,035	265
Denatured T2	15.0	0.5	4,200	270
Denatured calf thymus	45.6	4.7	9,200	180
Denatured *E. coli*	26.2	1.2	7,200	260
ϕX174	42.4	6.8	13,770	280
fd	29.3	6.5	10,800	300

[a]Each reaction mixture (0.25 ml) was prepared as described in the footnote to Table I with 20 nmoles of each DNA and 15 units (1.1 pmoles) of T3 polymerase. The molar concentrations of all other reaction components were the same as those described in the footnote to Table II. Incubation was at 37°C for 30 min. Incorporation of each of the $\gamma\text{-}^{32}$P-labeled nucleoside triphosphates was measured in separate reaction mixtures. RNA synthesis was measured by incorporation of $[^3\text{H}]$UTP. The amount of UMP incorporated was multiplied by a factor (ranging between 3.0 and 4.0) depending on the base composition of the DNA used to obtain total RNA synthesized in the reaction mixture.

produced only after net synthesis of RNA (11,12). An analysis of the product of the T3 RNA polymerase reaction with denatured DNA yielded similar results, as shown by the following experiments. First, the product generated from single-stranded templates was resistant to pancreatic RNase at concentrations that completely degraded RNA products formed with native T3 DNA (Fig. 4A). Heat denaturation of RNA products formed with denatured DNA as template rendered the RNA completely susceptible to RNase (data not shown). In addition, RNA products made with denatured DNA were susceptible to *E. coli* RNase H, an enzyme that specifically degrades RNA in DNA·RNA hybrids (Fig. 4B). Heat denaturation rendered the product insensitive to RNase H (data not shown). As a control, RNA formed with native T3 DNA as template, as expected, was insensitive to RNase H. Finally, ^{32}P-labeled RNA products made with ϕX174 DNA banded in

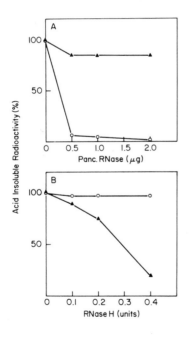

Fig. 4. Influence of pancreatic RNase and Escherichia coli RNase H on RNA products made by T3 RNA polymerase on native and denatured T3 DNA templates. A: Reaction mixtures (0.1 ml) contained 0.02 M tris-Cl buffer (pH 7.8), 0.04 M EDTA, 0.3 M KCl, 100 pmoles of ^{32}P-labeled RNA product (made either on native or denatured T3 DNA by T3 RNA polymerase), and increasing concentrations of pancreatic RNase. Incubation was at 37°C for 30 min, and reactions were terminated with 5% CCl_3COOH and the acid-insoluble radioactivity was determined by Millipore filtration. B: Reaction mixtures (0.1 ml) contained 0.02 M tris-Cl buffer (pH 7.8), 0.05 M KCl, 1 mM $MgCl_2$, 100 pmoles of ^{32}P-labeled RNA nucleotides, and increasing concentration of RNase H as indicated in the figure. RNase H was the kind gift of Dr. I. Berkower of Albert Einstein College of Medicine. One unit of RNase H is that amount of activity that released 1 pmole of RNA nucleotide from DNA·RNA hybrids under the conditions of the assay described by Berkower *et al.* (21). Incubation was at 37°C for 30 min. The reaction was terminated by adding ice-cold 5% CCl_3COOH, and the acid-insoluble ^{32}P radioactivity was determined by Millipore filtration. The RNA product labeled with ^{32}P in the internucleotide linkage was prepared by incubating a typical T3 RNA polymerase reaction mixture containing a-^{32}P-labeled ribonucleoside triphosphates and either native or heat-denatured T3 DNA. The ^{32}P-labeled RNA product was subsequently freed of unreacted nucleoside triphosphates and metal ions by passage through a Sephadex G50 column equilibrated with a solution containing 50 mM tris-Cl (pH 7.8) and 1 mM EDTA. ▲, RNA polymerase products made with denatured T3 DNA as template by T3 RNA polymerase; ○, RNA polymerase products made with native T3 DNA as template by T3 RNA polymerase.

Cs_2SO_4 equilibrium density gradient centrifugation in the region characteristic of DNA·RNA hybrids (Fig. 5). After heat denaturation, the [^{32}P]RNA product banded as free RNA in the heavier density region (data not shown).

Polyriboadenylate Formation

T3 RNA polymerase catalyzed poly(A) synthesis in a reaction analogous to that observed with *E. coli* RNA polymerase (13,14), as shown in Fig. 6. Polymer formation is dependent on the presence of both T3 RNA polymerase and denatured DNA (data not shown). Such homopolymer formation directed by denatured DNA is also specific for ATP. Other nucleoside triphosphates tested did not yield the corresponding homopolymers.

Fig. 5. Isopycnic banding in Cs_2SO_4 of RNA product made with T3 RNA polymerase and single-stranded $\phi X174$ DNA. ^{32}P-Labeled T3 RNA polymerase products were prepared with $\phi X174$ [^{14}C]DNA as template as follows. A typical T3 RNA polymerase reaction mixture containing a-^{32}P-labeled ribonucleoside triphosphates and $\phi X174$ [^{14}C]DNA was incubated at 37°C for 30 min. Subsequently, the reaction mixture was chilled, and the unreacted nucleoside triphosphates and metal ions were removed by passage through a column of Sephadex G50 equilibrated with a solution containing 50 mM tris-Cl (pH 7.8) and 1 mM EDTA. An aliquot of the isolated product containing 65,000 cpm of [^{14}C]-DNA and 22,000 cpm of [^{32}P]RNA in 3.0 ml was adjusted to a density of 1.516 by adding 1.9 g of solid Cs_2SO_4. The mixture was overlayed with paraffin oil and centrifuged for 50 hr in polyallomer tubes in a SW39 rotor at 20°C at 33,000 rpm. Twenty-four 10-drop fractions were collected and their refractive indices measured. Subsequently, ^{32}P and ^{14}C radioactivity content of each fraction was measured in Bray's solution in a liquid scintillation counter. The values reported were corrected for a 10% cross-contamination of ^{32}P counts in the ^{14}C channel. ●, [^{14}C]DNA; ○, [^{32}P]RNA.

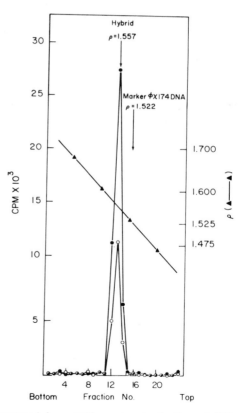

The requirements for poly(A) formation are shown in Table VI. The polymerization reaction required either Mg^{2+} or Mn^{2+} for activity, occurred maximally with denatured DNA, was abolished by DNase, and was unaffected by pancreatic RNase. The formation of poly(A) was not due to contamination of T3 RNA polymerase with *E. coli* RNA polymerase. Unlike *E. coli* RNA polymerase (Table VI, experiment B), reactions catalyzed by T3 RNA polymerase were unaffected by the antibiotics rifampicin and streptolydigin. In addition, with *E. coli* RNA polymerase Mn^{2+} was about twice as active as Mg^{2+} in poly(A) production, while with T3 RNA polymerase Mg^{2+} and Mn^{2+} were almost equally active.

The preferential utilization of denatured DNA templates by T3 RNA polymerase for poly(A) formation was observed with DNAs from widely differing sources (Table VII). The DNA preparations varied considerably in their ability to direct poly(A) synthesis, ϕX174 and calf thymus DNAs being the most efficient templates among the DNAs tested.

Some of the other properties of this reaction can be summarized as follows: (a) High concentrations of ATP are required to saturate the system. The apparent K_s for ATP was calculated to be 1.2×10^{-3} M—a value more than one order of magnitude higher than that for ATP in the T3 DNA directed RNA synthesis catalyzed by T3 RNA polymerase (7). (b) As in the *E. coli* RNA polymerase system, poly(A) formation catalyzed by T3 RNA polymerase was inhibited by relatively low concentrations of UTP, GTP, or CTP (data not shown).

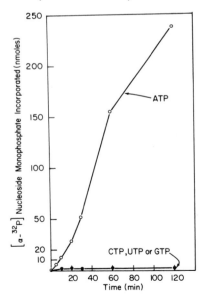

Fig. 6. Kinetics of poly(A) formation by T3 RNA polymerase. Each reaction mixture (0.2 ml) contained 50 mM tris-Cl (pH 7.8), 20 mM $MgCl_2$, 4 mM dithiothreitol, 500 nmoles of [a-^{32}P]ATP (1500 cpm/nmole), 20 μg of dialyzed bovine serum albumin, 10 nmoles of single stranded ϕX174 DNA, and 15 units of T3 RNA polymerase. Incubation was at 37°C. Aliquots (25 μl) were removed at various times as indicated, and the reaction was terminated by adding ice-cold 5% CCl_3COOH. The amount of radioactivity incorporated into an acid-insoluble polynucleotide product was determined by Millipore filtration. Where indicated in the figure, 500 nmoles of a-^{32}P-labeled CTP, UTP, or GTP replaced ATP as the ribonucleoside triphosphate substrate for homopolymer formation.

Table VI. Requirements for Poly(A) Formation by T3 RNA Polymerase[a]

Additions	AMP incorporated (nmoles/30 min)
Experiment A	
1. Complete system (with denatured calf thymus DNA)	6.2
2. Complete system, omit DNA	< 0.1
3. Complete system, omit T3 RNA polymerase	< 0.1
4. Complete system, omit Mg^{2+}	0.2
5. Complete system, omit Mg^{2+}, add Mn^{2+} (4 mM)	5.5
6. Complete system + DNase (5 μg)	< 0.1
7. Complete system + RNase (25 μg)	5.6
8. Complete system + rifampicin (2 μg) + streptolydigin (2 μg)	6.4
Experiment B	
1. Complete system with E. coli RNA polymerase	16.5
2. Complete system + rifampicin (2 μg) + streptolydigin (2 μg)	0.24
3. Complete system, omit Mg^{2+}, add Mn^{2+} (4 mM)	30.5

[a]Each reaction mixture (0.2 ml) was prepared as described in the caption of Fig. 6 except that heat-denatured calf thymus DNA was used instead of ϕX174 DNA and various additions or omissions were as described. [a-^{32}P]ATP was the substrate used. Experiment A was carried out with 4 units of T3 RNA polymerase and Experiment B with 3 units of E. coli RNA polymerase. Incubation was at 37°C for 30 min. Reactions were terminated by adding ice-cold 5% CC1$_3$COOH, and ^{32}P rendered acid insoluble was determined by Millipore filtration.

Table VII. Ability of DNA Preparations to Support Poly(A) Formation by T3 RNA Polymerase[a]

DNA added	[a-^{32}P] AMP incorporated (nmoles/30 min)	
	Native	Denatured
T2	0.4	3.7
T3	< 0.1	2.1
T7	< 0.1	4.3
Calf thymus	1.0	58.5
ϕX174	—	69.5
fd	—	18.5

[a]Reaction mixtures (0.2 ml) were prepared as described in the caption of Fig. 6 except that approximately 10 nmoles of the various DNA preparations was added. Incubation was at 37°C for 30 min with 15 units of T3 RNA polymerase. Reactions were terminated by adding ice-cold 5% CC1$_3$COOH, and ^{32}P rendered acid insoluble was determined by Millipore filtration.

Identification of Product as Poly(A)

The ^{32}P-labeled product made with [a^{32}-P] ATP, T3 RNA polymerase, and denatured DNA was identified as poly(A) by the following criteria: (a) The product was insensitive to pancreatic DNase, pancreatic RNase, and T1 ribonuclease but was completely sensitive to the action of *E. coli* RNase II, yielding 5'-AMP exclusively (data not shown). (b) Alkaline hydrolysis followed by high-voltage paper electrophoresis of the ^{32}P-labeled product resulted in the migration of all the ^{32}P with 2'(3')-AMP. No ^{32}P was detected in 2'(3')-UMP, GMP, or CMP regions (data not shown).

The synthesis of poly(A) catalyzed by T3 RNA polymerase is due to *de novo* synthesis of new chains that are not attached to the template DNA used to direct the reaction (Fig. 7). For this purpose, [^{32}P] poly(A) product was prepared using [^{14}C] fd DNA as template, and the reaction mixture, after denaturation with HCHO, was analyzed in a HCHO-sucrose gradient (Fig. 7). The [^{32}P] poly(A) product sedimented free of template fd DNA. Further substantiation of the *de novo* formation of poly(A) was obtained by the observation that [γ-^{32}P] ATP was incorporated into poly(A) products, indicating *de novo* synthesis of chains having nucleoside triphosphate at their 5' termini (Table VIII). From these experiments, it was cal-

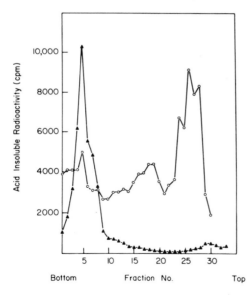

·*Fig. 7. Release of [^{32}P] poly(A) from fd[^{14}C] DNA.* Reaction mixtures (0.2 ml) were prepared with [a-^{32}P] ATP as described in the caption of Fig. 6 except that 12 nmoles of fd[^{14}C] DNA was used as the template. Incubation was for 30 min at 37°C with 12 units of T3 RNA polymerase. The reaction was terminated by adding EDTA to 50 mM and sodium dodecylsulfate to 0.5%. After incubation at 37°C for 2 min, the reaction mixture was chilled in ice and insoluble material was removed by centrifugation. Formaldehyde treatment to destroy RNA secondary structure was carried out by adding sodium phosphate buffer (pH 7.7) to 0.1 M and formaldehyde to 3% (v/v) and then heating the mixture at 65°C for 15 min followed by cooling to 20°C as described by Boedtker (22). Aliquots were layered onto 5 ml of a 5-20% linear sucrose gradient. Each gradient contained 0.1 M sodium phosphate buffer (pH 7.7), 0.2% sodium dodecylsulfate, 3% HCHO (v/v), and 1 mM EDTA. Tubes were centrifuged in a SW65 rotor for 3 hr at 60,000 rpm at 20°C. ▲, fd[^{14}C] DNA; ○, [^{32}P] poly(A).

culated that the average size of the poly(A) product is large (5000 nucleotides) and the average molecular weight is approximately 1.5×10^6. From HCHO-sucrose gradient centrifugation, the poly(A) products were found to be heterogeneous in size, ranging in molecular weight between 10^5 and 2.1×10^6 (Fig. 8).

Table VIII. Incorporation of $[\gamma\text{-}^{32}P]ATP$ into Poly(A) Chains by T3 RNA Polymerase[a]

Additions	Incorporation of ^{32}P (pmoles)
Complete system	12.3
Complete system, omit denatured DNA	0.5
Complete system, omit enzyme	0.4
Complete system + DNase (1 μg)	0.4
Complete system + RNase (2 μg)	15.2
Complete system with $[a\text{-}^{32}P]ATP$ in place of $[\gamma\text{-}^{32}P]ATP$	62,500

[a]Reaction mixtures (0.2 ml) were prepared as described in the caption of Fig. 6 except that 15 units of T3 RNA polymerase, 10 nmoles of ϕX174 DNA, and 400 nmoles of $[\gamma\text{-}^{32}P]ATP$ (1000 cpm/pmole) or $[a\text{-}^{32}P]ATP$ (1000 cpm/nmole) were used. Incubation was for 1 hr at 37°C. Reactions were terminated by adding ice-cold 5% CCl_3COOH, and ^{32}P rendered acid insoluble was determined.

Fig. 8. HCHO-sucrose gradient analysis of poly(A) product made with ϕX-174 DNA and T3 RNA polymerase. A reaction mixture (0.2 ml) was prepared with 400 nmoles of $[a\text{-}^{32}P]ATP$ as described in the caption of Fig. 6. Ten nanomoles of ϕX174 DNA and 20 units of T3 RNA polymerase were used. After incubation for 30 min at 37°C, the reaction was terminated and the ^{32}P-labeled RNA product formed was analyzed in HCHO-sucrose gradients exactly as described in the caption of Fig. 7. A gradient containing E. coli ribosomal RNA and tRNA similarly treated with sodium dodecylsulfate and formaldehyde was run in parallel to provide molecular weight markers. 23S, 16S, and 4S RNA are of molecular weights 1.1×10^6, 0.55×10^6, and 28,000, respectively.

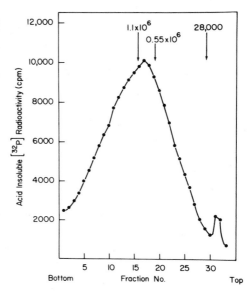

SUMMARY AND CONCLUSION

We may conclude that these studies with bacteriophage T3 induced RNA polymerase show that T3 RNA polymerase, upon copying its specific template, native T3 DNA, initiates RNA chains only with GTP. Pyrophosphate exchange studies and the direct determination of nucleotide sequence at the 5' end of RNA chains show that almost all RNA chains contain the sequence $pppGp(Gp)_n$ Ap at the 5'-triphosphate end, indicating a high degree of specificity of initiation of RNA chains by T3-induced RNA polymerase. In addition, studies of the polymerase reaction with native T3 DNA *in vitro* show that T3 RNA polymerase is able to terminate RNA synthesis with the release of RNA chains from the template DNA. Polymerase is also released in the process and, acting catalytically, reinitiates new RNA chains. Many moles of RNA chains are thus formed per mole of enzyme added to the reaction mixture.

RNA produced in the T3 RNA polymerase reaction contains all the sequences present in "late" mRNA isolated from T3 phage infected cells. Thus T3 RNA polymerase is involved in the synthesis of "late" mRNA formed in T3-infected cells. In addition, the T3 RNA polymerase product also contains sequences present in "early" mRNA.

Although T3 RNA polymerase possesses a highly specific template requirement and will copy only T3 DNA when native double-stranded template is used, the enzyme will transcribe a variety of single-stranded DNAs (heat-denatured T3, T7, calf thymus, and naturally occurring single-stranded circular DNAs such as ϕX174 and fd) at a markedly reduced rate. The product formed in a denatured DNA directed reaction is a DNA·RNA hybrid with more than 85% of RNA chains initiated with pppG. Some chains (approximately 10-15%) are initiated with pppA. The average chain length of RNA produced is considerably shorter (200-300 nucleotides) than that obtained in a native T3 DNA directed reaction (5000-6000 nucleotides).

With denatured DNA as template, T3 RNA polymerase is also able to carry out *de novo* synthesis of poly(A) chains. This reaction requires high concentrations of ATP and is inhibited by the presence of relatively low concentrations of other ribonucleoside triphosphates. Poly(A) chains formed are not attached to the template DNA, contain ATP at the 5' terminus, and are heterogeneous in size, ranging in molecular weight from about 10^5 to 2.1×10^6.

These denatured DNA directed reactions catalyzed by T3 RNA polymerase are analogous to those carried out by *E. coli* RNA polymerase and suggest that the high degree of template specificity of T3 RNA polymerase resides both in the enzyme and in the secondary structure of the template DNA used to direct the polymerase reaction.

ACKNOWLEDGMENTS

This work was supported by grants from the National Institutes of Health, The American Cancer Society, and The American Heart Association, Inc. U.M. is a recipient of the Faculty Research Award of the American Cancer Society. R.A.S. is a Fellow of the New York Heart Association, Inc.

REFERENCES

1. E. P. Geiduschek and R. Haselkorn. *Ann. Rev. Biochem.* **38**:647-676 (1969).
2. A. Travers. *Nature* **229**:69-74 (1971).
3. M. Chamberlin, J. McGrath, and L. Waskell. *Nature* **228**:227-231 (1970).
4. J. J. Dunn, F. A. Bautz, and E. F. K. Bautz. *Nature New Biol.* **230**:94-96 (1971).
5. U. Maitra. *Biochem. Biophys. Res. Commun.* **43**:443-450 (1971).
6. U. Maitra and H. Huang. *Proc. Natl. Acad. Sci. (USA)* **69**:55-59 (1972).
7. P. R. Chakraborty, P. Sarkar, H. Huang, and U. Maitra. *J. Biol. Chem.*, **248**:6637-6646 (1973).
8. J. J. Dunn, W. T. McAllister, and E. K. F. Bautz. *Virology* **48**:112-125 (1972).
9. U. Maitra and F. Barash. *Proc. Natl. Acad. Sci. (USA)* **64**:779-786 (1969).
10. R. L. Millette. *Proc. Natl. Acad. Sci. (USA)* **66**:701-708 (1970).
11. R. L. Sinsheimer and M. Lawrence. *J. Mol. Biol.* **8**:289-296 (1964).
12. M. Chamberlin and P. Berg. *J. Mol. Biol.* **8**:297-313 (1964).
13. A. Stevens. *J. Biol. Chem.* **239**:204-209 (1964).
14. M. Chamberlin and P. Berg. *J. Mol. Biol.* **8**:708-726 (1964).
15. U. Maitra, Y. Nakata, and J. Hurwitz. *J. Biol. Chem.* **242**:4908-4918 (1967).
16. U. Maitra, A. H. Lockwood, J. S. Dubnoff, and A. Guha. *Cold Spring Harbor Symp. Quant. Biol.* **35**:143-156 (1970).
17. A. P. Nygaard and B. D. Hall. *J. Mol. Biol.* **9**:125-142 (1964).
18. M. Gefter. Studies on methylated bases in bacteriophage DNA. Ph.D. thesis, Albert Einstein College of Medicine of Yeshiva University (1967).
19. E. T. Young and G. V. Houwe. *J. Mol. Biol.* **51**:605-619 (1970).
20. A. Guha and W. C. Szybalski. *Virology* **34**:608-616 (1968).
21. I. Berkower, J. Leis, and J. Hurwitz. *J. Biol. Chem.*, **248**:5914-5921 (1973).
22. H. Boedtker. *J. Mol. Biol.* **35**:61-70 (1968).

DISCUSSION

Question (Burma): How does the T3 enzyme recognize the promoter site?

Answer: In the T3 RNA polymerase reaction, all RNA chains formed in the native T3 DNA directed reaction contain the sequence $pppGp(Gp)_nA$--- at the 5' end. This shows a very high degree of specificity of initiation of RNA chains by T3 RNA polymerase. Thus recognition signals on the DNA template, in the form of unique nucleotide sequences and/or structural alterations, are probably responsible for recognition of initiation sequences on the DNA template.

Question (Burma): Is the same protein involved in recognition of promoter as well as for chain elongation?

Answer: Since T3 RNA polymerase used in our studies is electrophoretically pure and consists of a single polypeptide chain, it follows from the data I have presented here that

T3 RNA polymerase alone can bring about specific initiation, elongation, termination, and reinitiation of RNA synthesis.

Question (Mitra): Does T3 RNA polymerase exist in multimeric state?

Answer: Electrophoretically pure T3 RNA polymerase protein has been shown to be a single polypeptide chain of molecular weight 100,000 ± 5000. This is based on the observation that the molecular weight of the active enzyme in the native state as determined by glycerol-gradient centrifugation is approximately 105,000. The subunit molecular weight as determined by SDS-polyacrylamide gel electrophoresis is 100,000. Whether or not the polymerase can exist in multimeric state during the transcription process is not known.

12

Physical Mapping of Transcribing Regions on Coliphage fd DNA by the Use of Restriction Endonucleases

M. Takanami and T. Okamoto

Institute for Chemical Research
Kyoto University
Uji, Kyoto, Japan

In an RNA-synthesizing system consisting of *Escherichia coli* RNA polymerase holoenzyme and doubly closed replicative form (RF-I) DNA of phage fd, several species of RNA with unique starting sequences and size are transcribed from the "minus" strand of the template. Transcription of an RNA species starting with pppA proceeded to the size of about 26S and terminated, and the other RNA species starting with pppG had sizes of about 10S, 13S, and 17S (16). The results suggested that RF-I DNA provides sets of specific sites for initiation and termination of RNA transcription. As the transcription proceeds in the same direction, it is likely that the template provides a single termination site, so that RNA chains initiated at different loci proceed to the termination site, at which RNA synthesis ceases. However, there was no direct evidence supporting this model. In this chapter, experiments are described in which RF-I DNA was cleaved by endonucleases with cleavage-site specificities, and the template activity of the resulting unique fragments and the size of synthesized products were analyzed. As a result, we could map the approximate sites at which initiation and termination took place on RF-I DNA.

The procedures for preparing RF-I DNA from *E. coli* K38 cells infected with phage fd and *E. coli* RNA polymerase holoenzyme and the conditions used for labeling the starting termini of RNA have been described previously (14,15). For the preparation of endonucleases with cleavage-site specificities from the *Haemo-*

Table I. Specific Cleavage of fd RF-I DNA by Five
Different Endonucleases of the *Haemophilus* Group

Enzyme	Source	Number of cleavage sites
Endo Rd[a]	*H. influenzae* Rd	1
Endo AE[b]	*H. aegyptium*	11
Endo H-1	*H. influenzae* H-1	3
Endo GA	*H. gallinarum*	6
Endo AP	*H. aphirophilus*	13

[a] Endonuclease R of Smith and Wilcox (13).
[b] Endonuclease Z of Middleton *et al.* (10).

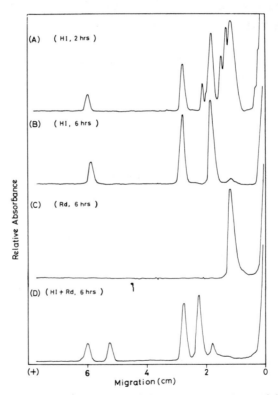

Fig. 1. Polyacrylamide gel electrophoresis of the digestion products of fd RF-I DNA by Endo H-1 and Rd(17). 0.3 OD $_{260}$ unit of RF-I DNA was incubated for 2-6 hr at 37°C with 10 units of enzyme in 0.2 ml of 7 mM tris (pH 7.6), 7 mM MgCl$_2$, 1 mM mercaptoethanol. The hydrolysates were layered on 3% gel columns (0.6 by 12 cm) and electrophoresed for 18 hr at 2 mA/tube. Gels were stained with 0.4% acridine orange and washed with 0.2 N acetic acid, and the color density was traced by a densitometer.

philus group, the plaque-forming abilities of RF-I DNA and the single-stranded DNA of phage fd were assayed on lysozyme-spheroplasts, and the fraction that preferentially destroys the infectivity of RF-I DNA was prepared. The specificity of the enzyme was then determined by resolving the hydrolysates of RF-I DNA on polyacrylamide gel electrophoresis (17).

SPECIFIC CLEAVAGE OF RF-I DNA

Restriction endonucleases, which degrade foreign DNA at a limited number of sites, have been prepared from several bacterial strains (4,6,9,10,13). These enzymes are known to attack double-stranded DNA by recognizing specific nucleotide sequences of DNA and to produce duplex cleavages (6,8). It is therefore possible to cleave DNA molecules at sites with such sequences (2,3,5, 7). The number of fragments produced from RF-I DNA by endonuclease R (abbreviated as Endo Rd) (13), endonuclease Z (abbreviated as Endo AE) (10), and three new enzymes isolated in our laboratory (abbreviated as Endo H-1, AP, and GA) (18) are listed in Table I (see Fig. 5).

Among these enzymes, Endo Rd cleaved RF-I DNA only at one specific site and Endo H-1 cleaved it at three different sites (17). Electrophoretic patterns of the hydrolysates are shown in Fig. 1. Incubation of DNA with Endo H-1 for a short period produced seven discrete peaks (Fig. 1A). Under the conditions for electrophoresis, RF-I DNA did not penetrate into the gel and RF-II DNA migrated in the vicinity of the slowest peak in Fig. 1A. On increasing the

Table II. Length of DNA Fragments Produced by Endo H-1 and Rd

	Length (μ)	Molecular weight[a] ($\times 10^6$)
RF-II DNA[b]	1.84 ± 0.07	3.5
Endo H-1 hydrolysate of RF-I DNA		
Fragment 1	1.14 ± 0.08	2.2
Fragment 2	0.58 ± 0.08	1.1
Fragment 3	0.23 ± 0.05	0.4
Endo Rd hydrolysate of fragment 1		
Fragment 4	0.86^c	1.7
Fragment 5	0.28^c	0.5

[a]Estimated assuming 1 μ corresponds to 1.92×10^6 daltons.
[b]Converted from RF-I DNA by introducing a nick.
[c]Estimated from relative mobilities on gel electrophoresis.

incubation period, three major peaks were obtained (Fig. 1B), and the pattern was not changed by further incubation. The additional peaks observed in Fig. 1A were therefore assumed to be intermediates of digestion. The lengths of the three fragments determined by electron microscopy are given in Table II. RF-II DNA, converted from RF-I DNA by introducing a nick, has the contour length of $1.84 \pm 0.07\ \mu$ (11). The sum of three fragments is about equal to the contour length of RF-II DNA. Assuming $1\ \mu$ corresponds to 1.92×10^6 daltons (11), molecular weights of the fragments were estimated as in Table II. In contrast to the pattern with Endo H-1, Endo Rd gave only a single peak with a slow mobility, and no smaller fragment was produced even after the incubation was prolonged (Fig. 1C). When RF-I DNA was treated by the combination of two enzymes, four peaks were obtained (fig. 1D). Among three fragments produced by Endo H-1, the species of $1.14\ \mu$ was cleaved into two, of which the lengths were estimated to be about $0.86\ \mu$ and $0.28\ \mu$ from the relative mobilities on gel electrophoresis. In the present study, most experiments were carried out with DNA cleaved by these two enzymes.

RNA SYNTHESIS ON CLEAVED DNA MOLECULES

The hydrolysates of RF-I DNA by Endo Rd and H-1 were added to RNA-synthesizing mixtures containing either $[\gamma\text{-}^{32}\text{P}]\text{ATP}$ or $[\gamma\text{-}^{32}\text{P}]\text{GTP}$ and the number of termini formed was determined. Both (pppA---)RNA and (pppG---) −RNA were synthesized with the cleaved DNA, though the efficiency of initiation with ATP considerably decreased. The formation of A termini on the Endo H-1 treated DNA was reduced to about 40% of the control and that on the Endo Rd treated DNA to about 70% of the control. On the other hand, the formation of G termini was less influenced by cleaving the DNA.

The size of the synthesized products was analyzed by band centrifugation on sucrose-density gradients. With the intact DNA molecule, (pppA---)RNA usually gives a single peak of about 26S and (pppG---)RNA three peaks of about 10S, 13S, and 17S (Fig. 2). When the Endo H-1 treated DNA was used as template, the sedimentation profile of (pppG---)RNA was essentially identical to that of intact DNA, though the height of the 17S peak became lower. The (pppA---)-RNA was much shorter than that formed on intact DNA and was estimated to be about 12S at the peak position. With DNA treated by Endo Rd, (pppG---)-RNA gave only two peaks, corresponding to the 10S and 13S components formed on intact DNA. The size of (pppA---)RNA was about 19S (Fig. 2).

RNA synthesized on the Endo Rd treated DNA was analyzed before deproteinization, using the conditions previously described (12). The 10S and 13S (pppG---)RNA formed on the cleaved DNA appeared apart from the DNA·enzyme complex, whereas the (pppA---)RNA was recovered at the complex region (Fig. 3). This observation implies that the termination of the two RNA species starting with GTP occurred normally on this template.

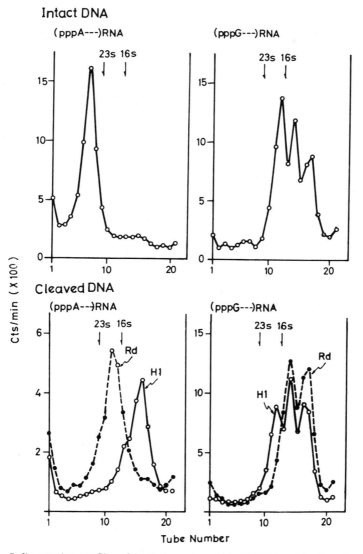

Fig. 2. Sedimentation profiles of RNA formed on fd RF-I DNA and its digestion products by Endo H-1 and Rd. The reaction mixture (1 ml) contained 8 mM MgCl$_2$, 40 mM tris (pH 7.9), 40 mM KCl, 0.1 mM dithiothreitol, 20 μM of [γ-^{32}P]ATP or [γ-^{32}P]GTP (about 10^4 cpm/pmole), 0.4 mM each of three other nucleoside triphosphates, 32 μg DNA, and 16 μg RNA polymerase. Following incubation for 5 min at 37°C, ATP or GTP was added to 0.4 mM, and incubation was continued for 20 min. The reaction was terminated by shaking with 80% phenol. The aqueous layers were passed through Sephadex G100 columns (1 by 20 cm), equilibrated with 0.14 M NaCl, 0.02 M tris (pH 7.6). RNA fractions eluted were layered on sucrose-density gradients and centrifuged for 6 hr at 38,000 rpm and 5°C. DNA hydrolysates were prepared as in Fig. 1.

The approximate molecular weights of these RNA chains were estimated as in Table III, using an empirical equation in which *E. coli* ribosomal RNA, tRNA, and phage RNA fit (1).

The hydrolysate of RF-I DNA by Endo H-1 was resolved by gel electrophoresis and the DNA fragments were eluted from the band regions. About equimolar amounts of the fragments were added to RNA-synthesizing mixtures containing either $[\gamma\text{-}^{32}\text{P}]$ ATP or $[\gamma\text{-}^{32}\text{P}]$ GTP. As shown in Table IV, (pppA---)-RNA was predominantly initiated on the $0.58\text{-}\mu$ fragment and (pppG---)RNA on the $1.14\text{-}\mu$ fragment.

PHYSICAL MAPPING OF THE INITIATION AND TERMINATION SITES

The $0.58\text{-}\mu$ fragment produced by Endo H-1 contains the promoter for (pppA---)RNA, and roughly two-thirds of this fragment is transcribed into RNA, as the size of (pppA---)RNA was about 12S. The size of (pppA---)RNA formed on the Endo Rd treated DNA would represent the approximate distance

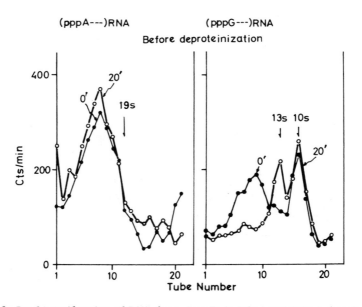

Fig. 3. *Band centrifugation of RNA formed on Endo Rd treated DNA before deproteinization.* Reaction mixtures containing Endo Rd treated DNA as template and $[\gamma\text{-}^{32}\text{P}]$ ATP or $[\gamma\text{-}^{32}\text{P}]$ GTP were prepared and incubated as in Fig. 2. At just before (0 min in figure) and 20 min after adding excess substrates, the reaction mixtures were passed through Sephadex G100 columns equilibrated with 8 mM MgCl$_2$, 20 mM tris (pH 7.6), layered on sucrose-density gradients, and centrifuged for 6 hr at 38,000 rpm and 5°C.

between the initiation site of this RNA species and the cleavage site by Endo Rd, and this cleavage site should be at about 25% of the distance from one end of the 1.14-μ fragment produced by Endo H-1. The 1.14-μ fragment would contain all of initiation and termination loci for (pppG---)RNA, because three (pppG---)-RNA species were formed on the Endo H-1 hydrolysate. The 17S (pppG---)RNA

Table III. Approximate Sizes of RNA Synthesized on fd RF-I DNA and Its Digestion Products by Endo H-1 and Rd

Template	S value		Molecular weight[a] ($\times 10^5$)
	(pppA-)RNA	(pppG-)RNA	
Intact DNA	26		15
		10	2.1
		13	3.5
		17	6.3
DNA cleaved by Endo H-1	12		3.0
		10	—
		13	—
		17	—
DNA cleaved by Endo Rd	19		8.0
		10	—
		13	—

[a]Estimated using an empirical equation(1).

Table IV. Initiation of RNA Synthesis on DNA Fragments Produced by Endo H-1[a]

	Nucleoside [γ-^{32}P] triphosphate incorporated (cpm)	
	ATP	GTP
Fragment 1 (1.14 μ)	709 (21%)	6095 (76%)
Fragment 2 (0.58 μ)	2430 (73%)	1187 (17%)
Fragment 3 (0.23 μ)	174 (5%)	750 (9%)

[a]The hydrolysate of RF-I DNA by Endo H-1 was resolved on gel electrophoresis as in Fig. 1. The gel was sliced, and extracts were prepared. The fragment regions were concentrated and added to RNA-synthesizing mixtures containing [γ-^{32}P]ATP or [γ-^{32}P]GTP (about 10^4 cpm/pmole), and P^{32} incorporated into RNA was determined as in Sugiura *et al.* (14).

was not formed on the Endo Rd hydrolysate. This suggests that the cleavage site by Endo Rd locates at or near the promoter of this RNA species. The 13S (pppG---)RNA was formed on both the Endo H-1 and Rd hydrolysates. Therefore, the origin of this RNA species would be in the larger piece produced by Endo Rd from the 1.14-μ fragment of the Endo H-1 hydrolysate.

These observations would provide enough informations to estimate the approximate sites for initiation and termination of all RNA species except for the smallest (pppG---)RNA. As schematically represented in Fig. 4, the data can be well explained with the model previously proposed, in which RNA chains initiated at the respective loci are terminated at a single termination site. The assignment of the 10S (pppG---)RNA is tentative, however. Our experiment does not rule out other possibilities such as RNA chains initiated at the promoter of the 13S RNA species being partially terminated at a site half way, producing the 10S fragment.

The size of the DNA fragments was directly determined by electron microscopy. However, estimation of the molecular weight of RNA is based on an empirical equation, and this would lead to considerable errors in calculations. For more accurate mapping, the size of RNA should be determined by other direct methods.

As demonstrated in the present study, initiation of RNA synthesis at specific sites appears not to be destroyed by cleaving DNA molecules with site-specific endonucleases, unless the cleavage site is in close proximity to the promoters. The action of these endonucleases is quite site specific, and the number of cleaved fragments appears to increase additively by the combination of enzymes with different cleavage-site specificities (Fig. 5). Therefore, it may be possible to

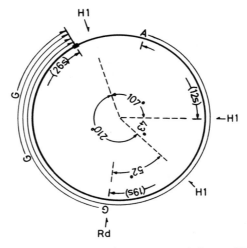

Fig. 4. Schematic representation of in vitro transcription on fd RF-I DNA.

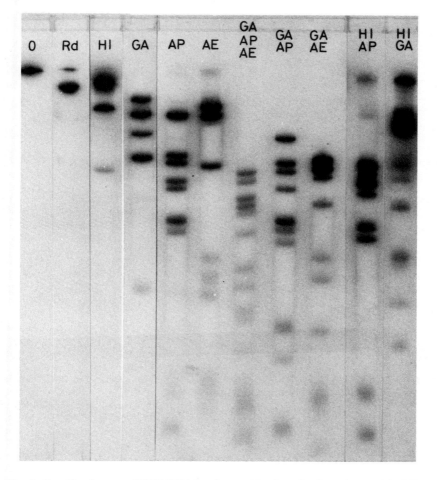

Fig. 5. Specific cleavage of RF-I DNA by the combination of endonucleases with different cleavage site specificities. RF-I [^{32}P]DNA was digested with enzymes indicated in the figure, and the hydrolysates were electrophoretically resolved as in Fig. 1, except that 5% gel columns were employed.

derive a more detailed transcription map and to obtain fragments containing the functional sites of DNA which are short enough for the determination of the nucleotide sequences.

ACKNOWLEDGMENT

We are greatly indebted to Dr. T. Oda of Okayama University Medical School for the size determination of DNA by electron microscopy.

REFERENCES

1. H. Boedtker. Molecular weight and conformation of RNA. In L. Grossman and K. Moldave (eds.), *Methods in Enzymology,* Vol. XII (1968), p. 429 Academic Press, New York.
2. K. Dana and D. Nathans. Specific Cleavage of SV 40 DNA by restriction endonuclease of *Hemophilus influenzae. Proc. Natl. Acad. Sci. (USA)* **68**:2913 (1971).
3. M. H. Edgell, C. A. Hutchison, III, and M. Sclair. Specific endonuclease R fragments of bacteriophage φX174. *J. Virol.* **9**:574 (1972).
4. B. Eskin and S. Linn. The DNA modification and restriction enzymes of *Escherichia coli* B. *J. Biol. Chem.* **247**:6183 (1972).
5. G. C. Fareed, C. F. Garon, and N. P. Salzman. Origin and direction of SV 40 DNA replication. *J. Virol.* **10**:484 (1972).
6. J. Hedgpeth, H. M. Goodman, and H. W. Boyer. DNA nucleotide sequence restricted by the R1 endonuclease. *Proc. Natl. Acad. Sci. (USA)* **69**:3448 (1972).
7. D. A. Jackson, R. H. Symons, and P. Berg. Biochemical method for inserting new genetic information into DNA of SV 40. *Proc. Natl. Acad. Sci. (USA)* **69**:2904 (1972).
8. T. J. Kelly and H. O. Smith. A restriction enzyme from *Hemophilus influenzae.* II. Base sequence of the recognition site. *J. Mol. Biol.* **51**:393 (1970).
9. M. Meselson and R. Yuan. DNA restriction enzyme from *E. coli. Nature* **217**:1110 (1968).
10. J. H. Middleton, M. H. Edgell, and C. A. Hutchison, III. Specific fragments of φX174 DNA produced by a restriction enzymes from *Haemophilus aegyptium,* endonuclease Z. *J. Virol.* **10**:42 (1972).
11. T. Oda, T. Nakamura, S. Watanabe, and M. Takanami. Electron microscopy of the replicative form DNA of coliphage fd. *J. Electron Micros.* **20**:67 (1971).
12. T. Okamoto, M. Sugiura, and M. Takanami. Length of RNA transcribed on the replicative form DNA of coliphage fd. *J. Mol. Biol.* **45**:101 (1969).
13. H. O. Smith and K. W. Wilcox. A restriction enzyme from *Hemophilus influenzae.* I. Purification and general properties. *J. Mol. Biol.* **51**:379 (1970).
14. M. Sugiura, T. Okamoto, and M. Takanami. Starting nucleotide sequences of RNA synthesized on the replicative form DNA of coliphage fd. *J. Mol. Biol.* **43**:299 (1969).
15. M. Sugiura, T. Okamoto, and M. Takanami. RNA polymerase σ factor and the selection of initiation site. *Nature* **225**:598 (1970).
16. M. Takanami, T. Okamoto, and M. Sugiura. The starting nucleotide sequences and size of RNA transcribed *in vitro* on phage DNA templates. *Cold Spring Harbor Symp. Quant. Biol.* **35**:179 (1970).
17. M. Takanami and H. Kojo. Cleavage site specificity of an endonuclease prepared from *Haemophilus influenzae* strain H 1. *FEBS Letters,* **29**:267 (1973).
18. M. Takanami. Specific cleavage of fd DNA by five different restriction endonucleases of *Haemophilus* genus. *FEBS Letters* **34**:318 (1973).

DISCUSSION

Question (Bautz): Do all RNA species produced on intact template occur in equimolar quantities?

Answer: About equimolar amounts of the 26S (pppA—)RNA, 17S (pppG—)RNA, and 13S (pppG—)RNA are usually formed on the intact fd RF-I DNA. But the amount of the 10S (pppG—)RNA varies with the reaction conditions.

Question (Mitra): Do chain termination and reinitiation on fd RF template by *E. coli* RNA polymerase require ρ protein?

Answer: There are two types of termination events on fd RF-I DNA: one is termination without ρ and the other is ρ-induced termination. RNA synthesis appears to be reinitiated without ρ.

Question (Burma): Isn't it true that similar experiments with SV40 show that there is a point of termination of RNA chains?

Answer: I do not know much about the SV40 DNA directed system. In the *in vitro* systems directed by phage DNAs such as ϕ80, λ, and T3, it has been shown that transcription is terminated at specific sites with or without ρ.

13

Transcriptional Control of the Expression of a Degradative Plasmid in *Pseudomonas*

A. M. Chakrabarty

Physical Chemistry Laboratory
General Electric Corporate Research & Development
Schenectady, New York, U.S.A.

Considerable attention has recently been directed toward studying the genetic basis of nutritional versatility in *Pseudomonas*. Unlike the enterobacteria, which grow on a limited number of complex organic compounds, the genus *Pseudomonas* is known for its ability to derive its carbon and energy from the dissimilation of a large number of organic compounds of varying complexities (1). The genetic and physiological regulation, the enzymology, and the biochemistry of a large number of catabolic pathways have therefore been extensively studied in this genus (2). The ability of the pseudomonads to degrade a number of complex organic compounds has been recently shown to be due to their possession of extrachromosomal elements that specify the entire enzyme complements of a particular degradative pathway. Thus the genes specifying enzymes responsible for the degradation of salicylate in a strain of *Pseudomonas putida* R1 are not part of the bacterial chromosome but are borne on extrachromosomal elements which are transmissible among a number of *Pseudomonas* species (3). Similarly, the camphor degradative pathway, comprised of a set of 15-20 inducible enzymes, is specified by genes that are also part of a transmissible plasmid (4). Another set of genes that code for enzymes responsible for the metabolism of octane is carried on yet another transmissible plasmid (5). We have proposed to term these naturally occurring plasmids "degradative plasmids" because of the selective nutritional advantage they offer to the host cells harboring them (6). All these degradative plasmids are highly specialized since they not only carry genes for their autonomous replication and transmission among a number of *Pseudomonas* species but also carry genes that are responsible for restriction of foreign DNA (A. M. Chakrabarty, unpublished observation) and genes that specify an array of enzymes that can convert a complex organic compound to a simple metabolite easily assimilated by the cell. The specialization of the genetic expression of the degradative plasmids is also evident from the fact that whereas the chromosomal genes seem to be fully expressed during the growth of *P. aeruginosa* at $42°C$, the expression of the degradative plasmid genes is inhibited at this temperature, although it is fully operational at permissible temperatures ($32°C$). In this chapter, we present some evidence that suggests that the inhibition of expression of the SAL plasmid at $42°C$ is due to an inhibition of the transcription of the plasmid genes, and not the translation of the preformed messenger RNA.

MATERIALS AND METHODS

Bacterial Strains. The composition of the synthetic medium and the growth conditions of strains of *P. putida* and *P. aeruginosa* have already been described (3).

Conjugational Transfer of Plasmids. Detailed methods describing the transmissibility of the degradative plasmids among different *Pseudomonas* species have already been described (3-5).

Enzyme Assays. Cells were harvested, and the enzymes of the *meta* pathway were assayed as described previously (3).

RESULTS

We have recently shown that the genes specifying enzymes responsible for the degradation of salicylate in *P. putida* strain R1 are tightly clustered and occur in the form of a transmissible plasmid (3). Thus it has been possible to transfer the genes for the entire salicylate degradative pathway to a number of *Pseudomonas* species such as *P. putida* strains PpG1 and PRS1, *P. fluorescens*, and *P. aeruginosa* PAO. The SAL plasmid is known to specify enzymes of the *meta* pathway, which can convert salicylate to pyruvate and acetate through intermediate formation of catechol and 2-hydroxymuconic semialdehyde (3). The *meta* pathway enzymes are induced by salicylate but not by catechol, 2-hydroxymuconic semialdehyde, or other intermediates of salicylate degradation. When the SAL plasmid was transferred to *P. aeruginosa* PAO, the resultant Sal$^+$ strain could grow well with salicylate as the sole source of carbon at $32°C$, but not at $42°C$. The parent salicylate-negative or the Sal$^+$ derivative of this strain can, however, grow well at $42°C$ with glucose or glutamate as the sole source of carbon (Table I). *P. putida* strains R1, PpG1, and PRS1 can grow at

Table I. Expression of SAL Plasmid at Different Temperatures

Strain	Carbon source	Growth temperature (°C)	Growth
Sal⁺ *P. putida*	Glucose	32	+
		40	-
Sal⁺ *P. putida*	Salicylate	32	+
		40	-
P. aeruginosa	Glucose	32	+
		42	+
Sal⁺ *P. aeruginosa*	Salicylate	32	+
		42	-
Sal⁺ *P. aeruginosa*	Glucose	32	+
		42	+

Table II. Expression of Several Degradative Plasmids at Different Temperatures in *P. aeruginosa*

Plasmid	Carbon source	Growth temperature (°C)	Growth
CAM	Camphor	32	+
		42	-
SAL	Salicylate	32	+
		42	-
CAM-OCT	*n*-Octane	32	+
		42	±[a]

[a]Slow growth with octane at 42°C.

32°C, but are incapable of growing at 42°C. The ability of Sal⁺ *P. aeruginosa* PAO to grow at 42°C with glucose as the sole source of carbon, but not with salicylate as the only carbon source, seems to suggest that some specific step in salicylate metabolism must be sensitive at higher temperature (42°C). In order to see if such a step is unique to salicylate metabolism or whether the expression of other degradative plasmids might also be affected at 42°C, two other degradative plasmids specifying enzymes of camphor and octane metabolism were introduced into *P. aeruginosa* PAO (4,5). The ability of Cam⁺ and Cam-Oct⁺ *P. aeruginosa* PAO (6) to grow with camphor or octane as the only source of carbon at 32°C and 42°C was then tested. It can be seen from the results in Table II that the expression of CAM plasmid remains inhibited at 42°C, while that of OCT is partially affected. This inhibition of the expression of CAM and OCT plasmids is not due to any general inhibitory phenomenon, since the CAM-OCT⁺ *P. aeruginosa* PAO could grow well at 42°C with glucose. While it is not clear whether the inability of Cam$^+$ or Cam-Oct$^+$ *P. aeruginosa* PAO to grow with camphor or octane as the sole carbon source at 42°C is due to any unique mechanism affecting expression of the degradative plasmids or whether there are unrelated single or multiple steps in the metabolism of these compounds that are particularly sensitive at 42°C, it appears that the phenomenon of inhibition of genetic expression at 42°C is rather common among these plasmids.

To see if the inability of Sal$^+$ *P. aeruginosa* to grow with salicylate as the only carbon source at 42°C is due to sensitivity of any particular enzyme of the *meta* pathway, the levels of *meta* pathway enzymes were determined in cells grown at 32°C and 42°C. Results in Table III clearly indicate that when cells were grown at 32°C, the levels of *meta* pathway enzymes were high. When grown at 42°C, the levels of all the enzymes were low. All the enzymes were, however, fully active at 42°C. These data suggest that the inability of Sal$^+$ *P. aeruginosa* PAO to grow at 42°C with salicylate as the sole source of carbon was not due to repression of the formation of any particular enzyme or to loss of activity of the enzymes at that temperature, but was due to failure of the formation of all the enzymes of the pathway.

The inability of Sal$^+$ *P. aeruginosa* PAO to produce all the *meta* pathway enzymes at 42°C seems to suggest that the expression of the entire plasmid might be inhibited at that temperature. Alternatively, the entire plasmid might be lost from the cells, since curing of plasmids at 42°C is a well-known phenomenon in other systems (7). It can be seen from the results in Table IV that the rate of segregation of the SAL plasmid from Sal$^+$ *P. aeruginosa* PAO at 42°C is not much different from that at 32°C. There is no appreciable increase in the rate of segregation of the SAL or CAM plasmids when the corresponding

Table III. Level of *Meta* Pathway Enzymes in Sal$^+$ *P. aeruginosa* Grown at 32°C and 42°C

	Specific activities[a]	
Enzymes	32°C-grown cells	42°C-grown cells
Catechol-2, 3-oxygenase	1.82	0.21
2-Hydroxymuconic semialdehyde hydro-lyase	0.18	0.05
4-Hydroxy-2-ketovalerate aldolase	0.031	0.005

[a]Cells were grown in a mineral medium containing 5 mM glutamate and 10 mM salicylate at 32°C or 42°C. Specific activities of the enzymes have been defined as micromoles of product formed or substrate used per minute per milligram protein.

Sal⁺ or Cam⁺ *P. aeruginosa* PAO cells are grown at 42°C in L broth or glucose-minimal medium. Thus the failure of Sal⁺ *P. aeruginosa* PAO to grow with salicylate at 42°C or that of Cam⁺ *P. aeruginosa* PAO cells to grow with camphor as the only carbon source at 42°C is not due to loss of the gene clusters from the cells.

Since the genetic information concerning salicylate metabolism persists at 42°C and since the cellular protein synthetic machinery seems perfectly func-

Table IV. Effect of Temperature on the Rate of Segregation of the Plasmids in *P. aeruginosa*

Plasmid	Growth medium	Growth temperature (°C)	Frequency of segregation (%)
SAL	L broth	32	0.7
		42	1.1
	Glucose minimal	32	< 0.5
		42	0.8
CAM	L broth	32	< 0.5
		42	< 0.5
	Glucose minimal	32	< 0.5
		42	< 0.5

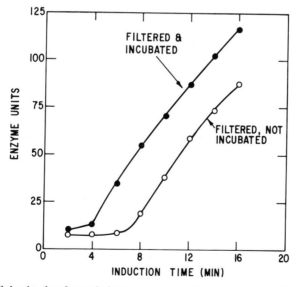

Fig. 1. Intracellular levels of catechol-2,3-oxygenase after exposure of cells to an optimal inducer for various times.

tional at this temperature, it is clear that the inability of Sal$^+$ *P. aeruginosa* PAO to produce any of the enzymes of the *meta* pathway must be due to an inhibition of the expression of the SAL plasmid. This inhibition might be due to an inhibition of the formation of the respective messenger RNAs (mRNAs) or to an inhibition of the translation of the corresponding mRNAs. The amount of mRNA specific for a particular enzyme can be measured by the "enzyme-forming potential" in the absence of the inducer under conditions optimal for protein synthesis. This can be seen more clearly from the results in Fig. 1, where the intracellular level of the enzyme catechol-2,3-oxygenase has been determined after harvesting cells exposed to an optimal inducer concentration for a varying length of time. The Sal$^+$ *P. aeruginosa* PAO cells were grown at 32°C in a minimal medium containing 5 mM glutamate, and at mid log phase 10 mM salicylate was added. Samples were taken at every 2 min, and the cells were quickly filtered through Millipore membrane filters and washed immediately with mineral medium without salicylate. The cells were then suspended in buffer, and the level of catechol-2,3-oxygenase was determined as described previously (see ref. 3; filtered, not incubated). In another experiment, the washed cells were resuspended in prewarmed mineral medium without salicylate but fortified with 1% Casamino acid. The cells were allowed to grow for 20 min at 32°C, and the level of catechol-2,3-oxygenase was determined (filtered and incubated). Results in Fig. 1 show that in the absence of the postfiltration incubation there is a lag of about 7 min, after which appreciable enzyme starts to form. On the other hand, if the cells are allowed to grow after filtration in the absence of salicylate, there is a lag of about 4 min, after which there is a rapid increase in the level of catechol-2,3-oxygenase. It is therefore clear that between 4 and 7 min there is an appreciable synthesis of mRNA, which is translated to the active enzyme during the postfiltration incubation.

The results in Fig. 1 enable us to study the genetic expression of the SAL plasmid in two separate phases. The amount of "enzyme-forming potential" (mRNA) can be suitably determined by measuring the increase in enzyme activity at 7 min before and after the postfiltration incubation. This would be a measure of the plasmid transcription phase. The "translation phase" would be the postfiltration incubation period itself, during which the "enzyme-forming potential" would be translated to the active enzyme. It was therefore possible to study the effect of high temperature (42°C) on these two processes separately. The results are shown in Table V. It can be seen that when the induction is carried out at the permissive temperature of 32°C and the postfiltration translation phase is carried out at either 32°C or 42°C, the amount of enzyme formed is almost the same. This suggests that the translation phase is not affected by incubation at the nonpermissive temperature (42°C). On the other hand, when the transcription phase is carried out at 42°C, and the translation phase at either 32°C or 42°C, very little active enzyme is formed. It is therefore clear that the

Table V. Inhibition of the Transcription of Catechol-2, 3-Oxygenase Gene in *P. aeruginosa* Grown at 42°C

Inducer[a]	Time of inducer addition (min)	Induction temperature (°C)	Filter (min)	Postfiltration incubation temperature (°C)	Enzyme activity units[b]
Salicylate	0	32	7	32	53
				42	47
Salicylate	0	42	7	32	8
				42	5

[a]The cells were grown at 32°C or 42°C in a mineral medium containing 5 mM glutamate, and at mid log phase 10 mM salicylate was added. After 7 min of growth, cells were quickly filtered and washed with mineral medium without salicylate. The cells were resuspended in prewarmed mineral medium without salicylate (but with 1% Casamino acid) at 32°C or 42°C and grown for 20 min. Catechol-2,3-oxygenase was then assayed as described before (3).

[b]One unit is the amount of enzyme that produces 1 nmole of 2-hydroxymuconic semialdehyde/min/mg protein.

absence of catechol-2,3-oxygenase formation when the cells are induced at 42°C in the presence of salicylate is due to an inhibition of the transcription phase, and not due to any inhibition of the translation phase. Exactly how incubation at 42°C affects the transcription phase is not clear as yet, but experiments are presently under way in our laboratory to find the site of action of such an inhibition.

DISCUSSION OF RESULTS

The inability of Sal$^+$ *P. aeruginosa* PAO to grow with salicylate as the only carbon source at 42°C appears to be due to low level of transcription of the plasmid genes at this temperature. This effect of 42°C on transcription has specifically been measured by determining the amount of "enzyme-forming potential" (mRNA) for catechol-2,3-oxygenase formed at 42°C. A better and perhaps easier method would be to estimate the amount of RNA formed at permissible temperatures such as 32°C and at the nonpermissible temperature of 42°C that would specifically be hybridizable to the plasmid DNA. Unfortunately, it has not been possible to isolate any of the degradative plasmid DNA free of chromosomal DNA, and hence any attempt to measure plasmid-specified RNA must await the physical isolation of the plasmid DNA. It must be stressed that our inference of low-level transcription of the plasmid DNA at 42°C is based on a measurement of low level of mRNA specific for catechol-2,3-oxygenase, and it is conceivable that the bulk of the other enzymes specified by the SAL plasmid are not produced due to an entirely different inhibitory mechanism operative at

42°C. This point can be resolved by comparing the amount of RNA hybridizable to the plasmid DNA at 32°C and at 42°C. Besides, it is not clear whether the inability of Cam$^+$ or Cam-Oct$^+$ *P. aeruginosa* PAO to grow with camphor or octane as the only carbon source at 42°C is also due to an inhibition of the transcription of the respective plasmids, or whether a different inhibitory mechanism might be operative at 42°C for these plasmids. The effect of incubation at 42°C on the formation of mRNA specific for some key enzymes in these pathways must be studied to pinpoint the effect of high temperature on the generalized inhibition of transcription of degradative plasmids in *Pseudomonas*.

The parent or Sal$^+$ *P. aeruginosa* PAO can grow well at 42°C with glucose or glutamate as the sole source of carbon, and all the cellular processes, such as the genetic transcription and translation and the protein synthetic machineries, are fully functional at this temperature. When the SAL plasmid is introduced to this strain, these cellular processes still remain fully operational, but the cells fail to specifically transcribe the plasmid DNA. This seems to suggest that additional factor or factors are needed for transcription of the plasmid DNA and the synthesis or activity of the factor(s) is presumably sensitive to higher temperatures such as 42°C. It is known that a specific protein factor is needed for transcription of T4 DNA by the cellular RNA polymerase and that modified RNA polymerases are needed for functional transcription of part of T7 phage DNA or the sporulation genes (8-10). It is conceivable that the cellular RNA polymerase might need some such protein factors for binding and for the initiation of transcription for the SAL plasmid DNA. Alternatively, the SAL plasmid DNA might specify an entirely different RNA polymerase specific for the transcription of the plasmid DNA only. It would be interesting to isolate RNA polymerase from Sal$^-$ and Sal$^+$ *P. aeruginosa* and analyze the subunit structures of such RNA polymerases and their ability to transcribe specifically the isolated plasmid DNA.

REFERENCES

1. R. Y. Stanier, N. J. Palleroni, and M. Doudoroff. *J. Gen. Microbiol.* **43**:159 (1966).
2. L. N. Ornston. *Bacteriol. Rev.* **35**:87 (1971).
3. A. M. Chakrabarty. *J. Bacteriol.* **112**:815 (1972).
4. J. G. Rheinwald, A. M. Chakrabarty, and I. C. Gunsalus. *Proc. Natl. Acad. Sci. (USA)* **70**:885 (1973).
5. A. J. Chakrabarty, G. Chou, and I. C. Gunsalus. *Proc. Natl. Acad. Sci. (USA)* **70**:1137 (1973).
6. A. M. Chakrabarty. *Proc. Natl. Acad. Sci. (USA)* **70**:1641 (1973).
7. J. W. May, R. H. Houghton, and C. J. Perret. *J. Gen. Microbiol.* **37**:157 (1964).
8. R. Losick. *Ann. Rev. Biochem.* **41**:409 (1972).
9. S. Ghosh and H. Echols. *Proc. Natl. Acad. Sci. (USA)* **69**:3660 (1972).
10. W. Summers and R. Siegel. *Nature (Lond.)* **228**:1160 (1970).

DISCUSSION

Question (Adhya): Can you pick up a mutant of SAL plasmid which can grow on salicylate as carbon source at $42°C$?

Answer: No; I have tried, but have failed to isolate any mutant that would grow at $42°C$ with salicylate as the sole carbon source.

Question (Ghosh): Does cometabolism between the plasmids exist?

Answer: If you are asking if the presence of two or more degradative plasmids in a single cell would allow the full expression of the plasmids simultaneously when the proper inducers are added, the answer is yes. Using suboptimal doses of appropriate inducers, we have shown that all the degradative pathways specified by the degradative plasmids are induced in the cell and lead to a higher rate of growth and a greater yield of cell mass.

Question (Ghosh): What is the real difficulty in isolating DNA from plasmids?

Answer: The real problem in isolating the plasmid DNA free of chromosomal DNA is the absence of satellite bands when the total DNA isolated from cells harboring one or more of the degradative plasmids is banded in a CsCl or CsCl - ethidium bromide gradient. We as yet do not know whether this is due to the fragile nature of the covalently closed circular plasmids or whether these plasmids are in fact linear molecules.

14

Studies on the Transcription
of Simian Virus 40 and Adenovirus Type 2

Joe Sambrook, Phillip A. Sharp,
Brad Ozanne, and Ulf Pettersson

Cold Spring Harbor Laboratory
Cold Spring Harbor, New York, U.S.A.

Both adenovirus 2 and simian virus 40 interact with cultured cells in two different ways. On the one hand, there is a productive or lytic response in which the great majority of the cells yield progeny virus and die, and on the other there is an incomplete infection in which little or no virus is produced and the cells survive. Some of these surviving cells assume a new set of stable properties that closely resemble the properties of cells derived from tumors. These cells are said to be "transformed." Which consequence virus infection produces is solely determined by the species of the host cell. Table I lists the cells that are commonly used in studies of lytic infection and transformation by adenovirus 2 and SV40.

Even though the two viruses provoke similar responses in the cells they infect, they have virtually no common properties. Adenovirus 2 is a large,

Table I. Cells Used for Lytic Infection and Transformation by Simian Virus 40 and Adenovirus Type 2

	Lytic infection	Transformation
Adenovirus 2	Human	Rat
SV40	Monkey	Mouse

architecturally complex virus (for review, see ref. 22). Its genome consists of a single piece of linear double-stranded DNA of molecular weight 29.9×10^6 (11,20,31). The DNA is neither circularly permuted (7) nor terminally redundant, but it has recently been shown that each of the two strands of adenovirus DNA contains complementary sequences at its ends (8,37). SV40 is a virus of simple structure whose genome consists of a molecule of closed circular double-stranded DNA, 3.4×10^6 daltons in mass (for review, see ref. 32).

Virus-specific RNA is found in cells transformed and lytically infected by adenovirus 2 and SV40, and in this paper we will survey some of the recent advances in our understanding of the transcription of these two viruses.

LYTIC INFECTION WITH SV40

During productive infection with SV40, there is no reduction in the rate of host cell RNA synthesis, and no method has been found to specifically inhibit host RNA metabolism. Therefore, the only way to examine the pattern of viral RNA synthesis in infected cells is by annealing DNA to RNA. Competition-hybridization experiments, published several years ago, showed that during productive infection certain viral RNA sequences appeared early and were synthesized throughout the virus growth cycle; others were detected only after the onset of viral DNA synthesis (2,4,16-18,28-30). Work in several laboratories during the past year has shown that these two classes of RNA are transcribed from different strands of the viral genome. It is impossible to prepare separated strands of SV40 DNA by the standard polymer binding techniques. However, Westphal (35), using *Escherichia coli* DNA-dependent RNA polymerase, showed that SV40 DNA is an efficient template for RNA synthesis. The product (cRNA) is highly asymmetrical, and Westphal suggested that it could be used to prepare separated strands of the viral DNA. When unit-length ^{32}P-labeled SV40 DNA is denatured and allowed to reanneal in the presence of excess cRNA, 50% of the radioactivity enters into the hybrid. These DNA·RNA hybrids can be separated from free single-stranded DNA by chromatography on hydroxylapatite (14,26), and control experiments show that the two fractions are in fact the separated strands of SV40 DNA. The strand that forms hybrids with cRNA is called "E DNA," the other is called "L DNA."

When the separated strands are annealed to RNA extracted from lytically infected cells at early times after infection, 30% of the sequences of the E strand enter into the hybrid (see Fig. 1). RNA extracted at late times after infection hybridizes to both strands of the DNA. At saturation, 30-35% of the E-strand and about 70% of the L-strand sequences anneal to RNA. These values agree well with those obtained from the competition-hybridization data, and they confirm the experiments of Martin and Axelrod (17) showing that at late times after infection 100% of the genome of SV40 is transcribed. In addition, these

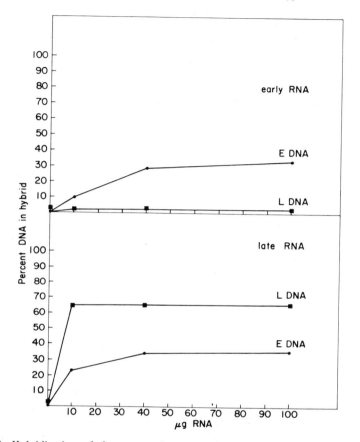

Fig. 1. Hybridization of the separated strands of SV40 DNA to RNA extracted from lytically infected cells at early and late times after lytic infection. Hybridization mixtures contained 2 ng of ^{32} P-labeled E- or L-strand DNA (specific activity 5×10^5 cpm/μg) and different amounts of RNA extracted from BS-C-1 cells by the hot-phenol method at 17 (early) and 48 hr (late) after infection by SV40. After incubation for 36 hr at 68°C, the samples were assayed by chromatography on hydroxylapatite. From Sambrook *et al.* (26).

experiments show that the "early" and "late" subsets of viral RNA are transcribed from different strands of SV40 DNA.

The factors that bring about the shift in patterns of viral RNA that occurs as cells pass from the early to the late stages of SV40 infection are unknown. Several explanations are possible: (a) There may be a change in the physical state of the viral DNA as a consequence of replication, so that a new promoter responsible for the initiation of late RNA synthesis becomes accessible to RNA polymerase. (b) Because viral RNA synthesis in nuclei isolated from infected cells at late times after infection is inhibited by α-amanitin, it seems likely that host RNA polymerase II is responsible for transcription of SV40 DNA (13). It is possible that during the course of infection there is a change in the specificity of this enzyme, which mediates the transition from the early to the late pattern of viral RNA synthesis.

Both of these orthodox explanations demand the presence of a promoter and a terminator on each of the viral DNA strands. However, there are less conventional models that eliminate these requirements: (c) It is known that SV40 DNA becomes integrated into host DNA during lytic infection (12), and it is possible that some classes of RNA are transcribed from the integrated viral sequences under the control of host promoters or terminators. (d) Finally, it is possible that control of the viral RNA species in infected cells is not accomplished at the transcriptional level. It may be that the primary RNA transcription product from SV40 DNA is the same at all stages of infection and that changes in post-transcriptional processing are responsible for the modulation of viral RNA expression. There is some evidence to support this hypothesis. Aloni (1) has shown that virus-specific, pulse-labeled RNA extracted from cells late in infection contains complementary sequences, whereas RNA extracted after long-term labeling does not. He interprets these results to mean that at least part of SV40 DNA is transcribed in a symmetrical fashion and that only part of the primary transcript is conserved into stable RNA species. Clearly, these experiments are of relevance not only to the specific control of viral RNA synthesis but also to the general mechanism of gene expression in mammalian cells. However, a large part of the difficulty in assessing the data is that we do not know whether the viral DNA that is transcribed into RNA is integrated or episomal or a mixture. It may be that shortlived viral RNA species are transcribed from integrated DNA and that stable species are synthesized from episomal templates. Because of these complexities, it is extremely difficult to design tight experiments that will provide fair tests for each of the possible models. Nevertheless, defined viral DNA sequences still represent the system of choice for study of gene expression in mammalian cells.

SV40 RNA SEQUENCES IN TRANSFORMED CELLS

Mouse cells transformed by SV40 contain viral DNA sequences in an integrated state (27). Different lines of cells contain different quantities of viral DNA (9,36). Some contain as few as one or two copies of viral DNA per diploid quantity of cell DNA (9); others contain as many as nine copies (19). Since the first demonstration by Benjamin (3), the existence of virus-specific RNA in transformed cells has never been questioned. However, there has been disagreement about the fraction of the genome that is transcribed. On the one hand, saturation-hybridization experiments have indicated that the whole viral genome is represented in RNA sequences (16,17); on the other, competition-hybridization experiments suggest that only the segment of the viral genome that is expressed early in lytic infection (which we now know to be 35% of the E strand) is found in RNA extracted from transformed cells (2,18,28-30).

We have used the separated strands of SV40 DNA, first, to measure the percentage of the viral sequences that are present in RNA extracted from different lines of transformed mouse cells and, second, to estimate the concentration of these sequences.

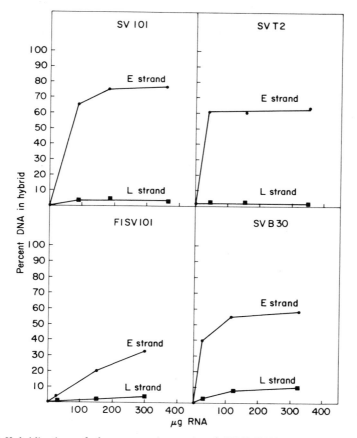

Fig. 2. Hybridization of the separated strands of SV40 DNA to RNA isolated from transformed cells. Hybridization mixtures contained 2 ng of ^{32}P-labeled E- or L-strand DNA (specific activity 8 × 10[5] cpm/μg) and different amounts of total RNA extracted from transformed cells by the hot-phenol method. The total volume of the reaction mixture was 0.125 ml, and the hybridization buffer consisted of 1 *M* NaCl, 0.2 m*M* EDTA, 1 m*M* tris (*p*H 7.5). After incubation for 36 hr at 68°C, the samples were assayed by hydroxylapatite chromatography. From Ozanne *et al.* (19).

Increasing amounts of RNA extracted from transformed cells were allowed to react with a constant amount of sheared ^{32}P-labeled DNA of each of the separated strands of SV40. Typical results from four lines of transformed cells are shown in Fig. 2. The amount of radioactivity that enters into the hybrid at saturating concentrations of RNA is a measure of the proportion of the sequences of the strand that are present in RNA. The hybridization conditions are exhaustive, so the amount of RNA that will just cause saturation must contain an amount of SV40 sequences equal to the weight of DNA in the hybridization mix that enters into the hybrid. For example, RNA extracted from the cell line SV101 (Fig. 2) contains sequences complementary to 75% of the E strand and to 3% of the L strand of SV40 DNA. About 150 µg of transformed cell RNA is required to saturate the DNA. From these data, we calculate that

$$\frac{(0.75 \times 2.0 \times 10^{-3})}{1.5 \times 10^2}$$

or one part in 10^5 of the total RNA extracted from the cells is complementary to SV40 DNA. A summary of the results obtained with RNA extracted from other lines of transformed mouse cells is shown in Table II.

There are several points of interest about these data. First, different lines of

Table II. Patterns of SV 40 RNA Present in Various Lines of Transformed Cells

Cell line	Phenotype	Percentage of viral genome present in RNA		Proportion of total cell RNA complementary to E strand
		E strand	L strand	
SV101	Transformed	75	3	1.0×10^{-5}
SV3T3 clone 9	Transformed	72	15	1.5×10^{-5}
SVT2	Transformed	58	0	2.5×10^{-5}
SVB30	Transformed	65	0	1.0×10^{-5}
SV*Py*11	Transformed	65	0	1.8×10^{-5}
SV*uv*30	Transformed	24	22	0.5×10^{-5}
F_1 SV101	Revertant	32[a]	3	$< 2.0 \times 10^{-6}$
CA^r30.4	Revertant	70	10	2.5×10^{-5}

[a]This figure is a minimum estimate because of difficulties in reaching saturating levels of RNA.

transformed cells display different hybridization patterns. The proportion of the E-strand DNA that is present in RNA varies from cell line to cell line, ranging from a low of 25% in the case of SVuv30 to a high of 75% in the case of SV101. Since only 30-35% of the E-strand DNA is represented in stable species of RNA during lytic infection, at least part of the viral RNA present in many transformants must consist of "anti-late" sequences. This result provides an explanation for the apparent discrepancy noted earlier between data obtained from saturation-hybridization and competition-hybridization experiments. "Anti-late" sequences would have been detected by the saturation technique but would not have been scored by competition hybridization.

Second, viral RNA sequences complementary to L-strand DNA can be detected in some lines of transformed cells. However, there is always difficulty in attaining saturation, and we conclude that RNA complementary to L-strand DNA is present in lower concentration than is RNA complementary to E-strand DNA. We do not know whether the RNA that binds to L-strand DNA is composed of true "late" or "anti-early" sequences, but whatever its origin it cannot play a role in maintaining the transformed state because it is not present in all transformed cell lines.

Third, virus-specific RNA accounts for about one part in 10^5 of the total RNA extracted from transformed cells.

Fourth, it is possible to isolate, from populations of SV40-transformed cells, revertants that have recovered at least some properties of normal cells (for review, see ref. 25). These revertants contain as much viral DNA as their transformed parents (19). Viral RNA can also be detected, and in many cases (e.g., the concanavalin-A resistant revertant CA^r30.4, Table II, and see ref. 19) the pattern of hybridization of this RNA to the separated strands of viral DNA is identical to that of RNA extracted from fully transformed cells. However, in cells of the line F_1SV101, isolated by Pollack *et al.* (23), the concentration of virus-specific RNA sequences is at least five times lower than in the parental transformed cell line. For this reason, we were never able to add enough RNA to estimate the proportion of the sequences of the viral genome that are represented in RNA. Clearly, it is attractive to think that the lower concentration of viral RNA is the reason for the cell's reversion to a normal phenotype. However, we cannot exclude the possibility that the reduced concentration of viral RNA is a consequence of reversion rather than the cause.

The simplest model that will account for all these data is that in order to preserve intact the functions necessary to maintain transformation the virus DNA integrates into host DNA with a break somewhere in its late genes, and that in different transformants the insertion point is located at different positions within the late region of the genome (see Fig. 3). The transcription of the integrated genome is under the control of a host promoter so that RNA molecules are synthesized that are considerably longer than a single strand of SV40 DNA and that contain covalently linked host and viral sequences. Such

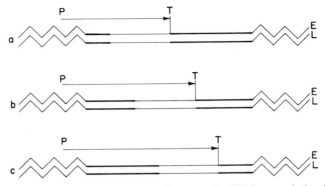

Fig. 3. Model for SV40 transcription in transformed cells. SV40 transcription in different transformants is represented by (a), (b), and (c). *P,* Promoter; *T,* terminator; broken lines, host DNA; light straight lines, early sequences of SV40; heavy straight lines, late sequences of SV40.

molecules have in fact been isolated from nuclei of SV40-transformed mouse cells (33). In order to account for the observation that the viral RNA sequences present in the cytoplasm of these cells are not attached to host sequences, it has been proposed that the primary transcription product undergoes processing during which polyadenylate residues are attached to the 3'-OH end of the molecule and the host sequences are removed from the 5' end (33). The SV40-specific sequences are transported into the cytoplasm, and it is these sequences that we measure in the hybridization reaction.

This model is not without deficiencies—for instance, it neglects the existence of the multiple copies of viral DNA in many lines of transformed cells and it does not predict whether control of viral gene expression occurs at the level of transcription or processing. Thus the point *T* in Fig. 3 could represent a true termination point for RNA synthesis. Alternatively, it may be that the primary transcription product contains the complete set of viral sequences and that *T* marks the site at which processing of RNA occurs. All those viral RNA sequences to the right of *T* would be degraded; all those to the left would be conserved.

Clearly, the easiest way to test this model is to ask whether the primary transcription product (i.e., virus-specific RNA labeled during a very short pulse of radioactivity) contains viral sequences that are not found in stable species of RNA.

TRANSCRIPTION OF ADENOVIRUS 2

Transcription of adenovirus-2 DNA during lytic infection, like that of SV40 DNA, seems to be divided into an "early" and a "late" phase; the shift from one pattern to another is coeval with the onset of viral DNA synthesis. The "early" sequences of RNA correspond to 10-20% of the sequences of adenovirus-2 DNA and are thought to be transcribed from segments of both strands of viral DNA (10). Several lines of evidence (5,15,24,34) indicate that both early and late species of viral RNA are synthesized by an RNA polymerase which is inhibited by α-amanitin and thus resembles RNA polymerase II of mammalian cells.

Recently, we have been able to study the pattern of strand switches that occur during RNA synthesis from adenovirus 2 in lytically infected cells, using specific fragments of the viral DNA.

It has been shown by Pettersson *et al.* (20) that the restricting endonuclease R·R$_I$ isolated from *E. coli* cleaves the DNA of adenovirus 2 into six unique fragments. These fragments can be separated by electrophoresis through agarose gels, and it is relatively simple to purify relatively large quantities of each of them. The molecular weights of the fragments are shown in Table III.

In order to examine the pattern of adenovirus-2 RNA synthesis, ^{32}P-labeled fragments were prepared, denatured, and allowed to reanneal in the presence of large quantities of unlabeled RNA extracted from lytically infected KB cells at 18 hr after infection. At this time, synthesis of both early and late species of viral RNA is in full swing. If RNA is present that is complementary to segments of both DNA strands of the fragment, then all the radioactivity will behave as hybrid when assayed by hydroxylapatite chromatography. However, if only one of the DNA strands is represented in RNA, not more than 50% of the radio-activity will act as hybrid. The results are shown in Fig. 4, in which a constant amount of ^{32}P-labeled DNA of each fragment was annealed to increasing quantities of 18-hr RNA. It can be seen (triangles) that at saturation consider-

Table III. Molecular Weights of the Fragments Generated by Cleavage of Adenovirus Type-2 DNA with Endonuclease R · R$_I$

DNA[a]	Molecular weight
Adenovirus 2	22.9×10^6
A	13.6×10^6
B	2.7×10^6
C	2.3×10^6
D	1.7×10^6
E	1.4×10^6
F	1.1×10^6

Data from Pettersson *et al.* (20).

[a]The order of the fragments along the viral genome is ABFDEC (Sharp, personal communication).

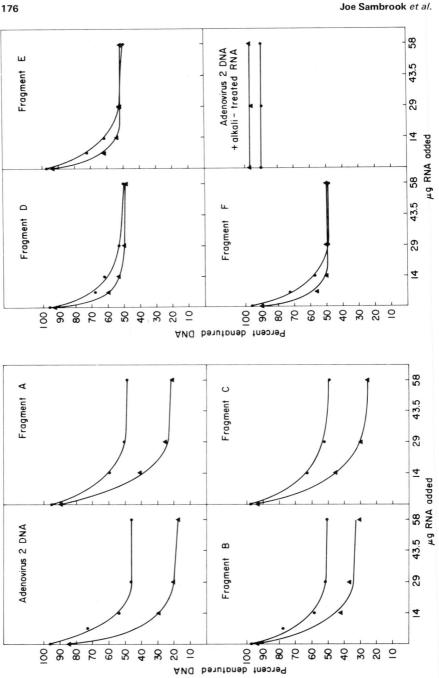

ably more than 50% of the radioactivity of fragments A, B, and C and complete adenovirus-2 DNA behaved as hybrid on hydroxylapatite. Exactly 50% of the radioactivity of fragments D, E, and F was converted to hybrid. These results mean that there are three or more strand switches during transcription of adenovirus-2 DNA, located in fragments A, B, and C.

When the fragments were sheared before hybridization to pieces of DNA about 700 nucleotides in length, 50% of the radioactivity of each of the fragments and whole adenovirus-2 DNA entered hybrid. This means that at 18 hr after infection the equivalent of one strand of viral DNA is present in RNA.

These results are exciting because they show that transcription of adeno-virus-2 RNA is more complicated than had been realized. Clearly, our picture of the pattern and control of this viral DNA is far from complete. However, the combination of analysis of DNA·RNA hybrids by chromatography on hydroxyl-apatite and the availability of specific fragments of the adenovirus-2 genome holds the promise of yielding rapid advances in our knowledge of gene regulation.

POSTSCRIPT

Our knowledge of the patterns of RNA synthesis directed by the two DNA tumor viruses adenovirus 2 and SV40 has recently increased greatly. The availability of specific DNA fragments of both viruses (6,20) means that detailed maps of the stable transcription products should soon be available. The DNA of both viruses becomes integrated into host cell DNA during transformation; thus mammalian cells are available that contain defined DNA sequences in a defined physical state. It does not seem too optimistic to hope that studies of adeno-virus-2 and SV40 transcription not only will tell us about the mechanisms of virus gene expression but also will yield information about the way in which host cells control their affairs.

Fig. 4. Hybridization of fragments of adenovirus-2 DNA to RNA extracted from lytically infected cells 18 hr after infection. ^{32}P-Labeled adenovirus-2 DNA (specific activity 5 × 10^5 cpm/μg) was prepared as described by Pettersson and Sambrook (21). Fragments of the DNA obtained by treating the DNA with endonuclease R·R$_I$ were purified by electrophoresis through 1.4% agarose as described by Pettersson *et al.* (20). The fragments were eluted electrophoretically from the gel. KB cells were infected were adenovirus 2 at a multiplicity of 20. Eighteen hours after infection, RNA was purified from the cells by the hot-phenol method as described by Sambrook *et al.* (26). Hybridization mixtures contained between 200 and 400 cpm of denatured DNA and increasing amounts of RNA in a total volume of 0.1 ml of 0.14 *M* phosphate buffer (*p*H 6.8). After incubation for 30 min at 68°C, the mixtures were analyzed by hydroxylapatite chromatography. In order to eliminate the possibility that there was adenovirus DNA in the RNA preparations, the RNA was hydrolyzed with 0.1 *N* NaOH for 16 hr at 37°C. When this RNA was used for hybridization, no ^{32}P-labeled DNA was converted to hybrid. ●, Sheared DNA; ▲, unit-length DNA.

ACKNOWLEDGMENTS

This work was supported by grants from the American Cancer Society and the National Cancer Institute. One of us (U. P.) is the recipient of an International Agency for Research on Cancer Fellowship.

REFERENCES

1. Y. Aloni. *Proc. Natl. Acad. Sci. (USA)* **69**:2404 (1972).
2. Y. E. Aloni, E. Winocour, and L. Sachs. *J. Mol. Biol.* **31**:415 (1968).
3. T. L. Benjamin. *J. Mol. Biol.* **16**:359 (1966).
4. R. I. Carp, G. Sauer, and F. Sokol. *Virology* **37**:214 (1969).
5. Y. Chardonnet, L. Gazzolo, and B. Pogo. *Virology* **48**:300 (1972).
6. K. J. Danna and D. Nathans. *Proc. Natl. Acad. Sci. (USA)* **68**:2913 (1971).
7. W. Doerfler and A. K. Kleinschmidt. *J. Mol. Biol.* **50**:579 (1970).
8. C. F. Garon, K. W. Barry, and J. Rose. *Proc. Natl. Acad. Sci. (USA)* **69**:2391 (1972).
9. L. D. Gelb, D. E. Kohne, and M. A. Martin. *J. Mol. Biol.* **57**:129 (1971).
10. M. Green, J. T. Parsons, M. Piña, K. Fujinaga, H. Caffier, and I. Landgraf-Leurs. *Cold Spring Harbor Symp. Quant. Biol.* **35**:803 (1970).
11. M. Green, M. Piña, R. C. Kimes, P. C. Wensink, L. A. MacHattie, and C. A. Thomas, Jr. *Proc. Natl. Acad. Sci. (USA)* **57**:1302 (1967).
12. K. Hirai and V. Defendi. *J. Virol.* **9**:705 (1972).
13. A. H. Jackson and B. Sugden. *J. Virol.* **10**:1086 (1972).
14. G. Khoury, J. C. Byrne, and M. A. Martin. *Proc. Natl. Acad. Sci. (USA)* **69**:1925 (1972).
15. N. Ledinko. *Nature New Biol.* **233**:247 (1971).
16. M. Martin. *Cold Spring Harbor Symp. Quant. Biol.* **35**:833 (1970).
17. M. A. Martin and D. Axelrod. *Proc. Natl. Acad. Sci. (USA)* **64**:1203 (1969).
18. K. Oda and R. Dulbecco. *Proc. Natl. Acad. Sci. (USA)* **60**:525 (1968).
19. B. Ozanne, P. A. Sharp, and J. Sambrook. *J. Virol.,* **12**:90 (1973).
20. U. Pettersson, C. Mulder, H. Delius, and P. A. Sharp. *Proc. Natl. Acad. Sci. (USA)* **70**:200 (1973).
21. U. Pettersson and J. Sambrook. *J. Mol. Biol.* **73**:125 (1973).
22. L. Philipson and U. Pettersson. *Advan. Exptl. Tumor Virus Res.* **18**:2 (1972).
23. R. E. Pollack, H. Green, and G. J. Todaro. *Proc. Natl. Acad. Sci. (USA)* **60**:126 (1968).
24. R. Price and S. Penman. *J. Virol.* **9**:621 (1972).
25. J. Sambrook. *Advan. Cancer Res.* **16**:141 (1972).
26. J. Sambrook, P. A. Sharp, and W. Keller. *J. Mol. Biol.* **70**:57 (1972).
27. J. F. Sambrook, H. Westphal, P. R. Srinivasan, and R. Dulbecco. *Proc. Natl. Acad. Sci. (USA)* **60**:1288 (1968).
28. G. Sauer. *Nature New Biol.* **231**:135 (1971).
29. G. Sauer and J. R. Kidwai. *Proc. Natl. Acad. Sci. (USA)* **61**:1256 (1968).
30. S. Tonegawa, G. Walter, A. Bernardini, and R. Dulbecco. *Cold Spring Harbor Symp. Quant. Biol.* **35**:823. (1970).
31. A. J. van der Eb, L. W. van Kestern, and E. F. J. Bruggen. *Biochim. Biophysl. Acta* **182**:530 (1969).
32. J. Vinograd and J. Lebowitz. *J. Gen. Physiol.* **49**:103 (1966).
33. R. Wall and J. E. Darnell. *Nature New Biol.* **232**:73 (1971).
34. R. D. Wallace and J. R. Kates. *J. Virol.* **9**:627 (1972).
35. H. Westphal. *J. Mol. Biol.* **50**:407 (1970).

36. H. Westphal and R. Dulbecco. *Proc. Natl. Acad. Sci. (USA)* **59**:1188 (1968).
37. J. Wolfson and D. Dressler. *Proc. Natl. Acad. Sci. (USA)* **69**:3054 (1972).

DISCUSSION

Question (Chakravorty): Does adenovirus pick up host DNA during continuous passage as SV40 does? If not, then it is a much cleaner system to work with.

Answer: There is no evidence that DNA molecules isolated from purified adenovirus particles contain host sequences. In our laboratory, adenovirus type-2 stocks are routinely prepared from a lysate which has been passed at high multiplicity for many generations, and we have never seen evidence of deletions or substitutions in the viral DNA.

Question (Chakravorty): During lytic infection of SV40, the viral DNA integrates with that of the host. I assume it is excised then. Is this correct?

Answer: The evidence that SV40 DNA integrates into the host genome during lytic infection is now very good. Although we don't know for sure whether the integrated viral sequences are ever excised, such excision could provide a mechanism to generate DNA molecules containing both host and viral sequences. We do not know whether or not integration of viral sequences is a necessary step for productive infection.

15

Transcription of Reovirus RNA

Amiya K. Banerjee, C. Martin Stoltzfus, Richard L. Ward, and Aaron J. Shatkin

Department of Cell Biology
Roche Institute of Molecular Biology
Nutley, New Jersey, U.S.A.

The diplornaviruses (1), so classified because they contain double-stranded RNA as their genetic material, are ubiquitous and infect bacteria (pseudomonad phage $\phi6$), fungi (*Penicillium* and *Aspergillus* virus), insects (cytoplasmic polyhedrosis virus), plants (rice dwarf virus, wound tumor virus), birds (avian reovirus), and mammals (blue tongue virus, African horse sickness virus), including man (Colorado tick fever virus and the three serotypes of reovirus) (2-7). The mammalian reoviruses include serotype 3, the prototype of the diplornaviruses (8). Its replication in mouse L cells in tissue culture has been investigated extensively (5-7), and this system provides an excellent model for studying the molecular biology of double-stranded RNA viruses and some general features of RNA transcription and translation as well.

STRUCTURE OF REOVIRUS

Reoviruses have a characteristic double-shell structure when examined in the electron microscope (Fig. 1a). The outer diameter is approximately 70 nm, and the inner core is approximately 50 nm. These cores or subviral particles (SVP) are resistant to digestion with proteolytic enzymes and can be exposed by treatment of virions with chymotrypsin (Fig. 1b). The SVP aggregate during chymotrypsin digestion, and their specific infectivity is 10^5-fold less than that of purified virions. SVP have a buoyant density in CsCl of 1.44 g/cm^3 and can be

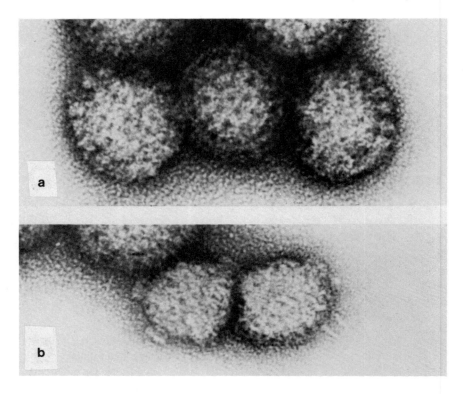

Fig. 1. Electron micrograph of reovirus (a) and reovirus cores (SVP) (b).

separated from undigested virions (ρ = 1.37 g/cm^3). The SVP contain the double-stranded RNA genome of total molecular weight about 15×10^6.

GENOME RNA

Extraction of the double-stranded genome RNA from purified reovirus type 3 releases a reproducible mixture of RNA fragments. By polyacrylamide gel electrophoresis, the mixture can be separated into distinct genome fragments, including three L (large), three M (medium), and four S (small) fragments (Fig. 2). These correspond to molecular weights of about 2.5, 1.4, and 0.7×10^6, respectively (9). An interesting question is whether the RNA within the virion is a long, linear double-stranded RNA that fragments to form distinct segments upon extraction. In fact, gentle lysis of virus particles with urea on an EM grid results in an occasional long RNA molecule of contour length 7 μ, the length expected for a double-stranded RNA of total molecular weight 15×10^6

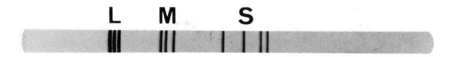

Fig. 2. *Polyacrylamide gel electrophoresis of isolated reovirus genome segments.* Twenty micrograms of double-stranded RNA from purified reovirus was analyzed in a 5% polyacrylamide gel. Electrophoresis was carried out at 4 ma for 20 hr at 20°C. The RNA was visualized by staining with methylene blue. Direction of migration is from left to right.

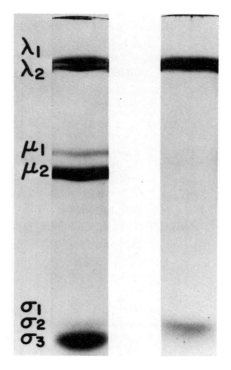

Fig. 3. *Electrophoretic patterns of structural proteins of virions and SVP.* Purified reovirus type 3 (left) or SVP (right) prepared by digestion of virus with an equal amount of chymotrypsin (2 hr at 37°C) were solubilized in 0.01 *M* tris buffer (*p*H 8) containing 8 *M* urea, 2% sodium dodecylsulfate, and 1% β-mercaptoethanol. The samples were dialyzed against 0.001 *M* phosphate buffer (*p*H 7.2) containing 8 *M* urea, 0.1% SDS, and 0.1% mercaptoethanol, and 20 μg of protein was applied to 10-cm 10% polyacrylamide gels. After electrophoresis in 0.1 *M* phosphate buffer (*p*H 7.2) containing 0.1% SDS for 22 hr at 4 ma/gel and 20°C, the gels were fixed and stained with 0.025% Coomassie blue in 10% trichloracetic acid and destained in 7% acetic acid.

(10,11). However, most of the molecules have lengths of 1.1, 0.6, or 0.3 μ, corresponding to molecular weights of 2.5, 1.4, and 0.7 $\times$ 10^6, respectively (10,12). These three classes of genome segments do not cross-hybridize, suggesting that they have different base sequences. The RNA extracted from the infected cell cytoplasm also includes ten single-stranded RNA species that hybridize with the corresponding genome segments (13,14). These results also indicate that the genome segments are unique, although they may be produced by specific cleavages at weak sites in a long duplex RNA molecule. As will be shown, the genome RNA segments are independently synthesized and exist as discrete molecules within the virion.

STRUCTURAL PROTEINS

Purified reovirus contains seven polypeptides that can be resolved when solubilized and electrophoresed in SDS-polyacrylamide gels (Fig. 3, left). Like the genome segments, the polypeptides are also separated into three size categories termed λ (large), μ (medium, and σ (small) with the following molecular weights: λ_1 = 155,000, λ_2 = 140,000, μ_1 = 80,000, μ_2 = 72,000, σ_1 = 42,000, σ_2 = 38,000, and σ_3 = 34,000 (15). Treatment with chymotrypsin selectively removes μ_1, μ_2, σ_1 and σ_3 (Fig. 3b). The remaining subviral particles consist of λ_1, λ_2, and σ_2.

The information content of the L, M, and S segments is sufficient to code for polypeptides of approximate molecular weight 150,000, 80,000, and 40,000. Table I shows that there is a striking correlation between the molecular weights of the structural proteins and the coding capacity of the genome RNA molecules. The results are consistent with a monocistronic function for the reovirus mRNAs. Eight gene products have been characterized, including six primary gene products in the viral capsid (16). Polypeptide μ_1 appears to be a precursor of μ_2. In the infected cell, two more virus-specific polypeptides have been found: μ_0 (mol wt 88,000) and σ_{2A} (mol wt 36,000) (17).

TRANSCRIPTASE WITHIN THE VIRION

Reovirus enters cells by phagocytosis, i.e., engulfment of the entire virion at the cell surface (18). Within the cytoplasm, a portion of the outer protein coat is stripped off by lysosomal hydrolases. Eight to ten hours after infection, ten

Table I. Molecular Weights of Reovirus mRNA and Proteins

RNA class	Number of segments	Mol wt observed	Protein class	Mol wt	
				Expected	Observed
L	3	1.3×10^6	λ	130,000	1. 155,000 (core)
					2. 140,000 (core)
					3. —
M	3	0.7×10^6	μ	70,000	1. 80,000
					2. 72,000
					3. —
S	4	0.4×10^6	σ	40,000	1. 42,000
					2. 38,000 (core)
					3. 34,000
					4. —

distinct single-stranded messenger RNAs corresponding to ten double-stranded genome RNA segments are found (13,14). It was observed that viral mRNA synthesis proceeds in cells treated with cycloheximide from the beginning of infection (19). This observation suggested the presence of a preformed viral RNA polymerase, and it was subsequently found that the purified reovirus subviral particles contain an RNA-dependent RNA polymerase. The activity of this transcriptase was only discernible when the purified virus was treated with chymotrypsin (20) or heated briefly to 60°C (21). The transcript products are single-stranded RNAs with a characteristic trimodal distribution (Fig. 4). The sedimentation coefficients for the large (l), medium (m), and small (s) mRNA species are approximately 25, 19, and 12S, respectively. The RNA species in each size class are unique molecules and not degradation products. The l species hybridizes specifically with the L segments, m with the M, and s with the S segments. Thus, *in vitro,* the virion-associated polymerase synthesizes ten RNA species corresponding to the ten double-stranded RNA genome segments. The synthesis of RNA *in vitro* continues linearly for hours with manyfold net synthesis of the template RNA. There is no self-annealing of the *in vitro* RNAs, suggesting that only one strand of the double-stranded genome RNA is being transcribed. Furthermore, the double-stranded template RNA labeled with ^{32}P was completely conserved and remained tightly bound to the core proteins during many rounds of transcription (22-24).

Fig. 4. Sedimentation of RNA products in glycerol gradients. Virus was digested with chymotrypsin or heated (60°C for 1 min) and incubated under standard assay conditions. The mixture consisted of 60 mM tris buffer (pH 8.0), 6 mM MgCl$_2$, 2 mM phosphoenolpyruvate, 1.4 μg of pyruvate kinase, and 1 mM each of ATP, CTP, UTP, and GTP. The radioactive precursor was [^{3}H]GTP (specific activity 7000 cpm/nmole). After incubation, the mixture was made 1% in sodium dodecylsulfate and sedimented for 16 hr at 75,000 × g in a 5-30% glycerol gradient (0.02 M tris buffer, pH 8, containing 0.1 M NaCl and 0.005 M EDTA). Fractions were precipitated with 5% trichloroacetic acid containing 0.02 M PPi, collected on Millipore filters, and counted. Arrows indicate the positions of *E. coli* ribosomal and soluble RNA centrifuged under the same conditions.

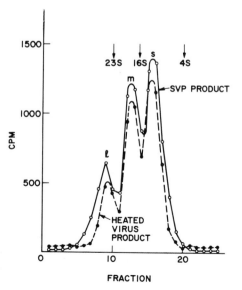

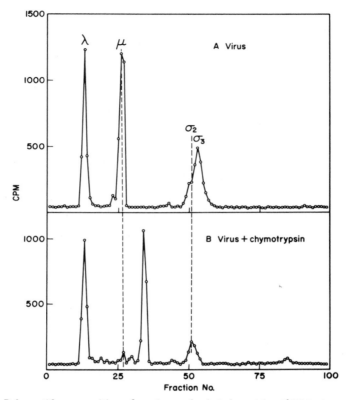

Fig. 5. *Polypeptide composition of reovirus and subviral particles.* [³H] Amino acid - labeled reovirus before (A) and after (B) digestion for 1 hr at 40°C with 200 μg of chymotrypsin/ml in phosphate-buffered saline was solubilized and analyzed on 10% polyacrylamide gels as described in Fig. 3.

IN VITRO PRODUCTION OF INFECTIOUS SUBVIRAL PARTICLES

Transcription of the reovirus double-stranded genome RNA is temporally controlled in virus-infected L cells (19). Viral mRNA synthesized in cyclo-heximide-treated, infected cells (early mRNA) is copied predominantly from four of the ten genome segments. At later periods, all genome segments are transcribed. The mechanism of this temporal control of RNA synthesis *in vivo* is not known, but it could be mediated by a viral-specific protein or a host function. It was of interest to test whether the control phenomenon could be reproduced *in vitro*. As described above, infectious reovirus can be converted into subviral particles after exhaustive digestion with chymotrypsin. The resulting particles

synthesize ten single-stranded mRNA molecules *in vitro*. However, when particles were degraded with chymotrypsin to a limited extent, thus mimicking the
fate of the parental virus particles early in infection (25,26), infectious subviral
particles (SVPi) were produced (27). The SVPi have an active RNA-dependent
transcriptase and are similar in composition to the partially uncoated virions

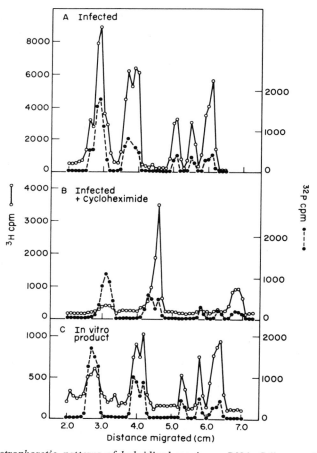

Fig. 6. Electrophoretic patterns of hybridized reovirus mRNA. Cells were infected with
infectious subviral particles (SVPi) (50 PFU/cell) and labeled with [³H]uridine from 1.5 to
12 hr after infection in the presence (B) or absence (A) of 20 μg of cycloheximide/ml. RNA
was extracted with phenol, denatured with dimethylsulfoxide, and annealed with reovirus
genome RNA. ³²P-Labeled genome RNA was added to the annealed RNA as a marker, and
the mixture was analyzed by electrophoresis in 5% polyacrylamide gels as described in Fig.
3. The infectious subviral particles were also concentrated and incubated for 1 hr in a
reaction mixture designed for the synthesis of viral RNA. The *in vitro* product was
extracted, hybridized, and analyzed (C).

isolated from infected L cells. SVPi have a buoyant density of 1.40 g/cm^3 in Cs Cl and sediment at approximately 420S as compared to 1.37 g/cm^3 and approximately 630S for purified virions. They consist of 30% less protein and include the polypeptides of the inner structural layer λ_1, λ_2, and σ_3, and a polypeptide of apparent molecular weight 60,000 derived by cleavage of μ_2, a constituent of the outer shell (Fig. 5). In addition to its high specific infectivity, the SVPi synthesized all ten mRNA species *in vitro* (Fig. 6C). To test whether polypeptides μ_1, σ_3, and intact μ_2 are required for the regulation of early mRNA synthesis, cells were infected with SVPi in the presence and absence of cycloheximide. The virus yield increased from 4 PFU/cell at 90 min to 360 PFU/cell at 24 hr after infection in the untreated samples. The cycloheximide-treated cultures decreased from 4 PFU/cell to 0.2 PFU/cell during the same interval. Viral mRNA labeled between 90 min and 12 hr after infection was isolated, hybridized to genome RNA, and analyzed by polyacrylamide gel electrophoresis. The mRNA from cells productively infected with SVPi gave the same gel pattern as mRNA from virus-infected cells, consistent with the transcription of all genome segments (Fig. 6A). However, early mRNA formed in the presence of cycloheximide hybridized predominantly with one M and two S genome segments and to a very limited extent with L segments (Fig. 6B). The results indicate that the pattern of virus mRNA synthesis is unaltered in cells infected with SVPi, particles that have lost μ_1 σ_2, and one-fifth of the length of polypeptide μ_2. This strongly suggests that the host cell plays a role in the regulation of reovirus transcription. Since cycloheximide was present during infection with SVPi, it seems likely that preformed host protein(s) may be involved in the early control of viral mRNA synthesis.

INITIATION OF mRNA SYNTHESIS *IN VITRO*

Reovirus SVP or SVPi are thus composed of viral "chromosomes" and structural proteins that can carry out transcription of mRNA *in vitro*. The ten single-stranded mRNA species are not the result of cleavage of a long RNA molecule but are unique transcript products representing specific segments of the double-stranded RNA genome. We studied the incorporation of β,γ-^{32}P-labeled ribonucleoside triphosphates, which specifically label the 5' termini of the RNA chains. If the *in vitro* synthesized RNA were a long molecule of 7.5×10^6 daltons that is subsequently cleaved to yield ten fragments, one would expect to find one 5'-polyphosphate terminus per RNA chain of 7.5×10^6. On the other hand, if the synthesis of ten mRNA molecues were due to the transcription from ten unique regions of the double-stranded genome RNA, one would expect to obtain ten 5'-polyphosphate termini in the transcription products.

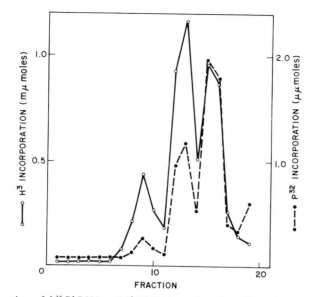

Fig. 7. *Separation of [³²P] RNA and [³H] RNA products in a glycerol gradient.* Incubation of purified reovirus type 3 and an equal amount of chymotrypsin was carried out for 2 hr at 37°C in 0.25 ml of a standard assay mixture as in Fig. 4, except that $[\beta,\gamma\text{-}^{32}P]$ GTP (specific activity = 500 cpm/pmole) was also included in the reaction mixture. Gradient centrifugation was carried out as in Fig. 4.

Table II. 5′ Termini of RNA Products

RNA product	Number of segments	Value of S	Average chain length	[³H]GMP incorporated[a] (nmole)	$[\beta,\gamma\text{-}^{32}P]$ GTP incorporated (pmole ³² ppG) Expected	Observed[a]
l	3	25	3500	0.5	0.6	0.5
m	3	19	2000	1.2	2.6	2.6
s	4	12	1000	1.1	4.2	4.3

[a]Values tabulated from Fig. 7.

mRNA synthesis was carried out by purified reovirus in the presence of chymotrypsin and four ribonucleoside triphosphates including $[\beta,\gamma\text{-}^{32}P]$ GTP and [³H] GTP (28). The RNA products were separated in a 5-30% glycerol gradient (Fig. 7). It was found that the three classes of mRNA, l, m, and s, contained both ³H and ³²P. The ³²P was present only at the 5′ termini, since treatment of the products with alkaline phosphatase converted all the ^{32}P to inorganic phosphate. In contrast, the ^{3}H counts which were incorporated into internal positions remained acid precipitable. This indicated that the RNA products have 5'-polyphosphate guanosine ends. However, no detectable ^{32}P was incorporated into the RNA products when the $[\beta,\gamma\text{-}^{32}\text{P}]$GTP was replaced by $[\gamma\text{-}^{32}\text{P}]$GTP, showing thereby that the γ-phosphate of the RNA chains is removed during RNA synthesis. The resulting diphosphate ends at the 5' termini were confirmed to be ppGp by high-voltage paper electrophoresis after alkaline digestion. The γ-phosphate is cleaved by an SVP-associated phosphohydrolase (29,30). From the extent of synthesis of 1, m, and s products and their respective chain lengths estimated from the sedimentation studies, the expected pmoles of ^{32}ppG termini can be calculated. The observed pmoles of termini formed are in excellent agreement with the calculated values, indicating that all ten mRNA species have ppG at the 5' termini (Table II).

The synthesis of both total RNA and 5' termini continued at a linear rate for 2 hr or longer. To confirm that reinitiation of RNA chains occurred, synthesis was allowed to proceed with unlabeled ribonucleoside triphosphates for 30 min, the time required for net synthesis to occur. After the 30-min incubation, the reaction mixture was pulsed with $[^3\text{H}]$GTP and $[\beta,\gamma\text{-}^{32}\text{P}]$GTP, and the incubation was continued for 2 hr. As shown in Table III, both ^{3}H and ^{32}P incorporation proceeded linearly as expected for a reinitiating reaction (34).

In order to characterize the 5' penultimate nucleotide, RNA products synthesized with $[\beta,\gamma\text{-}^{32}\text{P}]$GTP and $[^3\text{H}]$GTP were digested with pancreatic RNase and the resulting oligonucleotides were separated on a DEAE-cellulose column (Fig. 8). The ^{32}P-labeled oligonucleotides comprising the 5' ends eluted as a single peak. On the basis of its elution position, a structure of ppG-Yp (Y - pyrimidine nucleoside) was assigned to the oligonucleotide. The penultimate residue was confirmed to be at least 90% Up by observing that alkaline digestion

Table III. Initiation and Reinitiation of RNA Chains

	Incorporation			
	$[^3\text{H}]$GMP (nmoles)		$[\beta,\gamma\text{-}^{32}\text{P}]$GTP (pmoles)	
Preincubation (min) +	0	30	0	30
Incubation (min) ↓				
30	1.5	1.5	3.8	3.6
60	3.0	3.2	8.0	7.8
120	6.4	6.6	16.4	16.2
240	12.1	–	31.2	–

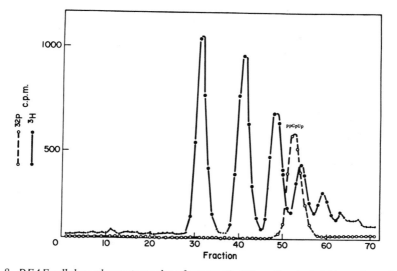

Fig. 8. DEAE-cellulose chromatography of pancreatic RNase digest of RNA products. RNA synthesized in the presence of [³H]GTP and [β,γ-³²P]GTP as in Fig. 7 was purified by gel filtration, mixed with 1.5 mg of yeast tRNA in 0.1 *M* tris buffer (*p*H 8) containing 100 μg of pancreatic RNase in a total volume of 0.5 ml, and incubated for 8-10 hr at 37°C. The digest was diluted with an equal volume of H₂O and applied to a DEAE-cellulose column 20 by 1 cm. The oligonucleotides were eluted with a linear gradient of 0.05-0.5 *M* NaCl in 0.05 *M* tris buffer (*p*H 8) and 7 *M* urea. The absorbance profile (not shown) was measured continuously by absorbance at 260 nm. Radioactivity was determined by counting 0.1 ml of each 2.0-ml fraction in 5 ml methylcellosolve and 8 ml toluene-based scintillation fluid.

of products synthesized with [α-³²P]UTP released ppG³²p. Ten percent of the terminal nucleotides were also recovered as ppG³²p when the precursor was [α-³²P]CTP, a finding consistent with the presence of penultimate Cp in the 5′ termini of one of the mRNA species (31). However, most of the mRNA species synthesized *in vitro* by the reovirion-associated polymerase terminate predominantly with ppG-Up at the 5′ ends.

The above results clearly indicate that correct initiation and termination of RNA chains occur *in vitro*. All ten mRNA products are independently initiated, presumably by the virion polymerase transcribing from ten promoter sites. As shown below, these sites correspond to the termini of the ten duplex segments (32).

EVIDENCE OF A SEGMENTED GENOME WITHIN THE VIRION

To demonstrate that the reovirus double-stranded genome RNA exists as segments *in situ*, we analyzed the 5′ termini of the viral RNA. If the genome is a continuous linear duplex molecule, it would contain two 5′-polyphosphate termini per 15×10^6 daltons. On the other hand, if the genome RNA exists as distinct segments within virions, all ten duplex molecules would bear unique 5′ termini, i.e., twenty 5′-polyphosphate ends per 15×10^6 daltons.

The ^{32}P-labeled purified double-stranded reovirus RNA was denatured by dimethylsulfoxide treatment and degraded to its constituent oligonucleotides by exhaustive digestion with pancreatic RNase. The resulting products were analyzed on a DEAE-cellulose column. Eight peaks marked I-VIII were clearly discernible (Fig. 9). The recovery of radioactivity from the column was quantitative.

In order to determine which of the oligonucleotides contained the 5′ termini, peaks III-VIII were further analyzed. Alkaline digests of I and II would not be expected to contain 5′ termini since the double-stranded RNA segments

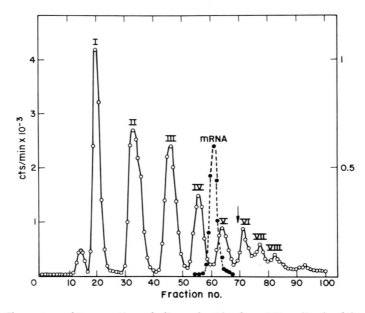

Fig. 9. Chromatographic separation of oligonucleotides from RNase digests of denatured, double-stranded RNA and 5′-terminally labeled reovirus RNA. Dimethylsulfoxide-denatured, uniformly ^{32}P-labeled double-stranded RNA was digested with pancreatic RNase and applied to a DEAE-cellulose column. Samples of 0.02 ml were counted for fractions 1-70. As indicated by the arrow, the samples were increased to 0.04 ml for fractions 71-100. Reovirus mRNA was synthesized *in vitro* in the presence of $[\beta,\gamma\text{-}^{32}P]$GTP in order to label the 5′ termini as described in Fig. 7. The mRNA was isolated, digested with pancreatic RNase, and analyzed in a DEAE-cellulose column under conditions identical to those used for double-stranded RNA. Samples of 1 ml were counted. ○, Double-stranded RNA, left scale; ●, mRNA, right scale.

are known to have at least one phosphate at the 5' ends (33). The 5'-terminal nucleotide released by alkaline treatment would therefore have a minimum charge of −4(pRp;R = purine nucleotide) and would elute with peak III or later. Therefore, the fractions comprising peaks III-VIII were hydrolyzed with alkali. Each digest was chromatographed on a DEAE-cellulose column previously calibrated with authentic ppG, pppG, and pppGp. Peaks III, VI, VII, and VIII did not liberate any radioactivity that eluted with any of the markers. Only peaks IV and V liberated radioactivity upon alkaline digestion that cochromatographed with authentic ppGp. Table IV lists the amount of radioactivity liberated as ppRp by alkaline hydrolysis of peaks III-VIII. On the basis that there are ten double-stranded genome segments (twenty 5' termini) including three large, three medium, and four small segments of average chain lengths 3500, 2000, and 1000 nucleotides (28), respectively, it can be calculated that the 5'-ppGp liberated after alkaline hydrolysis should contain 0.15% of the RNA phosphate. As shown in Table IV, 6596 cpm, 97.8% of the expected value, was found equally distributed in peaks IV and V. Thus reovirus genome RNA contains twenty 5' termini as ppRp. The nucleotides containing the 5' termini elute between peaks IV and V, a position identical to the elution profile of the 5' fragment released by pancreatic RNase digestion of the *in vitro* synthesized mRNA (Fig. 8). Thus, the 5'-end sequence of all ten genome segments is ppR-Yp. The purine residue was found to be guanosine in a separate experiment; genome RNA labeled with [³H]guanosine was hydrolyzed with alkali and chromatographed on DEAE-cellulose. The expected amount of [³H]ppGp was recovered (32).

Table IV. 5'-Terminal Nucleotide Recovered from the Alkaline Digests of Separated Oligonucleotides

Peak	ppRp	
	Cpm[a]	Percent
III	0	0
IV	3428	50.8
V	3168	47.0
VI	0	0
VII	0	0
VIII	0	0

[a]Total cpm applied = 4.5×10^6; ppGp cpm expected = 6750.

It was of interest to compare the 3' termini of the genome RNA and the mRNA species synthesized *in vitro*. Accordingly, purified double-stranded RNA and single-stranded mRNAs were treated with potassium periodate and reduced with potassium [³H] borohydride (34). The labeled 3'-nucleoside from both the genome and mRNA was identified as cytosine. The 3' ends of the double-stranded genome RNA were analyzed further, and all were found to contain the unique sequence . . . Y-A-A-C (35).

ADENINE-RICH RNA IN REOVIRIONS

In addition to ten double-stranded genome RNA segments, purified reovirus contains 40-50% of its total RNA as single-stranded oligonucleotides rich in adenine (A-rich RNA) (36,37). ³²P-Labeled RNA was extracted with phenol from purified reovirus, and the A-rich RNA was separated by gel filtration in

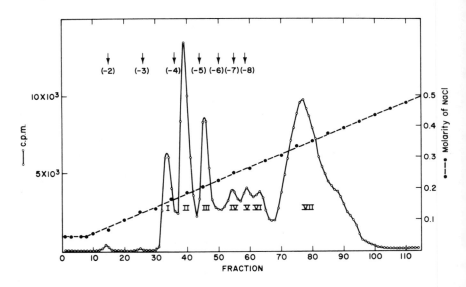

Fig. 10. Chromatography of oligonucleotides from reovirus on DEAE-cellulose column. ³²P-Labeled reovirus (2.2 × 10⁶ cpm) was extracted with phenol, and the A-rich RNA (0.9 × 10⁶ cpm) was separated from the double-stranded RNA on a Sephadex G100 column. Fractions containing the A-rich RNA were combined and lyophilized. To the dried sample was added 0.5 ml 0.05 *M* tris-HCl (*p*H 8.0), 0.05 *M* NaCl, 7 *M* urea. The samples were applied to a DEAE-cellulose column (1 × 16 cm) and eluted with a linear NaCl gradient (0.05-0.5 *M*, 120 ml each) in 0.05 *M* tris-HCl (*p*H 8.0) and 7 *M* urea. Fractions of 2 ml were collected, and aliquots (1 ml) were counted for radioactivity. The salt concentration of the fractions was determined by conductivity measurements. Shown in the figure are positions of oligonucleotides with increasing net negative charge obtained from pancreatic ribonuclease digestion of ³²P-labeled reovirus RNA.

Sephadex G100. A-Rich RNA was further resolved into seven peaks of radio-activity by DEAE-cellulose chromatography (Fig. 10). The percent of radioactivity in each peak was constant in several different preparations of purified virus from mouse, hamster, and human cells. Each peak was isolated and its sequence determined as shown in Table V.

The A-rich RNA is composed of two classes (38,39): (a) oligomers containing $5'$-ppGp with predominantly pyrimidines as the internal residues (peaks I-III) and (b) oligomers containing pAp with adenine as the only base (peak VII). It was calculated that there are, on the average, 2500 molecules of class (a) and 1200 molecules of class (b) oligonucleotides per virion. The origin of such a large number of oligomers and the mechanism by which they are packaged within reovirus are unclear. However, the following speculations can be made on the basis of the structure of these oligomers: (i) The oligonucleotides in class (a) terminate with ppGp, the same $5'$-polyphosphorylated base as found in the reovirus mRNA synthesized both *in vivo* and *in vitro*. Presumably, they are synthesized by the virion-associated polymerase. The sequence ppG-C, ppG-U, ppG-C-C, ppG-C-U-A may be abortive products whose synthesis is initiated at different sites on the double-stranded RNA; (ii) The class (b) oligonucleotides are composed entirely of adenine, but have a monophosphate group at the $5'$ termini. The presence of the monophosphate group suggests that they may be derived by cleavage of a phosphodiester bond rather than by an initiation process. The class (b) oligonucleotides may be covalently linked to viral-specific RNA during some stage of the viral replicative cycle.

Table V. Structure of Oligonucleotides from Reovirions

Peaks	5' end	3' end	Percent Pi release	Major NMP (internal)	Proposed structures	Number per virion
I	ppGp	U C	70	—	ppG-C ppG-U	560
II	ppGp	U C	50	Cp	ppG-C-C ppG-C-U	1060
III	ppGp	A	50	Cp Up	ppG-C-U-A	600
IV-VI	ppGp	C A U	27	Ap Cp Up	—	725
VII	pAp	A	9	Ap	$p(Ap)_{10-15}A$	1200

ABSENCE OF POLY(A) SEQUENCES IN REOVIRUS mRNA *IN VIVO*

Covalently linked poly(A) sequences have been found in many viral RNAs and mRNAs isolated from infected and uninfected eukaryotic cells (40). An exception is histone mRNA (41). Studies on normal cells in culture have shown that poly(A) may be a post-transcriptional modification that is involved in the transport and/or stability of mRNA. The function of poly(A) in viral RNA is unknown.

In an attempt to determine whether the reovirus class (b) oligonucleotides arise by cleavage of poly(A) from viral mRNA, reovirus mRNA was isolated from L cells after pulsing with radioactive precursors of RNA at different times after infection. The labeled viral mRNA was digested with pancreatic and T1 RNase and electrophoresed in a 20% polyacrylamide gel. As shown in Fig. 11, no RNase-resistant fragment was liberated from reovirus mRNAs. In contrast, 35S poliovirus RNA isolated from infected HeLa cells liberated a heterogeneous peak of radioactivity which migrated with the 4S tRNA marker. Poliovirus RNA contains 80-90 adenine residues at the 3' end (42).

Reovirus mRNA isolated from infected cells did not bind to nitrocellulose filters, poly(U)-containing filters, and poly(dT)-cellulose, in contrast to polio-

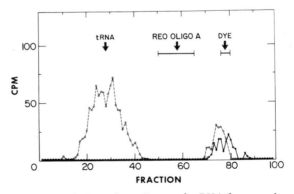

Fig. 11. Gel electrophoresis of ribonuclease digests of mRNA from reovirus- or poliovirus-infected cells. Reovirus mRNA labeled with ^{32}P from 3 to 8 hr (early mRNA) and from 9 to 13 hr (late mRNA) was isolated from infected cell cytoplasm by phenol-chloroform extraction. ^{32}P-Labeled reovirus single-stranded early mRNA (●) or [^{3}H]adenosine-labeled poliovirus single-stranded RNA (○) was digested with RNase A and RNase T1 at an enzyme:substrate ratio of 1:10 and 1:100, respectively, for 1 hr at 37°C. The resistant material was precipitated with ethanol in the presence of 100 μg yeast tRNA, redissolved, and electrophoresed in 20% polyacrylamide gels containing 8 *M* urea (44). Arrows indicate the positions of tRNA, reovirus oligo(A), and bromphenol blue. Similar results were obtained with late mRNA or mRNA isolated after a 30-min pulse with [^{3}H]adenosine, 7.5 hr after infection. Direction of migration is from left to right.

Table VI. Percent of Radioactive RNA Bound to
Poly(U) and Nitrocellulose Filters

Type of RNA	Poly(U)[a]	Nitrocellulose[b]
Poly(A)	86	94
Reo oligo(A)	93	5.2
Reo mRNA (early)	3.0	3.4
Reo mRNA (late)	3.2	3.6
Reo mRNA (30-min pulse)	1.5	ND
Polio RNA	68	83
L-cell ribosomal RNA (18S)	0.5	2.6
Reo RNA (double-stranded)[c]	0.6	ND

[a]Poly(U) filters were prepared and assay was carried out according to Sheldon et al. (45).

[b]Binding assays were carried out in the presence of 0.5 M KCl according to Lee et al. (46).

[c]Reovirus double-stranded RNA was denatured with Me_2SO, precipitated, and redissolved in binding buffer.

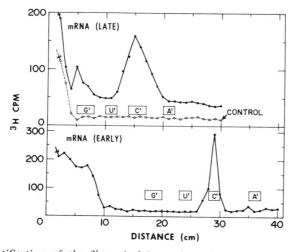

Fig. 12. Identification of the 3'-terminal base of reovirus mRNA from infected cells. ^{32}P-Labeled reovirus early or late mRNA was isolated from infected cells as in Fig. 11. The mRNAs were hybridized to unlabeled double-stranded reovirus genome RNA with oxidized-reduced 3'-terminal ends. The hybrid molecules were separated from the unhybridized ^{32}P-labeled single-stranded mRNA, unlabeled ribosomal RNA, and tRNA by cellulose CF11 chromatography. The purified hybrid molecules contained unreacted hydroxyl groups at the 3' ends only in the mRNA strands. These free groups were oxidized by KIO_4 and reduced by ^{3}H-labeled KBH_4. The labeled 3'-terminal base was identified by paper chromatography following alkali hydrolysis. Control: KB^3H_4 labeling of oxidized-reduced double-stranded genome RNA followed by alkaline hydrolysis and paper chromatography.

virus RNA (Table VI). Short tracts of adenine insufficient to result in binding also are not present at the 3′ end of reovirus RNA. mRNA isolated early and late after reovirus infection was specifically labeled as follows. Reovirus double-stranded genome RNA, purified free of A-rich RNA, was oxidized with potassium periodate (KIO_4) and reduced with unlabeled sodium borohydride ($NaBH_4$). ^{32}P-Labeled reovirus mRNA from infected cells was then hybridized with the oxidized-reduced double-stranded RNA. The resulting hybrid molecules were separated from the single-stranded mRNA by cellulose CF11 chromatography. These hybrid molecules thus contained one strand with oxidized-reduced 3′ ends (contributed by the genome RNA) and a complementary strand with a free 3′-hydroxyl group (the ^{32}P-labeled mRNA). The isolated duplex molecules were further oxidized with KIO_4 and reduced with radioactive KB^3H_4 to label the free 3′-hydroxyl group of the ^{32}P-labeled strand. The 3′-nucleoside was identified as cytosine for both early and late mRNA (Fig. 12). Thus reovirus mRNA isolated from infected cells contains cytosine as the 3′-terminal base.

SUMMARY OF FINDINGS

The findings for reovirus genome transcription and replication may be summarized as follows:

a. All ten double-stranded RNA segments isolated from purified reovirus contain ppGp at the 5′ termini and pY-A-A-C at their 3′ ends.

b. The presence of 20 unique 5′-terminal diphosphates per 15×10^6 daltons of double-stranded RNA indicates that the viral genome *in situ* consists of segments that are synthesized as discrete units in infected cells.

c. The penultimate base is a pyrimidine. This 5′-sequence, ppG-Yp, is identical to that in the ten reovirus mRNA species synthesized *in vitro*. The 3′-terminal base is also the same, i.e., cytosine. Thus, the double-stranded RNA segments are perfect duplexes that are transcribed end-to-end by the virion-associated polymerase.

d. Single-stranded RNA species have been shown to be the precursors of double-stranded RNA (43). Each species of mRNA apparently is transcribed and replicated independently. By an unknown but intriguing mechanism, ten double-stranded segments are correctly packaged to form mature virions.

e. A common sequence, pY-A-A-C, at the 3′ termini of the double-stranded RNA may be the recognition site of the virion-associated polymerase or involved in linking the genome segments within the virion.

f. In addition to the double-stranded segments, purified virions contain a large amount of two types of single-stranded oligomers: class (a) oligomers all having ppGp and class (b) consisting of $p(A)_{10-15}A$. Their function remains to be elucidated.

g. Reovirus mRNA, like histone mRNA but in contrast to many viral and cellular mRNAs, contains no poly(A).

REFERENCES

1. D. W. Verwoerd. *Progr. Med. Virol.* **12**:192 (1970).
2. J. S. Semancik, J. L. Van Etten, and A. K. Vidaver. *Proc. Am. Soc. Microbiol.,* **p. 220** **(1972).**
3. G. T. Banks, K. W. Buck, E. B. Chain, J. E. Darbyshire, and F. Himmelweit. *Nature* **222**:89 (1969).
4. G. T. Banks, K. W. Buck, E. B. Chain, J. E. Darbyshire, F. Himmelweit, T. J. Sharpe, and D. M. Planterose. *Nature* **227**:505 (1970).
5. A. J. Shatkin. *Advan. Virus Res.* **14**:63 (1969).
6. C. J. Gauntt and A. F. Graham. In H. B. Levy (ed.), *The Biochemistry of Viruses,* M. Dekker Inc., New York, p. 259 (1969).
7. W. K. Joklik and H. J. Zweerink. *Ann. Rev. Genet.* **5**:297 (1971).
8. P. J. Gomatos, I. Tamm, S. Dales, and R. M. Franklin. *Virology* **17**:441 (1962).
9. A. J. Shatkin, J. D. Sipe, and P. Loh. *J. Virol.* **2**:986 (1968).
10. C. Vasquez and A. K. Kleinschmidt. *J. Mol. Biol.* **34**:137 (1968).
11. N. Granboulan and A. Niveleau. *J. Microsc.* **6**:23 (1967).
12. P. J. Gomatos and W. Stoeckenius. *Proc. Natl. Acad. Sci. (USA)* **52**:1449 (1964).
13. A. R. Bellamy and W. K. Joklik. *J. Mol. Biol.* **29**:19 (1967).
14. Y. Watanabe and A. F. Graham. *J. Virol.* **1**:665 (1967).
15. W. K. Joklik. *J. Cell Physiol.* **76**:289 (1971).
16. H. J. Zweerink and W. K. Joklik. *Virology* **41**:501 (1970).
17. H. J. Zweerink, M. J. McDowell, and W. K. Joklik. *Virology* **45**:716 (1971).
18. S. Dales. *Progr. Med. Virol.* **7**:1 (1965).
19. Y. Watanabe, S. Millward, and A. F. Graham. *J. Mol. Biol.* **36**:107 (1968).
20. A. J. Shatkin and J. D. Sipe. *Proc. Natl. Acad. Sci. (USA)* **61**:1462 (1968).
21. J. Borsa and A. F. Graham. *Biochem. Biophys. Res. Commun.* **33**:895 (1968).
22. A. K. Banerjee and A. J. Shatkin. *J. Virol.* **6**:1 (1970).
23. J. J. Skehel and W. K. Joklik. *Virology* **39**:822 (1969).
24. D. H. Levin, N. Mendelsohn, M. Schonberg, H. Klett, S. Silverstein, A. M. Kapular, and G. Acs. *Proc. Natl. Acad. Sci. (USA)* **66**:890 (1970).
25. C. T. Chang and H. J. Zweerink. *Virology* **46**:544 (1971).
26. S. C. Silverstein, C. Astell, D. H. Levin, M. Schonberg, and G. Acs. *Virology* **47**:797 (1972).
27. A. J. Shatkin and A. LaFiandra. *J. Virol.* **10**:698 (1972).
28. A. K. Banerjee, R. Ward, and A. J. Shatkin. *Nature New Biol.* **230**:169 (1971).
29. A. M. Kapular, N. Mendelsohn, N. Klett, and G. Acs. *Nature (Lond.)* **225**:1209 (1970).
30. J. Borsa, J. Grover, and J. D. Chapman. *J. Virol.* **6**:295 (1970).
31. J. L. Nichols, A. J. Hay, and W. K. Joklik. *Nature New Biol.* **235**:105 (1972).
32. A. K. Banerjee and A. J. Shatkin. *J. Mol. Biol.* **61**:643 (1971).
33. S. Millward and M. Nonoyama. *Cold Spring Harbor Symp. Quant. Biol.* **35**:773 (1970).
34. A. K. Banerjee, R. Ward, and A. J. Shatkin. *Nature New Biol.* **230**:169 (1971).
35. A. K. Banerjee and M. A. Grece. *Biochem. Biophys. Res. Commun.* **45**:1518 (1971).
36. A. J. Shatkin and J. D. Sipe. *Proc. Natl. Acad. Sci. (USA)* **59**:246 (1968).

37. A. R. Bellamy and W. K. Joklik. *Proc. Natl. Acad. Sci. (USA)* **58**:1389 (1967).

38. C. M. Stoltzfus and A. K. Banerjee. *Arch. Biochem. Biophys.* **152**:733 (1972).

39. J. L. Nichols, A. R. Bellamy, and W. K. Joklik. *Virology* **49**:562 (1972).

40. A. J. Shatkin. *Ann. Rev. Biochem.* (1974)

41. M. Adesnik and J. E. Darnell. *J. Mol. Biol.* **67**:397 (1972).

42. Y. Yogo and E. Wimmer. *Proc. Natl. Acad. Sci. (USA)* **69**:1877 (1972).

43. M. Schonberg, S. C. Silverstein, D. H. Levin, and G. Acs. *Proc. Natl. Acad. Sci. (USA)* **68**:505 (1971).

44. G. R. Molloy, W. L. Thomas, and J. E. Darnell. *Proc. Natl. Acad. Sci. (USA)* **69**:3684 (1972).

45. R. Sheldon, C. Jurale, and J. Kates. *Proc. Natl. Acad. Sci. (USA)* **69**:417 (1972).

46. S. Y. Lee, J. Mendecki, and G. Brawerman. *Proc. Natl. Acad. Sci. (USA)* **68**:1331 (1971).

47. R. Spendlove, M. E. McClain and E. H. Lennette, *J. Gen. Virol.* **8**:83 (1970).

48. M. Nonoyama, Y. Watanabe and A. F. Graham, *J. Virol.* **6**:226 (1970).

DISCUSSION

Question (Chakravorty): The maturation of reovirus is really a mystery. Is it possible that the ten pieces of RNA are wrapped up in a random fashion and that the particles which possess at least one copy of those ten RNA pieces are infective? Are the rest all noninfective particles, because PFU are usually 1/100 of the actual particle number?

Answer: I do not think the genome segments are wrapped up in a random fashion for the following reasons: (a) there is a report in the literature that some chymotrypsin-resistant strains of reovirus have a particle/PFU ratio of 1 (47); (b) if one sediments purified reovirus to equilibrium in CsCl, the virus collected from all regions of the band contains the same molar ratios of large, medium, and small genome segments; (c) defective, noninfectious reovirus has been obtained which lacks the largest genome segment (48). Thus it seems that all reovirus particles have ten segments in the same molar ratio.

16

Initiation and Regulation of Transcription in Coliphage Lambda

Waclaw Szybalski

McArdle Laboratory for Cancer Research
University of Wisconsin
Madison, Wisconsin, U.S.A.

This chapter is an extended and updated but largely unreferenced summary of previous reviews (18-22). It discusses the transcriptional controls active during development of the bacteriophage λ. This phage provides a model system which permits critical study of the detailed mechanisms regulating gene expression.

BACTERIOPHAGE λ

Coliphage λ is a conventional phage of medium size, the head of which contains a linear DNA molecule of molecular weight 30.8×10^6, corresponding to 46,500 nucleotide pairs (5). Upon phage infection, λ DNA is injected into the *Escherichia coli* host cell through the flexible phage tail. After entering the bacterial cell, the linear DNA molecule is converted into a circular form (Fig. 1) by the covalent joining of its two single-stranded cohesive ends, each composed of 12 complementary deoxynucleotides, employing the DNA ligase of the host.

Depending on the phage strain and the physiological state of the bacterial host, λ infection may lead to either a *lytic* or a *lysogenic* response. In the *lytic* response, λ functions become sequentially expressed, λ DNA replicates, heads and tails are synthesized, and ultimately a new crop of mature phage progenies is produced, resulting in death and lysis of the host cell. In the *lysogenic* response, the host cell survives, and the circular λ genome is linearly inserted into the bacterial genome, as shown in Fig. 1. This is possible because phage λ produces the Int enzyme(s), which mediates the insertion, and because it can elicit

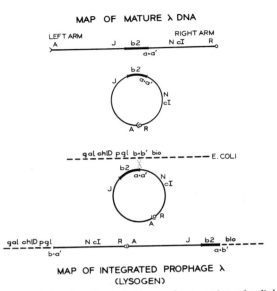

Fig. 1. Campbell's model for the circularization and integration of coliphage λ DNA into the genome of Escherichia coli. The symbols a·a' and b·b' indicate the attachment sites on the viral (solid line) and bacterial (broken line) genomes, respectively. From Szybalski et al. (21).

synthesis of the λ repressor, the product of gene cI, which blocks all the lytic λ functions. The lysogenic response can occur if the repressor is produced early enough to block lytic development and, thus, to prevent death of the infected host cell.

In the lysogenic state, the phage genome, now denoted "prophage," can be considered as a cluster of "bacterial" genes which comprises about 1% of the host DNA. Since the λ prophage is an integral part of the bacterial genome, it is vertically inherited by all the bacterial progeny cells, a very effective and harmless form of symbiotic propagation of the viral genome. However, prophage propagation by this means would be terminated in the event of death of the lysogenic host cell. To ensure its survival, the λ prophage developed a mechanism for sensing impending death of the host and for entering the lytic cycle, which leads to production of a crop of mature phage. Conversion from the lysogenic (prophage) state into the lytic cycle is denoted "induction," and its first step is the inactivation of the λ repressor protein. This inactivation is normally accomplished by certain bacterial products that accumulate in the early stages of the slowdown of DNA synthesis, one of the first symptoms of cell death.

In this summary, I shall first discuss the transcriptional controls in the repressed λ prophage and then describe the chain of events that ensues after induction of the lysogenic cell.

TRANSCRIPTION IN THE PROPHAGE STATE

In the prophage state, in which the λ genome exists as an innocuous component of the bacterial chromosome, only one major operon of λ is transcribed. The host RNA polymerase recognizes the p_c promoter (*prm*) and produces mRNA for genes *cI* and *rex,* copying the *l* strand of λ DNA (Fig. 2a). This *cI-rex* mRNA is translated into the λ repressor protein and the *rex* product. The repressor interacts with the o_L and o_R operators and blocks expression of all the major λ genes. Thus in the prophage state only about 4% (74.3-78.4%λ; Fig. 2a) of the prophage genome is transcribed. The λ repressor confers immunity against infection by λ phage, whereas the *rex* function blocks the development of certain mutants of the unrelated coliphages T4 and T5. Thus prophage λ

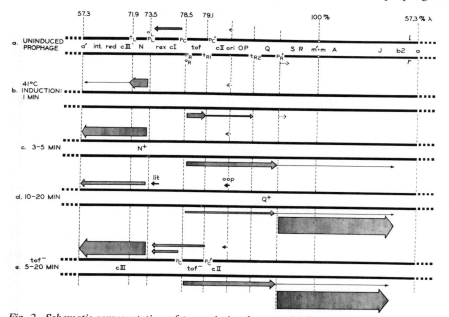

Fig. 2. Schematic representation of transcriptional events. (a) Transcription in λ prophage. (b-d) Transcription at various stages of development after thermal induction of λcI857. (e) The uncontrolled transcription in the induced *tof⁻* mutant of λ. The maps of the λ prophage are not drawn to scale, and the immunity region is expanded. The numbers in the top line indicate the positions of various sites in respect to the ends of the mature λ DNA molecule (5): *att* (57.3%λ), the t_L terminator (about 71.6%λ), the left end of *imm*434 between s_L and p_L-o_L (73.5%λ), a site between p_c and p_R-o_R (about 78.5%λ), the right end of *imm*434 next to the t_{R_1} terminator (79.1%λ), the *ori* site (about 81%λ), the t_{R_2} site(s) (between 84 and 89%λ), the p'_R (or p_Q) late promoter (near 92–93%λ) for the 198 nucleotide-long minor rightward RNA (dotted rightward arrow) which is extended by the Q product into the "late" mRNA (very wide rightward arrow). Based on studies reviewed by Szybalski *et al.* (21,22) and Szybalski (19,20).

pays tribute to the host by offering limited protection against several phages, a factor of possible evolutionary significance.

The cI-*rex* transcription corresponds to about 90% of the total λ prophage transcription, with the remainder assigned to a few other sites, including regions *oop* (traces of an 81-nucleotides-long RNA) and *int* on the *l* strand and a 198-nucleotides-long RNA in the p'_R region on the *r* strand. However, these very minor transcriptions (also in the b2 region) appear to be of no physiological importance to the maintenance of the prophage state.

Under special circumstances, lysogeny can be maintained even in the absence of the functional repressor or when the λ genome remains as a plasmid, i.e., not integrated into the bacterial chromosome.

INACTIVATION OF THE REPRESSOR

To induce phage development, it is necessary first to inactivate the λ repressor. To simplify this task, many λ mutants were isolated in which the cI protein is thermosensitive. Heating such λcI*ts* lysogens to about 41°C inactivates the repressor but does not otherwise interfere with phage development. This *direct* method of inactivation of repressor is commonly practiced in the laboratory, since it results in synchronous and almost instantaneous induction.

The *indirect* method of prophage induction is based on the fact that transient interference with the host DNA synthesis by, for instance, irradiation, base analogs, or mitomycin treatment, results in accumulation of some bacterial product which interacts with the ind^+-coded site on the repressor and converts it into inactive form. This indirect process requires over ½ hr and is inoperative if the bacteria carry a *rec*A or *lex* mutation or if the phage has an ind^- mutation in gene cI. Since the active repressor has an oligomeric structure, its inactivation must often be associated with dissociation into cI subunits of molecular weight about 27,000 (13). This indirect method of repressor inactivation permits induction of many kinds of lysogenic strains as found in nature, and as already mentioned is probably of evolutionary significance because it permits rescue of the prophage genomes from the "sinking" host by converting them into mature and infective phage particles.

Induction can also ensue when the genome of the lysogen is transferred into a repressor-free receptor cell. This phenomenon is called "zygotic" induction.

IMMEDIATE-EARLY TRANSCRIPTION AFTER PROPHAGE INDUCTION

Inactivation of the λ repressor and its removal from the o_L and o_R operator sites permits the host RNA polymerase to initiate the leftward and rightward transcriptions at the p_L and p_R promoters (Fig. 2). The leftward transcription, however, does not proceed very far (about 1.5 %λ), the bulk of it being terminated at the t_L terminator. Similarly, most of the rightward transcription is blocked at the t_{R1} terminator, with only about 0.5 %λ length (240 nucleotide pairs) being transcribed, and the remainder of the t_{R1} readthrough is probably stopped at the t_{R2} terminator[1] (Fig. 2B). The host factor denoted ρ is instrumental in blocking transcription at the t sites (15). Immediate-early leftward transcription yields mRNA for gene N, and the bulk of the immediate-early rightward mRNA codes for the product of gene *tof*.

DELAYED-EARLY TRANSCRIPTION

The product of gene N acts as the antitermination factor (ref. 15 and H. A. Lozeron, unpublished). It interacts with the host RNA polymerase and abolishes the ρ-imposed termination at the t sites. The N product of λ appears to be specific for the t sites[1] on the λ DNA. In this manner, the leftward transcription extends from the p_L site to gene *int*, and the rightward transcription, which originates at p_R, covers genes *tof, O, P, Q*, and beyond (Fig. 2c).

LATE TRANSCRIPTION

Although the p_R-initiated delayed-early transcription appears to extend beyond gene Q,[1] it yields very little mRNA for genes A to J, which code for major structural components of the phage head and tail. This amount of

---

[1] The specificity of antitermination at the tandem set of terminator sites might be more complex. To explain a so-called λ*imm*21 paradox (when the early rightward transcription, which originates in the *imm*21 region, can pass through the λ-specific t_{R2} terminator, although phage λ*imm*21 does not code for the N product of λ, and the N-like product of λ*imm*21 cannot antiterminate at t_{R2} of λ*imm*λ; refs. 3 and 8), I proposed in 1971 the "t_1 training model," which could be summarized as follows: In the case of several *cis*-arranged terminators (t_1, t_2, t_3, . . ., t_n), the successful antitermination event depends on the specificity of the N product for only the first t_1 terminator. The complex of the host RNA polymerase and the antitermination product of N or a N-like gene (N+RNApol complex) "locks into a passing t_1-trained conformation" by initiating transcription at the specific promoter - startpoint locus and then traversing the first N-specific t_1 terminator. Such a "t_1-trained" N+RNApol complex could now traverse the consecutive t terminators (t_2, t_3, . . ., t_n and maybe some other polar mutations and even U_6A-OH), even in the absence of t_2-t_n-specific N-like factors. However, in the case where the t_1 terminator is deleted or bypassed by a new promoter located between t_1 and t_2, the t_2 terminator (which now assumes a role of the "t_1" terminator) must be N-specific, or acquire this specificity, in order to permit the N+RNApol complex to traverse it. Furthermore, one should realize that the N+RNApol complex might have somewhat different characteristics than the nonmodified host RNA polymerase. Actually, there appears to be evidence (9) that the N+RNApol complex may be more efficient than the host RNA polymerase in initiating transcription at the p_L and p_R promoters. One could also postulate (D. I. Friedman, personal communication) that the N+RNApol complex may sometimes acquire its N-specific antitermination properties already at the N-specific promoter site. One could summarize our model by stating that the N-RNApol complex becomes unresponsive to the *subsequent* terminator signals (loses termination specificity) after successfully crossing the *first* terminator-associated, N-specific, recognition site during transcription of the particular DNA molecule.

transcription would be barely enough to produce protein components for one phage particle per cell. To amplify the transcription in the *S-R-A-J* region, the following regulatory mechanism is provided: The product of gene Q permits the RNA polymerase to extend the p'_R-initiated minor rightward RNA, with a resulting massive rightward transcription of the *S-J* region (Fig. 2d). Thus enough products are provided for about 100 or more phage particles per cell.

This orderly and sequential chain of transcriptional events results in expression of all the λ genes and should lead to production of a healthy crop of progeny phage. However, further controls are required to make the process more efficient and more responsive to environmental factors.

REGULATION OF EARLY TRANSCRIPTION

Under *in vivo* conditions, the p_L promoter appears to be more active than the p_R promoter, with resulting massive early leftward transcription after prophage induction. The product of gene N permits antitermination, as already discussed, and the products of the gene cluster *int* and *xis* direct the excision and circularization of the λ genome, which in this manner becomes an autonomous plasmid-like entity. Since these events occur early, a mechanism evolved that curbs the powerful leftward transcription when it is no longer needed. The product of gene *tof* acts as the "second repressor" and by its action near the o_L operator reduces the leftward transcription by a factor of 5-10 (compare Figs 2c and 2d). Although acting at the same or almost the same site, the repression by the *tof* product appears to be less efficient than that by the product of gene *cI*, the "first" λ repressor. The *tof* product has two more effects: it appears to depress somewhat the rightward p_R-promoted transcription by acting near the o_R operator, and at the same time it blocks the *cI-rex* transcription, as will be discussed in the next section. The unrestricted transcription in the absence of the *tof* product is schematically shown in Fig. 2e.

The negative control of the p_R-initiated rightward transcription by the *tof* product is an example of autorepression, because in this case the *tof* gene regulates its own expression. This phenomenon might be quite important for λ DNA replication since genes O and P, which control λ DNA replication, are a part of the same operon. For instance, $\lambda N^- cI^-$ or its p_R-O-P fragments, denoted λdv, can persist as autonomous plasmids and replicate in concert with the host. I believe that this is possible because of the autorepressive control of the λ replication genes by the *tof* product, since such a mechanism would permit maintaining a precise and self-regulating balance between the replication of the λ plasmids and that of the carrier cells.

CONTROL OF IMMUNITY TRANSCRIPTION

The *cI-rex* transcription initiated at the p_c promoter must be carried out by the host RNA polymerase, but it probably requires some additional factors since transcription of this operon appears not to be initiated *in vitro* by the purified RNA polymerase (1). The *in vivo* p_c-*cI-rex* transcription can be turned off by the product of gene *tof* (*cro*), which therefore was named "antirepressor" (12). How then can gene *cI* be transcribed and repressor produced after phage infection, when the antagonistic *tof* product is one of the earliest λ products? This is accomplished by activation of the alternative mode of transcription of genes *cI* and *rex*, which is promoted at the p'_c site (*pre*) activated by the products of genes *cII* and *cIII* (14) (Fig. 2e). This mode of λ repressor expression appears to be still sensitive to the *tof* product (compare Fig 2b,c and e) but somehow manages to produce enough repressor to establish lysogeny.

About 5-10 min after thermal induction of the λ*tof*[+] prophage, a short RNA molecule denoted *lit* (*l*ate *i*mmunity *t*ranscription; Fig. 2d) becomes synthesized in the *rex* region of the λ genome (7). Its synthesis is coordinate with the *oop* RNA, as will be discussed in the next section. It is not known whether the *lit* RNA is of any significance for λ development.

All these factors exemplify the complexity of the immunity controls, with two or even three modes of expression of the genes within the *cI-rex* region and a special controlling element, the product of gene *tof*, also called "second repressor" or "antirepressor." Other possible control factors include the counter-current transcription in the p_c-p_R-*tof*-p'_c region from both the *l* and *r* strands of DNA, the effect of the multiplicity of infection, and other elements not discussed here.

TRANSCRIPTION AS RELATED TO λ DNA REPLICATION

λ DNA replication starts 3-4 min after thermal induction at the site designated *ori* (*ori*gin of DNA replication) and is bidirectional. Its initiation requires the λ products *O* and *P* and the intact *ori* site (6). It also requires host products coded by genes *dna*B, *dna*E, and *dna*G (7,23). Moreover, for the initiation of the λ DNA replication fork two kinds of RNA transcripts are required: the rightward RNA transcription in the *ori-O-P* region (6) and a strong augmentation of the synthesis of the 81-nucleotides-long *oop* RNA (Fig. 2). Synthesis of *oop* RNA depends on the λ elements *ori*, *O*, and *P* and on the products of the host genes *dna*B and *dna*G, but not on *dna*E (7). There appear to be two phases of λ DNA synthesis: (a) early bidirectional replication of the λ DNA circles, and (b) late, predominantly leftward replication leading to formation of the long λ DNA concatemers which are cut by the Ter function of λ and packaged into the phage heads. One might speculate that a processed fragment of the ordinary p_R-*O-P* transcript serves as a primer for the early rightward DNA replication, whereas the self-terminating *oop* RNA, which carries a U_6A-OH 3'-terminal sequence, is a special primer for both the early and late leftward λ DNA synthesis.

IN VITRO SYNTHESIS OF λ RNA

To simplify the determination of the 5′-terminal sequences of the λ transcripts, we synthesized very short RNA chains using a λb2 template and purified RNA polymerase in a reaction lasting only 5-24 sec at 25°C (1). Under these conditions, RNA synthesis starts at only four sites. The bulk of the RNA is initiated at the startpoints designated s_L and s_R, located a short distance downstream from the corresponding $p_L o_L$ and $p_R o_R$ sites. Thus the initially surprising observation was made that neither the promoter nor the operator site was transcribed into RNA. The distance between the $p_L o_L$ promoter-operator site and the s_L startpoint was carefully measured by a combination of the electron microscopy of heteroduplexes, novel genetic mapping, and sequence analysis, and most recent data indicate that it should be at least 20 to 30 nucleotide pairs long (ref. 2 and measurements of M. Fiandt and E. H. Szybalski). Several implications of this finding are discussed by Blattner *et al.* (2), and the model is summarized in Fig. 3.

The p_L and p_R RNAs correspond to about 50 and 40%, respectively, of the *in vitro* transcripts produced in a 24-sec reaction. The remainder of the RNA belongs to two minor transcripts, one coded by the *l* strand in the vicinity of the *ori* site and the other transcribed from the *r* strand in the *Q-R* region. Whereas the p_L and p_R RNAs can be extended into very long messengers during a longer-lasting RNA polymerase catalyzed reaction (ref. 15 and K. Carlson, unpublished), the minor leftward RNA remains 81 nucleotides long (4) and the minor rightward RNA 198 nucleotides long (10). Both contain a 3′-terminal sequence U_6A-OH, which appears to be associated with this "natural" termination of transcription, independent of ρ factor.

One might summarize these observations by saying that *in vitro* RNA synthesis on a λb2 template DNA starts at only four sites, producing four RNAs, one with the pppG 5′-terminus (minor leftward RNA) and three initiated with

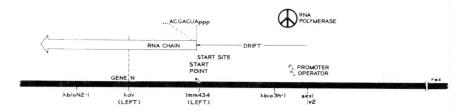

Fig. 3. Physical map of the beginning of the leftward operon of phage λ, *modified from Blattner et al.* (2). The RNA polymerase enters the DNA at the promoter site, "drifts" toward the start site without producing RNA transcripts, receives at start site a signal for initiation of RNA synthesis, and begins the RNA synthesis at the s_L startpoint. The approximate positions of the indicated endpoints, as measured from the left terminus (0 %λ) of mature λ DNA (5) are 73.05 %λ for λ*bio*N2-1, 73.25 %λ for λdv, 73.53 %λ for *imm*434 and 73.55 %λ for λ*bio*3h-1.

pppA. Two initiations are quite effective and lead to the synthesis of long p_L and p_R mRNAs, whereas two other starts result in synthesis of short, self-terminating RNAs.

COMPARISON OF *IN VIVO* AND *IN VITRO* INITIATION OF RNA SYNTHESIS

Since the p_L and p_R RNAs were sequenced for a distance of over 150 nucleotides (Dahlberg and Blattner, unpublished) and the two minor RNAs were sequenced completely (4,10), the obvious question arose whether these *in vitro* RNAs are identical to the *in vivo* transcripts. The ^{32}P-labeled 5'-terminal fragment of the p_L-*N-int* mRNA was isolated by a combination of the fractionation and hybridization procedures and was found to have exactly the same sequence, including the 5'-pppA terminus, as the p_L RNA synthesized *in vitro* (11). Lozeron *et al.* (in preparation) have found that the three remaining *in vitro* transcripts have their *in vivo* counterparts with identical 5'-terminal sequences.

One may conclude, therefore, that the *in vitro* initiation of λ RNA synthesis exhibits a complete fidelity for the four transcripts. These are the p_L- and p_R-promoted major λ mRNAs, the *oop* RNA, and the minor rightward RNA in the p'_R region. However, the *in vitro* RNA polymerase catalyzed reaction did not lead to initiation of synthesis for several mRNAs observed *in vivo,* namely, the p_c- and p'_c-promoted transcripts of the *cI-rex* operon, the *lit* RNA, and the p'_R-promoted, very long late RNA (Fig. 2e). Probably, these initiation events require some other factors in addition to the purified RNA polymerase of *E. coli.* One might speculate that the minor rightward RNA is initiated at the p'_R promoter and, although terminated at its U_6A-OH sequence, it can be extended into the "late" mRNA region by the antiterminating activity of the product of gene Q. As determined by Blattner *et al.* (unpublished), the positions of the p'_R promoter and of the minor rightward RNA are indistinguishable, as mapped with a series of λ deletion mutants, including λgalM3 (cut near the right terminus of gene Q) and λp4 (cut to the right of p'_R) (ref. 5). Some of these minor rightward RNAs could serve as primers for one of the Okazaki-type pieces of newly synthesized λ RNA (16) or might have no obvious biological role.

CONCLUDING COMMENTS

We have presented merely an idealized overview of the transcriptional controls operating during the development of a relatively simple virus. In actuality, these controls are more complex and are complemented by post-transcriptional controls, including the programmed processing and degradation of RNA transcripts (11), and by many translational and post-translational controls. One can only marvel how through evolution there emerged such a complex system of controls in a creature as simple as bacteriophage λ. Beyond that, the imagination is staggered by the prospect of a complete analysis of the regulatory mechanisms in more complex organisms, as, for instance, the *E. coli* host with 100 times more genetic information, needless to say a human cell with 100,000 times more DNA than bacteriophage λ.

REFERENCES

1. F. R. Blattner and J. E. Dahlberg. RNA synthesis startpoints in bacteriophage λ: Are the promoter and operator transcribed? *Nature New Biol.* **237**:227 (1972).
2. F. R. Blattner, J. E. Dahlberg, J. K. Boettiger, M. Fiandt, and W. Szybalski. Distance from a promoter mutation to an RNA synthesis startpoint on bacteriophage λ DNA. *Nature New Biol.* **237**:232 (1972).
3. M. Couturier, C. Dambly, and R. Thomas. Control of development in temperate bacteriophages. V. Sequential activation of the viral functions. *Mol. Gen. Genet.* **120**: 231 (1973).
4. J. E. Dahlberg and F. R. Blattner. Sequence of a self-terminating RNA made near the origin of DNA replication of phage lambda. *Fed Proc.* **32**:664 abst. (1973). *In vitro* transcription products of lambda DNA: nucleotide sequences and regulatory sites. In C. F. Fox and W. S. Robinson (eds.), *Virus Research* Academic Press, New York, pp. 533-543 (1973).
5. N. Davidson and W. Szybalski. Physical and chemical characteristics of lambda DNA. In A. D. Hershey (ed.), *The Bacteriophage Lambda,* Cold Spring Harbor Laboratory, Cold Spring Harbor, New York, pp. 45-82 (1971).
6. W. F. Dove, H. Inokuchi, and W. F. Stevens. Replication control in phage lambda. In A. D. Hershey (ed.), *The Bacteriophage Lambda,* Cold Spring Harbor Laboratory, Cold Spring Harbor, New York, pp. 747-771 (1971).
7. S. Hayes and W. Szybalski. Possible primer for DNA replication in coliphage lambda. *Fed. Proc.* **32**:529 abst. (1973). Synthesis of RNA primer for lambda DNA replication is controlled by phage and host. In B. A. Hamkalo and J. Papaconstantinou (eds.), *Molecular Cytogenetics*, Plenum Press, New York, pp. 277-283 (1973). Control of short leftward transcripts from the immunity and *ori* regions in induced coliphage lambda. *Molec. Gen. Genet.* **126**: 275 (1973).
8. I. Herskowitz and E. Signer. Control of transcription from the *r* strand of bacteriophage lambda. *Cold Spring Harbor Symp. Quant. Biol.* **35**:355 (1970).
9. S. Kumar, E. Calef, and W. Szybalski. Regulation of the transcription of *Escherichia coli* phage λ by its early genes N and *tof. Cold Spring Harbor Symp. Quant. Biol.* **35**:331 (1970).
10. P. Leibowitz, S. M. Weissman, and C. M. Radding. Nucleotide sequence of a ribonucleic acid transcribed *in vitro* from λ phage deoxyribonucleic acid. *J. Biol. Chem.* **246**:5120 (1971).
11. H. A. Lozeron, M. L. Funderburgh, J. E. Dahlberg, B. P. Stark, and W. Szybalski. Identity of *in vitro* and *in vivo* initiation of phage lambda mRNA: Analysis of *in vivo* cleavage products. *Abst. Ann. Meet. Soc. Microbiol.,* p. 237 (1972).
12. A. B. Oppenheim, Z. Neubauer, and E. Calef. The antirepressor: A new element in the regulation of protein synthesis. *Nature* **226**:31 (1970).
13. M. Ptashne. Repressor and its action. In A. D. Hershey (ed.), *The Bacteriophage Lambda,* Cold Spring Harbor Laboratory, Cold Spring Harbor, New York, p. 221 (1971).
14. L. Reichardt and A. D. Kaiser. Control of λ repressor synthesis. *Proc. Natl. Acad. Sci. (USA)* **68**:2185 (1971).

15. J. F. Roberts. The "rho" factor: Termination and anti-termination in lambda. *Cold Spring Harbor Symp. Quant. Biol.* **35**:121 (1970).
16. A. Sugino, S. Hirose, and R. Okazaki. RNA-linked nascent DNA fragments in *Escherichia coli. Proc. Natl. Acad. Sci. (USA)* **69**:1863 (1972).
17. W. Szybalski. Initiation and patterns of transcription during phage development. In *Canadian Cancer Conference* (Proceedings of the Eighth Canadian Cancer Research Conference, Honey Harbor, Ont., 1968), Vol. 8, Pergamon Press, New York, pp. 183-215 (1969).
18. W. Szybalski. Various controls of transcription in coliphage lambda. In L. Silvestri (ed.), *RNA Polymerase and Transcription,* Lepetit Colloquia on Biology and Medicine 1, North-Holland, Amsterdam, pp. 209-217 (1970).
19. W. Szybalski. Controls of transcription and replication in coliphage lambda. Karl-August-Forster Lectures: *Informationsgesteuerte Synthese,* Akad. Wiss. Literat. Mainz, Mathem. Naturwiss. Klasse, Vol. 6, F. Steiner Verlag, Wiesbaden, Germany, pp. 1-45 (1971).
20. W. Szybalski. Transcription and replication in *E. coli* bacteriophage lambda. In L. Ledoux (ed.), *Uptake of Informative Molecules by Living Cells,* North-Holland, Amsterdam, pp. 59-82 (1972).
21. W. Szybalski, K. Bøvre, M. Fiandt, A. Guha, Z. Hradecna, S. Kumar, H. A. Lozeron, V. M. Maher, Sr., H. J. J. Nijkamp, W. C. Summers, and K. Taylor. Transcriptional controls in developing bacteriophages. *J. Cell Physiol.* **74**:33 (Suppl. 1) (1969).
22. W. Szybalski, K. Bøvre, M. Fiandt, S. Hayes, Z. Hradecna, S. Kumar, H. A. Lozeron, H. J. J. Nijkamp, and W. F. Stevens. Transcriptional units and their controls in *Escherichia coli* phage λ: Operons and scriptons. *Cold Spring Harbor Symp. Quant. Biol.* **35**:341 (1970).
23. J. A. Wechsler and J. D. Gross. *Escherichia coli* mutants temperature-sensitive for DNA synthesis. *Mol. Gen. Genet.* **113**:273 (1971).

DISCUSSION

Question (Murthy): For *in vitro* initiation of λ transcription of the immunity region of λ, do you need any special factors and λ-specific polymerase?

Answer: Most probably, we need some specific factor(s) for the initiation of *cI-rex* mRNA synthesis at the p_c promoter, since we do not observe any RNA in this region when purified RNA polymerase and a λ DNA template are used.

Question (Mandal): What is the half-life of *E. coli* RNA polymerase and how long after lytic induction of λ does the host continue to make its own RNA polymerase?

Answer: As far as I know, *E. coli* RNA polymerase is a very stable protein and must survive λ induction, since synthesis of RNA is very active and remains rifampicin sensitive.

Question (Sambrook): The Dahlberg and Blattner experiments were done with limiting triphosphates: is it possible that this provides an explanation for the four starts that you find *in vitro* compared with the nine that exist *in vivo*?

Answer: In addition to the seven RNA starts shown in Fig. 2, there are leftward starts in the *int* and b2 regions, and rightward start(s) in b2, altogether ten or more *in vivo* starts. *In vitro,* there are four starts on the λb2 template, but at least two more starts are seen in the b2 region when λ⁺ DNA template is used. Under special conditions, Dr. Karin Carlson in our laboratory did observe the *lit* start (Fig. 2). The starts controlled by the p_c and p'_c, and extension of the start controlled by the p'_R promoter (Fig. 2) most probably require special factors, including the products of λ genes *cII, cIII,* and *Q.*

Question (Sambrook): About the *oop* RNA, if it is indeed involved in initiation of λ DNA synthesis it must be a "late" function. Why then do you find it transcribed *in vitro* by *E. coli* RNA polymerase?

Answer: The *in vitro* synthesis of *oop* RNA most probably reflects the very low constitutive level of this RNA, as indicated by the dotted arrows in Fig. 2a-c. Only after this transcription is stimulated fifty- to a hundred fold above the prophage level by the products of genes *O, P, dna*B, and *dna*G does the amount of *oop* RNA seem to become sufficient to serve as a primer for the initiation of λ DNA replication.

17

Termination and Antitermination in Transcription: Control of Gene Expression

Sankar Adhya, Max Gottesman, and Benoit de Crombrugghe

Laboratory of Molecular Biology
National Cancer Institute
National Institutes of Health
Bethesda, Maryland, U.S.A.

The expression of many, if not all, genes in microbial systems is regulated according to the "operon" model proposed by Jacob and Monod (1). Regulation occurs at the step of initiation of transcription of genes or operons, as was originally outlined by these authors (2). In known cases, this is accomplished by a specific repressor molecule interacting at the operator site to inhibit transcription from the cognate promoter locus (negative control) or a positive factor(s) stimulating transcription (positive control) or both (3,4). The *in vitro* controlled transcription of certain specific operons has already been demonstrated using purified RNA polymerase holoenzyme. The essential feature of these systems is that transcription is initiated by the correct initiating signals, i.e., promoters. For the *lac* and *gal* operons of *Escherichia coli*, correct initiation depends on the presence of additional positive control elements: cyclic AMP and its recepter protein (CRP) (5-7). In case of the immediate early operons of bacteriophage λ, however, correct transcription occurs just with RNA polymerase holoenzyme alone (8,9). In all of the above three systems, purified *lac, gal,* or λ repressor specifically inhibits the transcription of its respective operon (8-11).

Under the framework of the model of Jacob and Monod (2), the operons behave as discrete transcriptional units; for this to occur, it is imperative that transcription terminate at the promoter-distal end of these units. Although our knowledge about the mechanics of transcriptional termination is still meager, it is already becoming evident (12) that the control of transcription termination at the end of a gene would also control the expression of promoter-distal genes or operons. In what follows, we present some results obtained both *in vivo* and *in vitro* to elucidate, first, the genetic sites involved in termination and, second, the control of termination of transcription. For obvious reasons, we have studied two model systems: prophage λ and its chromosomal neighbor, the *gal* operon of *E. coli.*

TERMINATION FACTOR ρ

The termination of transcription *in vitro* can be influenced by a variety of factors (12-16). The addition of a protein factor, ρ (17), purified from *E. coli,* to an *in vitro* transcription system results in the synthesis of homogeneous RNA products. Transcripts made from λ, T4, and T7 DNA templates in the presence of this factor correspond to natural messenger RNA in both size and nucleotide sequence. It has been suggested that ρ reacts catalytically with RNA polymerase to produce termination, at specific sites, without influencing the initiation process (12,14). We shall discuss the capacity of ρ to terminate transcription of bacterial DNA templates. We have found that the *gal* operon of *E. coli* contains ρ-sensitive termination sites (7,22). We shall also discuss certain polar mutations of the *gal* operon caused by the insertion of a foreign piece of DNA containing a ρ-sensitive termination site (22).

EFFECT OF ρ ON *gal* OPERON

The *gal* operon of *E. coli* K12 consists of three structural genes, *K, T,* and *E,* with the operator-promoter region (*O-P*) situated at the *E* end (18,19). It is convenient for the study of *gal* transcription to use nondefective transducing phage carrying various segments of the *gal* operon (λp*gal*) (20). Their genetic structures are shown in Fig. 1. Controlled transcription of the *gal* operon has been achieved *in vitro* using the DNA from λp*gal*$_8^+$ phage, which carries an intact *gal* operon (7). As mentioned before, correct initiation of *gal* mRNA synthesis depends on the presence of RNA polymerase holoenzyme, cyclic AMP, and its receptor. The *gal* operon is transcribed from the *l* strand both *in vivo* and *in vitro* (7,21). The *gal*-specific mRNA is detected by exhaustive prehybridization of the *in vitro* RNA products with λ DNA (to remove λ mRNA) followed by hybridization with separated *l* strands of λp*gal* DNA. *Gal*-specific transcription is repressed by the addition of purified *gal* repressor, which binds to the cognate operator (11).

The effect of ρ on *in vitro* *gal*-specific transcription has been studied by analyzing the size of the RNA products. This involves sedimentation in linear

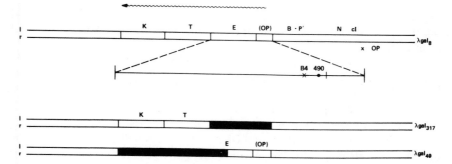

Fig. 1. Genetic map of λpgal DNAs used either as templates in the gal transcription reactions or as detectors in the DNA · RNA hybridization reactions. 490 is the insertion mutation, and B4 is the ochre. The dark areas correspond to the deleted segment.

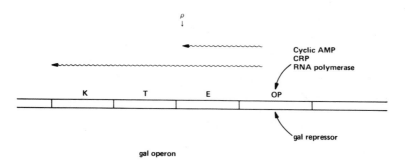

Fig. 2. Structure of the wild-type gal operon showing the extent of transcription in the presence and absence of ρ.

sucrose gradients and subsequent hybridization of each fraction to various segments of *gal* DNA (22). Most of the *gal* RNA products, made in the presence of 0.1 *M* KCl and absence of ρ, are very large molecules. These molecules contain λ-specific RNA sequences (corresponding to the *l* strand of the λ genes *J* through *A*, due to readthrough of transcription initiated from the *gal* promoter) (7). When 8 μg/ml of ρ is added to the incubation mixture, *gal*-specific RNA sequences sediment as a symmetrical peak with an S value of 14. This transcript is apparently pure *galE* mRNA; its length corresponds to the size of the *E* gene (about 1100 bases) and it is complementary only to *galE* DNA; i.e., it hybridizes to λp*gal*$_{49}$ (*E*) but not to λp*gal*$_{317}$ (*KT*) (see Fig. 1 and ref. 22). This indicates the presence of a ρ-sensitive transcription stop at or near the end of *E*, the first structural gene of the operon (Fig. 2). At low concentrations of ρ (0.5 μg/ml), *gal* RNA molecules ranging in size from 22-25S to 12-15S are synthesized. The polarity that ρ produces *in vitro* suggests that intraoperonic transcriptional termination may be the cause of "natural polarity" (synthesis of more polypeptide chains encoded by operator-proximal cistrons than by operator-distal ones) found in certain bacterial operons, including *gal* (D. Wilson, personal communication).

POLAR EFFECT OF INSERTION MUTATIONS

Some structural gene mutations in the *gal* operon reduce the expression of genes operator-distal to the mutated one (23-26). Of these polar mutations, one class originates by the insertion of a DNA piece of about 800 or 1400 base pairs of unknown origin (27-29). The insertion mutations are considerably more polar than polypeptide chain-terminating amber or ochre mutations. We believe that this extreme polarity is the consequence of transcription termination at the site of the insertion. Our conclusion rests on results obtained in the purified transcription system for *gal* mRNA synthesis using as template λp*gal*$^+_8$ DNA and derivatives of this phage that carry various polar mutations in the *gal* operon (Fig. 1). The presence of a polar ochre mutation (mutation B4 in the operator-proximal segment of *E*) in the template has no detectable effect on transcription; in this system, stimulation of *gal* mRNA synthesis by cyclic AMP and inhibition by ρ are seen for both wild-type and ochre template. The selective inhibition of distal RNA (*KT* region) relative to operator-proximal RNA (*E* gene) by ρ is also identical in the two templates (22). We have also studied the effect of an insertion mutation, designated 490,[1] on *gal* transcription. In the

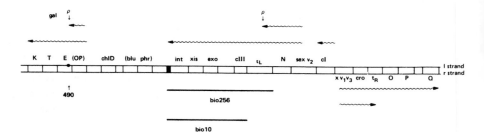

Fig. 3. Genetic map of the prophage λ *and adjacent genetic region of* Escherichia coli *K12 chromosome. K, T, E, O,* and *P* constitute the *gal* operon, *chlD, blu,* and *phr* are bacterial genes located between *gal* and λ with unknown directions of transcription. *sex* and v_2 are promoter and operator for transcription of the *l* strand (genes *N, c*III*, exo,* and *xis,* for example) and *x* and $v_1 v_3$ are for transcription of the *r* strand (genes *cro, O,* and *P,* for example) of λ DNA. The wavy lines indicate the orientation and direction of transcriptions. Note the position of gene *N.*

---

[1] The insertion mutation 490 maps in the operator-proximal end of the *E* cistron (Adhya, unpublished observations) and is composed of about 1400 nucleotide pairs (29).

absence of ρ, both the insertion and the mutant *gal* operon are transcribed normally. However, the addition of ρ completely inhibits cyclic-AMP-dependent *gal* transcription. The inhibition of transcription is the consequence of ρ-mediated termination of transcription at the site of insertion, which is early in the *E* gene. Transcription appears to terminate within the insertion itself. Furthermore, unlike the termination of transcription at the end of the *E* gene in the wild-type *gal* operon, very low concentrations of ρ (0.5 μg/ml) suffice to terminate transcription within the insertion (22). These results strongly support the idea that the insertion contains a transcription termination signal, dependent on ρ. The strong polar effect *in vivo* of such a mutation may also be the result of ρ-mediated termination of transcription.

ρ AND λ

Infection of *E. coli* K12 with bacteriophage λ or induction of cells lysogenic for a λ prophage leads to a regulated sequence of phage gene expression. First, the immediate early genes *N* and *cro* are expressed (for review, see ref. 30). Gene *N* is transcribed from the *l* strand of DNA starting from the *sex* promoter, and *cro* is transcribed from the *r* strand initiating at the *x* promoter (see the genetic map of prophage in Fig. 3). Next, the delayed-early genes located to the left of *N* and genes *O* and *P* to the right of *cro* are expressed. The product of gene *N* is needed for the expression of these functions (31). RNA synthesized *in vitro* from wild-type λ DNA by RNA polymerase holoenzyme contains RNA transcripts originating from the two early promoters, *sex* and *x,* but transcription proceeds beyond *N* and *cro,* respectively, to yield larger heterogeneous molecules (12). When incubations are carried out in the presence of ρ and 0.1 M KCl, transcription stops at t_L and t_R, termination signals to the left of *N* and right of *cro,* respectively (Fig. 3). The two products, a 12S RNA molecule corresponding to gene *N* and a 7S molecule corresponding to *cro,* are comparable to transcripts made *in vivo* by an *N* mutant (31). The observation that ρ-sensitive termination signals exist distal to genes *N* and *cro* and that *N* product is needed for efficient expression of genes beyond these signals led Roberts (12) to propose that *N* functions as an antiterminator factor in transcription; i.e., *N* product counteracts ρ, preventing transcription termination at t_L and t_R. The strongest support for this hypothesis is the observation that *N* stimulates the expression of delayed-early genes (*exo* and *O*) only when RNA synthesis is initiated at the promoters, for the immediate-early genes *sex* and *x* (32-34). When these promoters are inactivated by repression or mutation, no stimulation of delayed-early transcription by *N* product occurs. Furthermore, immediate-early transcription is independent of *N* (31).

ANTITERMINATION AND ESCAPE SYNTHESIS

We have tested the antitermination hypothesis of N product by studying its effect on the ρ-sensitive transcription termination sites introduced by the 490 insertion of the *gal* operon, described above. The results are shown in Table I. The *gal* operon is normally inducible by D-galactose or D-fucose (35); the addition of fucose to exponentially growing wild-type cells increased galacto-kinase levels after 90 min more than fourfold above that found in the absence of the inducer (lines 1 and 2). However, the amount of galactokinase made in cells carrying the *galE* insertion mutation 490 was undetectable in either the presence or the absence of fucose (lines 3 and 4). In another experiment, galactokinase was assayed in fucose-grown *galE*490 cells, after infection with phage λ. If the N protein of the infecting phage antagonized the action of ρ at the 490 site, the infected cells, as opposed to uninfected cells, would synthesize galactokinase. As shown in line 5, no detectable level of the enzyme was observed after infection.

Table I. Escape Synthesis of Galactokinase[a]

Experi-ment	Genotype of cell	Addition of 10^{-3} M fucose	Induced for	Temperature (°C)	Specific activity
1	$K^+T^+E^+$	-		32	1.4
2	,,	+	90 min	32	6.3
3	K^+T^+E490	-		32	0.1
4	,,	+	90 min	32	0.1
5[b]	,,	+	30 min	32	0.1
6	$K^+T^+E^+$ (λcI857xis6P3)	-		32	1.5
7	,,	+	30 min	32	3.2
8	,,	-	,,	41	7.2
9	,,	+	,,	41	10.4
10	K^+T^+E490 (λcI857xis6P3)	-		32	0.1
11	,,	+	30 min	32	0.1
12	,,	-	,,	41	5.9
13	,,	+	,,	41	5.3

[a]Galactokinase was assayed as described by Wilson and Hogness (36). The enzyme unit is nmoles of [^{3}H]galactose-phosphate formed per minute per 10^9 cells. Cells were grown at 32°C in M56 minimal medium supplemented with 0.3% glycerol plus 0.1% Casamino acid and treated with D-fucose or heated to 41°C to induce the prophage or both for indicated period of time. Cells were then chilled, and enzyme was extracted after centrifugation and treatment with 0.6 mg/ml of egg-white lysozyme in the presence of 7×10^{-3} M EDTA in 0.1 M tris-C1 (pH 8.0).

[b]In experiment 5, cells were infected with λcI857 at zero time.

Thus either λ N function cannot suppress the 490 termination signal or the experimental conditions are inappropriate for demonstrating this effect.

We shall demonstrate that λ N function can in fact suppress the 490 insertion and that this suppression has the same requirement as the N-mediated suppression of t_L, namely, an active *sex* promoter *cis* to the *gal* operon.

The *gal* operon is derepressed by the induction of a λ prophage (37,38). Although other models have been proposed to explain this "escape synthesis" of *gal* enzymes (39), it is now clear that it is the sum of two different processes (Adhya and Gottesman, in preparation; Buttin, unpublished): (a) uncontrolled replication of the *gal* operon along with prophage DNA (dependent on λ replication genes O and P) with the resultant titration of the cellular *gal* repressor (replicational escape); and (b) transcription originating at the *sex* promoter and extending through the *gal* operon (transcriptional escape). It is already known that transcription originating from an upstream promoter is insensitive to its normal repressor (40). Note that the *sex*-promoted transcription of *gal* follows the same strand and direction as that initiated at the *gal* promoter (Fig. 3). This second component of escape synthesis was applied to study the antitermination role of N.

Bacterial strains lysogenic for phage λ carrying an excision-defective mutation (*xis*) to amplify the *sex*-promoted transcriptional escape and a replication-defective mutation (P) to eliminate replicational escape were used. The prophage also carries a thermolabile repressor (*c*I857) to facilitate induction of the prophage. When a *gal*$^+$ cell, lysogenic for this prophage, is induced by heat, the level of galactokinase is increased from a low basal level by about fivefold in 30 min (lines 6-9). This level can be further increased by the addition of an inducer of the *gal* operon, fucose. A similar lysogen, but carrying the ρ-sensitive insertion mutation 490 in the E gene, also makes a large amount of kinase when the prophage is heat induced (lines 10-13). Addition of fucose, however, does not further derepress the operon, suggesting that only transcription from the *sex* promoter can penetrate the polar insertion. Further experiments have shown that the suppression of polarity by transcriptional escape from the *sex* promoter has an absolute requirement for N function. Given these conditions, all polar mutations in the *gal* operon that we have tested (long and short insertions as well as ochres) can be suppressed. This suggests that all polarity involves termination of transcription by ρ factor.

CONCLUSION

It has been shown, in a purified system, that the protein factor ρ can profoundly affect transcription of a bacterial operon. It can terminate transcription not only at the end of an operon but also at the end of the first structural gene of the operon. These effects of ρ *in vitro* may parallel those *in vivo*—the former explaining how operons can behave as transcriptional units, while the latter may account for natural polarity. Another example of the effects of ρ is the severe reduction of the expression of distal genes caused by insertion of a DNA site strongly sensitive to ρ within the operon. ρ-sensitive sites (t_L and t_R) are also present in the wild-type DNA of phage λ. Roberts proposed that N stimulates the expression of the genes located beyond t_L and t_R by antagonizing ρ-mediated transcription termination at these sites (17). Our observation that N product, under given conditions, can overcome the ρ-dependent transcriptional terminators present in the insertion mutations of the *gal* operon supports that hypothesis.

REFERENCES

1. F. Jacob and J. Monod. *J. Mol. Biol.* **3**:318 (1961).
2. F. Jacob and J. Monod. *Cold Spring Harbor Symp. Quant. Biol.* **26**:193 (1961).
3. W. Epstein and J. Beckwith. *Ann. Rev. Biochem.* **37**:411 (1968).
4. H. Echols. In A. D. Hershey (ed.), *The Bacteriophage Lambda,* Cold Spring Harbor Laboratory, New York, p. 247 (1971).
5. R. Perlman, B. Chen, B. de Crombrugghe, M. Emmer, M. Gottesman, H. Varmus, and L. Pastan. *Cold Spring Harbor Symp. Quant. Biol.* **35**:419 (1970).
6. R. Arditti, L. Eron, G. Zubay, G. Tocchini-Valentini, S. Connaway, and J. Beckwith. *Cold Spring Harbor Symp. Quant. Biol.* **35**:437 (1970).
7. S. P. Nissley, W. Anderson, M. Gottesman, R. Perlman, and I. Pastan. *J. Biol. Chem.* **246**:4671 (1971).
8. P. Chadwick, V. Pirrotta, R. Steinberg, N. Hopkins, and M. Ptashne. *Cold Spring Harbor Symp. Quant. Biol.* **35**:283 (1970).
9. A. Wu, S. Ghosh, M. Willard, J. Davison, and H. Echols. In A. D. Hershey (ed.), *The Bacteriophage Lambda,* Cold Spring Harbor Laboratory, New York, p. 589 (1971).
10. B. de Crombrugghe, B. Chen, W. Anderson, P. Nissley, M. Gottesman, I. Pastan, and R. Perlman. *Nature New Biol.* **231**:139 (1971).
11. S. Nakamshi, S. Adhya, M. Gottesman, and I. Pastan. *Proc. Natl. Acad. Sci. (USA),* **70**:334 (1973).
12. J. Roberts. *Cold Spring Harbor Symp. Quant. Biol.* **35**:121 (1970).
13. U. Maitra, A. Lockwood, J. Dubnoff, and A. Guha. *Cold Spring Harbor Symp. Quant. Biol.* **35**:143 (1970).
14. A. Goldberg. *Cold Spring Harbor Symp. Quant. Biol.* **35**:157 (1970).
15. C. Goff and E. Minkley. In L. Silvestri (ed.), *Lepetit Colloquium on RNA Polymerase and Transcription,* North-Holland, Amsterdam, p. 124 (1970).
16. A. Travers. *Nature* **225**:1009 (1970).
17. J. Roberts. *Nature* **224**:1168 (1969).
18. G. Buttin. *J. Mol. Biol.* **7**:183 (1963).
19. J. Shapiro and S. Adhya. *Genetics* **62**:249 (1969).
20. M. Feiss, S. Adhya, and D. Court. *Genetics* **71**:189 (1972).
21. A. Guha, M. Tabaczynski, and W. Szybalski. *J. Mol. Biol.* **35**:207 (1968).
22. B. de Crombrugghe, S. Adhya, M. Gottesman, and I. Pastan. *Nature,* **241**:260 (1973).
23. S. Adhya and J. Shapiro. *Genetics* **62**:231 (1969).
24. J. Shapiro and S. Adhya. *Genetics* **62**:249 (1969).

25. E. Jordan and H. Saedler. *Mol. Gen. Genet.* **100**:283 (1967).
26. E. Jordan, H. Saedler, and P. Starlinger. *Mol. Gen. Genet.* **100**:296 (1967).
27. J. Shapiro. *J. Mol. Biol.* **40**:93 (1969).
28. E. Jordan, H. Saedler, and P. Starlinger. *Mol. Gen. Genet.* **102**:353 (1968).
29. M. Fiandt, W. Szybalski, and M. Malamy. *Mol. Gen. Genet.,* **119**:223 (1972).
30. W. Szybalski. In R. K. Zahn and R. Blasberg (eds.), *Informational Directed Synthesis,* Vol. 6, p. 9, F. Steiner Verlag, Wiesbaden, Germany (1972).
31. P. Kourilsky, M. Bourguignon, M. Bouquet, and F. Gros. *Cold Spring Harbor Symp. Quant. Biol.* **35**:305 (1970).
32. P. Kourilsky, L. Marcaud, P. Shildrick, D. Luzzati, and F. Gros. *Proc. Natl. Acad. Sci. (USA)* **61**:1013 (1968).
33. S. Kumar, K. Bovre, A. Guha, Z. Hradecna, V. Maher, and W. Szybalski. *Nature* **221**:823 (1969).
34. S. Heinemann and W. Spiegelman. *Cold Spring Harbor Symp. Quant. Biol.* **35**:315 (1970).
35. G. Buttin. *J. Mol. Biol.* **7**:164 (1963).
36. D. Wilson and D. Hogness. In E. Neufield and V. Ginsburg (eds.), *Methods in Enzymology, Vol. 8,* pp. 229-240 (1966).
37. G. Buttin, F. Jacob, and J. Monod. *Compt. Rend. Acad. Sci.* **250**:2471 (1960).
38. M. Yarmolinsky and H. Wiesmeyer. *Proc. Natl. Acad. Sci. (USA)* **46**:1626 (1960).
39. H. Echols, B. Butler, A. Joyner, M. Willard, and L. Pilarski. In J. Colter (ed.), *Molecular Biology of Viruses,* Academic Press, New York, p. 125 (1967).
40. K. Krell, M. Gottesman, J. Parks, and M. Eisenberg. *J. Mol. Biol.* **68**:69 (1972).

DISCUSSION

Question (Kumar): In your *in vitro* system, do you get an effect of ρ on the size of *gal* mRNA if the template is such that genes E and T are fused by an internal deletion?

Answer: We have just been able to isolate such a strain and are currently doing the experiment.

Question (Kumar): You have shown that N product can suppress an ochre mutation in *e*. How do you explain the existence of ochre mutations in λ?

Answer: We have shown that N product can suppress the polar effect of an ochre mutation and not the mutation itself.

18

Control of Transcription in *Neurospora crassa*

P. R. Mahadevan
Chief of Research and Development
Antibiotics Plant
Virbhadra, U.P., India

and

A. S. Bhagwat
Biology and Agriculture Division
Bhabha Atomic Research Centre
Trombay, Bombay, India

Gene expression can be assessed by the amounts and types of RNA synthesized at any growth period. No differences were observed in the polynucleotide sequences of DNA from different organs, although large differences were noted among the rapidly labeled RNAs isolated from these tissues (1). The method of molecular hybridization has permitted measurement of the extent of gene activity. This technique has also helped in the identification of tissue-specific RNA by means of competition-hybridization experiments (2,3). All these studies indicated the existence of regulated gene activity as expressed by differential gene expression. Such a regulation has been suggested as a basic molecular event behind the processes of cell differentiation and morphogenesis.

Several chemical factors influence *in vitro* RNA synthesis by DNA-dependent RNA polymerase of *Escherichia coli* (4). Some stimulate transcription by the enzyme (5), and others such as rifamycin (6), Streptovaricin, and B_{44} (7,8) inhibit enzyme activity. Basic proteins isolated from nuclei of eukaryotes also cause inhibition of *in vitro* RNA synthesis normally occurring in the presence of the RNA polymerase of *E. coli* (9). However, the physiological significance of this type of inhibition is still unknown. A trypsin-sensitive, template-selective inhibitor of RNA polymerase has been isolated from *spo*I-infected *Bacillus subtilis* (10). Proteins that can bind to DNA that are produced at specific stages of the cell cycle in HeLa cells have also been identified recently. However, their action on RNA polymerase is not known. A definite possibility is indicated that *in vivo* transcriptional control can be due to some of these factors.

In this chapter, we report experimental results that show the extent of and differences in gene activity during three stages of growth of *Neurospora* and the presence of two proteins that inhibit *in vitro* polynucleotide synthesis by the DNA-dependent RNA polymerase of *Neurospora crassa* and *E. coli*. These proteins, which are produced only at a specific stage of the life cycle, have the capacity to bind to *Neurospora* DNA and seem to be selectively complexed to some regions of the DNA. They thus show some properties of *in vivo* repressors of transcription.

RESULTS

Hybridizable mRNA During Various Growth Periods

Nonribosomal, rapidly labeled RNA species from *Neurospora* after growth periods of 8, 16, and 24 hr were labeled with [^{3}H]uridine and used for hybridization with DNA. Figure 1 shows the maximum hybridizable RNA present in the RNA samples isolated after these growth periods. It is clear that the saturation values are different for the different growth periods. This perhaps

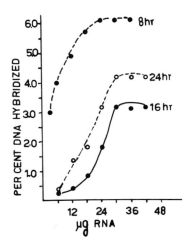

Fig. 1. Saturation level for hybridization of mRNA from 8-, 16-, and 24-hr growth periods. Each point is an average of three separate experiments.

Table I. Hybridization Values for Total
Pulse-Labeled RNA with DNA[a]

Total RNA from growth period[b] (hr)	Percent DNA hybridized (three separate experiments)		
	1	2	3
8	9.8	9.7	9.82
16	6.4	6.48	6.35
24	7.6	7.8	7.49

[a]Hybridization experiments were carried out essentially according to the method of Gillespie and Spiegelman (11). The optimum conditions for such hybridization with preparations from *Neurospora* were reported earlier (12). DNA was isolated from lyophilized mycelia using Marmur's method (13). RNA was isolated by a modification of Kirby's method (14). The isolation and characterization of mRNA species have been described earlier (11).

[b]Specific activity of the RNA: 8 hr, 850 cpm/μg; 16 hr, 352 cpm/μg; 24 hr, 690 cpm/μg.

shows that the number of genes active during the three growth periods differs, being highest at 8 hr.

The RNA isolated and characterized as messenger RNA showed template activity *in vitro* and did not show any competition with the ribosomal RNA isolated after the same growth periods.

The total RNA extracted from a culture pulse-labeled with [^{3}H] uridine was also used for hybridization experiments. The results are presented in Table I, which shows the total hybridizable rapidly labeled RNA from these three growth periods. The highest saturation value for 8-hr RNA is still evident.

Another experiment was done in which DNA was first hybridized with unlabeled transfer and ribosomal RNAs, both purified by methylated albumin - kieselguhr chromatography. Duplicate samples were treated with RNase to remove loosely bound RNA from the membrane filter. Then one set was further exposed to labeled tRNA and rNA to show that the sites on DNA for these species are occupied by unlabeled tRNA and rRNA. The other set was allowed to hybridize with a pulse-labeled RNA preparation. This was done for samples from all three growth periods. Table II shows the hybridization levels with pulse-labeled total RNA after saturating the sites for tRNA and rRNA. The values for hybridization of 7.55, 3.55, and 3.9 for 8-, 16-, and 24-hr cultures, respectively, seen in this experiment are close to the data obtained as hybridization values for isolated mRNA species (12). This clearly shows that the satura-

Table II. Hybridization Values for Pulse-
Labeled RNA After Saturation of DNA
Sites with tRNA and rRNA[a]

Total RNA from growth period (hr)	Percent DNA hybridized	
	1	2
8	7.55	7.6
16	3.55	3.52
24	3.9	4.1

[a]Purified DNA samples free of any protein or
RNA contamination were dissolved in 0.24 M
phosphate buffer (pH 6.8). DNA samples (10
mg/ml) were then sheared by ultrasonic dis-
integration at 20 kc/sec for 1 min, and the
buffer strength was diluted to 0.12 M with
distilled water. DNA was denatured in a boiling-water bath for 15 min and transferred immediately to an ice bath.

tion values obtained in the earlier experiments with isolated nonribiosomal RNA
have no contribution from tRNA and rRNA. The techniques and complete data
leading to these conclusions were published earlier (12).

Hybridizable RNA or DNA Isolated from Different Growth Periods (Hydroxylapatite Chromatography)

Hybridization of ^{32}P-labeled DNA was carried out with ^{3}H-labeled RNA by
hydroxylapatite chromatography (16). The RNA·DNA hybrids were separated
from single-stranded DNA and RNA by chromatography of the sample on a
hydroxylapatite column at elevated temperature. In this system, the amount of
labeled DNA that remained adsorbed to the column and eluted only at a higher
molarity of phosphate buffer (0.48 M) was considered as the amount hybridized
to RNA. The percent hybridization was expressed as the percent of the input
DNA that remained in the form of hybrid with RNA. The amount of input DNA
was kept constant in all the experiments. From the specific activity of the DNA
preparation, the amount of DNA hybridized to RNA was calculated. These data
are presented in Table III after correction for self-reassociation. This was
achieved by hybridizing ^{32}P-labeled *Neurospora* DNA to nonhomologous *E. coli*
DNA (unlabeled). The hybridizable DNA was 9.9, 5.2, and 6.0% (experiment 1)
for 8, 16, and 24 hr growth, respectively. It should be noted that the values are
quite comparable to those obtained by the membrane technique as the amount

of RNA hybridized and by an independent verification of the saturation values obtained earlier (see Table I).

Competition-Hybridization Experiments (Membrane Techniques)

To test whether or not similar species of mRNA were produced during the three growth periods, competition hybridization was done. The amount of radioactivity in hybrids using 8-hr RNA in the presence of increasing amounts of 16-hr RNA was gradually reduced (Fig. 2, left) until it leveled off at 66% of the original hybridizable level. This indicated that between 8 and 16 hr the RNA has homology to some extent (up to 34%); at the same time, new species were present at 8 hr that were not seen at 16 hr. The reciprocal experiment (Fig. 2, right) also showed that at 16 hr there were common species (up to 42%) with 8 hr, while the rest were new species characteristic of 16 hr. Figure 3 presents the data for such an experiment between 8-hr and 24-hr DNA. This also shows the presence of new species at 24 hr and common species or homology (up to 68%) in 8-hr and 24-hr DNA.

In all hybridization experiments using membranes, the controls were those wherein hybridization was done using labeled RNA in the presence of unlabeled RNA from the same culture (growth period), and the competition was nearly 100%.

Table III. Amount of $[^{32}P]$DNA Hybridizable to RNA (Hydroxylapatite Chromatography)[a]

Total RNA from growth period[b] (hr)	Percent DNA hybridized 1	2	Comparable data from Table I[c]
8	9.9	9.88	9.8
16	5.2	5.15	6.4
24	6.0	6.02	7.6

[a]In hybridization experiments 5 μg of ^{32}p-labeled DNA was incubated in 0.12 M phosphate buffer with 250 μg of ^{3}H-labeled RNA (pulse-labeled total RNA) for 52 hr at 30°C in a water bath. After the incubation period, the sample was immediately frozen and kept until it was analyzed on the column. The hydroxylapatite column was prepared according to the method of Miyazawa and Thomas (15). The chromatography was done according to the method of Kohne (16).

[b]Specific activity of RNA: 8 hr, 2244 cpm/μg; 16 hr, 1982 cpm/μg; 24 hr, 800 cpm/μg.

[c]Data from molecular hybridization by the membrane technique.

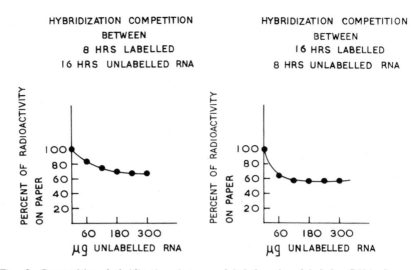

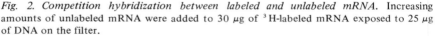

Fig. 2. Competition hybridization between labeled and unlabeled mRNA. Increasing amounts of unlabeled mRNA were added to 30 μg of ³H-labeled mRNA exposed to 25 μg of DNA on the filter.

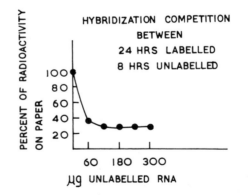

Fig. 3. Competition hybridization between 24-hr labeled mRNA and 8-hr unlabeled mRNA. Amounts of DNA and labeled RNA were the same as in Fig. 2.

Presence of RNA Synthesis Inhibitor in *Neurospora*

Crude extract from a 9-hr culture of *Neurospora* when added to a reaction mixture of polynucleotide synthesis resulted in inhibition of RNA synthesis to a significant extent (Fig. 4 and Table IV). In this experiment, the DNA was incubated with the crude extract for 10 min before the reaction was initiated;

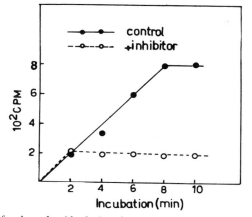

Fig. 4. Synthesis of polynucleotide during the time of incubation of the reaction mixture with or without the inhibitor. The inhibitor was present with the DNA before the reaction was started by addition of other components.

Table IV. Inhibition of Polynucleotide Synthesis[a]

Sample	[^{14}C] ATP incorporated into acid-insoluble precipitate (cpm)		
	1	2	3
Control	1462	572	406
Same, but DNA was incubated with crude *Neurospora* extract[b]	728	266	200

[a]The strain of *N. crassa* used in these experiments was RL 3-8-A (Rockefeller wild type). The fungus was grown from a conidial inoculum for 9 hr in 100 ml of 2% sucrose, minimal salt solution in a conical flask placed on a rotary shaker at 30°C. The mycelial mass was homogenized with sand in tris buffer (0.04 M tris at pH 8.1, 0.001 M β-mercaptoethanol, 0.2 mM EDTA, 0.01 M MgCl$_2$), and the supernatant obtained after contrifugation for 30 min at 30,000 X g was concentrated by lyophilization and resuspended in a small volume of buffer after extensive dialysis against the same buffer. The concentrated crude extract was used as a source of the inhibitor. The procedure of the assay and the components of the incubation mixture were basically similar to those described by Maitra and Hurwitz (17).

[b]DNA used as template was incubated with *Neurospora* extract for 10 min before other components were added to start the reaction.

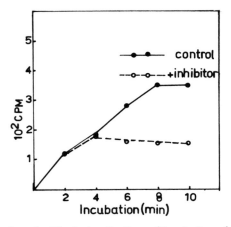

Fig. 5. Synthesis of polynucleotide during the time of incubation of the reaction mixture with or without the inhibitor. The inhibitor was added to DNA along with all other components.

the same amount of nonspecific protein (albumin) when added to the reaction mixture failed to show any inhibition of RNA synthesis, indicating that the inhibition is caused by some specific proteins. However, addition of the crude extract along with all other components for *in vitro* RNA synthesis produced no inhibition during the first 4 min but no further increase in RNA synthesis thereafter (Fig. 5). In both experiments, polynucleotide synthesis was demonstrated every 2 min during 10 min of incubation.

Binding of Inhibitor to DNA

Experiments with this inhibitor described in the previous paragraph indicated that it probably binds to DNA before inhibiting RNA synthesis. This possibility was checked by experimental tests that could show complex formation of the inhibitor molecule with DNA and dissociation of such a complex after purification.

The binding proteins inhibitory for *in vitro* RNA synthesis were purified by DNA-cellulose column chromatography (18). This step resolved these proteins into two distinct peaks (Fig. 6) which were eluted from the column with 0.15 and 0.6 *M* NaCl, respectively. These two peaks were pooled and loaded on Sephadex G75 column. From Fig. 7, it can be seen that again these proteins resolved into two peaks. All the fractions were checked for their inhibition of polynucleotide synthesis.

These fractions were pooled and dialyzed to remove sodium chloride. The concentrated samples were tested for their inhibitory activity toward *in vitro* RNA synthesis using *N. crassa* or *E. coli* polymerase (Table V). It is evident from

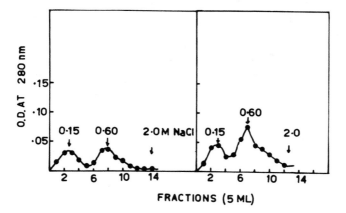

Fig. 6. Chromatography of Neurospora extract on a DNA-cellulose column. The ordinate gives optical destiny eluted in each fraction. *Neurospora* mycelia grown for 9 hr were homogenized with acid-washed sand in a solution containing 0.04 M tris-Cl (pH 8.1), 0.001 M β-mercaptoethanol, 0.2 mM EDTA, and 0.01 M MgCl$_2$. The homogenate was centrifuged for 45 min at 16,000 rpm. The supernatant was dialyzed against a buffer containing 0.02 M tris-Cl, 0.001 M β-mercaptoethanol, 0.2 mM EDTA (pH 8.1). DNA-cellulose was prepared using *Neurospora* DNA. A column containing 2 g of cellulose (1.2 mg of DNA bound per g of cellulose) was equilibrated with the same buffer but without Mg^{2+}; in addition, 10% glycerol and 0-5 mg/ml bovine serum albumin (rinse buffer) were used. Approximately 20 mg of cell proteins was added to the column. After the extract had passed into the DNA-cellulose, the flow was shut off for 15 min. Flow was then resumed, and the column was washed with 15 vol of rinse buffer without Mg^{2+} and then 25 vol of rinse buffer without albumin. The bound proteins were eluted with 7 vol each of 0.15, 0.6, and 2.0 M NaCl. Fractions of 1.3 ml were collected, and fractions were scanned at 280 nm.

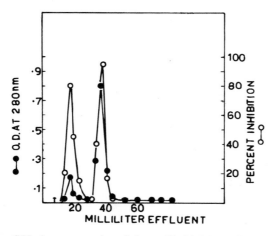

Fig. 7. Sephadex G75 chromatography of the purified inhibitor from DNA-cellulose chromatography. A Sephadex column 1.3 by 20 cm was loaded with 1 mg of protein and eluted with dilute NaCl solution. Each fraction was assayed for inhibitory activity.

Table V. Inhibition of RNA Polymerase by Proteins
That Bind to DNA (as Determined by DNA-
Cellulose Chromatography)

[^{14} C] ATP incorporated into acid-insoluble precipitate (cpm)

	E. coli polymerase		*Neurospora* polymerase	
	1	2	1	2
Control (complete reaction mixture)	287	286	278	661
Reaction mixture with DNA-binding protein	42	101	73/86[a]	126/86[a]

[a]Duplicates.

Table VI. Inhibition of Polynucleotide Synthesis by
Proteins Using Different DNAs as Template[a]

	[^{14} C] ATP incorporated into acid-insoluble precipitate (cpm)	
Template DNA from	Control	With inhibitor protein
1. *N. crassa*	279	42
2. *E. coli*	310	72
3. Calf thymus	290	31

[a]Values are average of two experiments.

Table V and Fig. 6 that proteins having a binding affinity for DNA caused the inhibition of RNA synthesis.

Both peaks obtained by Sephadex chromatography were pooled and were used for further experiments. These proteins showed no specificity with respect to the DNA used, since inhibition was observed even if the DNA was from *E. coli* or calf thymus (Table VI).

Nature of the Inhibitor

The protein nature of the inhibitor was indicated by (a) the loss of activity upon Pronase treatment (Table VII), (b) the incorporation of [^{14} C] leucine into purified inhibitor, and (c) the separation of purified inhibitor proteins into two discrete protein bands on acrylamide gel electrophoresis at pH 8.3 (Fig. 8). The

Table VII. Pronase Reversal of Inhibition[a]

Sample	[14 C] ATP incorporated into acid-insoluble precipitate (cpm)
Control	963
Same, but with partially purified inhibitor	101
Same, but inhibitor was Pronase-treated before use[b]	512[c]
	484[c]

[a]RNA polymerase from *Neurospora* was prepared from the nuclei of the fungus. Crude extract prepared according to the method of Roeder and Rutter (19) was fractionated on a DEAE-Sephadex column. All the fractions showing enzyme activity were pooled and used as a source of the enzyme.

[b]Partially purified inhibitor was treated with 50 µg/ml of nuclease-free Pronase in 0.01 M phosphate buffer (pH 7.0) for 1 hr.

[c]Duplicates.

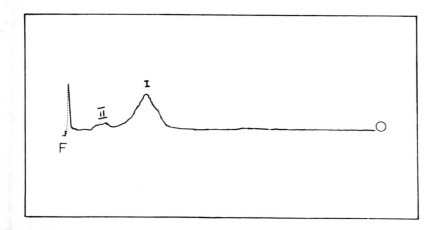

Fig. 8. Polyacrylamide gel electrophoresis on 7% standard gel of proteins eluted from the DNA-cellulose column. Gels were scanned in a densitometer. The electrophoresis was based on the method of Davis (20).

proteins hardly migrated from the origin in an acid gel at pH 4.3, suggesting a nonbasic nature. This is interesting because histones have been shown to be absent in *Neurospora* (21), also, (d) the inhibitor did not degrade the product of RNA polymerase assay systems; therefore, we believe that this inhibitor is not a nuclease (Table VIII). The crude extract was dialyzed in buffer containing no

Table VIII. Effect of Inhibitor Protein on the
Preformed Product (Polynucleotide)[a]

	[^{14}C] ATP incorporated in acid-insoluble portion (cpm)
Complete reaction mixture (control)	387
Inhibitor protein added at 0 min of reaction	97
Inhibitor added after 10 min of enzymatic synthesis (20 min incubation with the inhibitor)	367

[a]Values are the average of two different experiments.

divalent cations, and the elution from the DNA-cellulose column was also achieved by the same buffer. Under these conditions, no DNase was adsorbed to the column (less than 0.05%), eliminating the possibility of the inhibitor being a DNase.

Specificity of the Binding

The binding of these proteins indicated a high affinity for DNA, because after saturating the DNA-cellulose column with 0.5% albumin about 1.35% of the total input *Neurospora* proteins remained bound to DNA and could be eluted only with 0.15 and 0.6 M NaCl.

Furthermore, it was checked as to whether the proteins have any specificity to some regions of DNA. This was done by isolating the rRNA cistron of DNA and determining the ability of these proteins to form complexes with these DNA fragments as compared to the total DNA region. Lack of binding to ribosomal cistrons of *N. crassa* is shown by the data presented in Table IX. Ribosomal cistrons purified by hydroxylapatite column chromatography (16) did not show any binding to the purified proteins, as seen by the insignificant amount of complex trapped on the filter (22). In the control where total DNA regions were used, there was significant binding and the complex could be trapped in the filter.

Isolated rDNA cistrons were demonstrated to be functional in serving as a template for RNA synthesis (Table X). When rDNA was used as a template for RNA synthesis, these inhibitor proteins did not show any inhibition of RNA

Table IX. Comparison of Binding of Inhibitor Protein to Ribosomal Cistron and Total DNA[a]

	Cpm on the paper after reaction and DNase treatment of complex	
	1	2
[32]P-labeled rRNA cistron + protein	305	449
[32]P-labeled total DNA + protein	2047	3102
[^{32}P] DNA only (blank)	142	149

[a]The reaction was carried out as detailed earlier. The same amounts of DNA and protein were taken for binding studies in rRNA cistron and total DNA, i.e., 10 μg of DNA + 20 μg of protein and 20 μg of serum albumin in tris buffer. Specific activity of rRNA cistron was 1600 cpm/μg and total DNA 1430 cpm/μg. Ribosomal RNA cistrons were purified according to the method of Kohne (16), Ribosomal RNA was purified through a MAK column. Ribosomal RNA cistrons were characterized by reassociation kinetics and their *in vitro* ability to serve as template for ribosomal RNA synthesis. The inhibitor activity was assayed according to the method of Riggs *et al.* (22), slightly modified. In the method, 20 μg of purified protein was added to 0.5 ml of an assay mixture containing 10 μg of ^{32}P-labeled rRNA cistrons or denatured [^{32}P]DNA, 20 μg bovine serum albumin, 10 mM tris-Cl (pH 7.9), 10 mM MgCl$_2$, 0.1 mM dithiothreitol, 0.1 mM EDTA, and 0.5 mM KCl. Duplicate samples were incubated at 30°C for 15 min and the free DNA was digested by 25 μg/ml of DNase I for 20 min. The DNase-resistant complex was then precipitated with the addition of 10% trichloroacetic acid and carrier DNA. Samples were filtered through a Millipore filter, washed three or four times with 50% acid, and dried. The radioactivity on the paper was determined in a liquid scintillation spectrometer using BBOT (0.4%) in toluene as scintillation fluid.

Table X. *In Vitro* RNA Synthesis Using Isolated rDNA (^{32}P-Labeled)[a]

	[^{3}H]ATP incorporated into acid-insoluble precipitate (cpm)
1. rDNA (control)	682
2. rDNA + inhibitor	652
3. rDNA + actinomycin D	282

[a]Conditions of incubation were the same as described in the footnote to Table IX.

synthesis (Table X). This observation indicates that these proteins do not bind to the rDNA region and so fail inhibition of RNA synthesis.

Presence of Inhibitor in the Cytoplasm

The presence of the inhibitor was checked by using a cell-free extract from 9- and 16-hr cultures. The data presented in Table XI show that the inhibitor is present in the cytoplasm of a 9-hr culture but not in that of a 16-hr culture.

Table XI. Presence of Inhibitor at 9 and 16 hr of Growth

| | Radioactivity incorporated into polynucleotide (cpm)[a] | | |
	1	2	3
1. Complete reaction mixture (no crude extract)	572	1462	2536
2. With 9-hr extract	259	728	910
3. With 16-hr extract	693	1135	2430

[a]Conditions of incubation were the same as Table IV.

Table XII. Effect of Activator (Fv) on *In Vitro* RNA Synthesis in the Presence of the Inhibitor[a]

| Experiment | Acid-insoluble counts on the paper | | |
	1	2	3
Blank	154		
Control (no inhibitor)	834	830	865
Inhibitor + Fv added simultaneously	524	513	512
Fv added to DNA 5 min before the repressor was added	614	609	609

[a]The incubation mixture (0.6 ml) contained 20 μM tris buffer (pH 8.1), 5 μM mgSO$_4$, 8 μM mercaptoethanolamine, 3 μM spermidine, 60 μg calf thymus or *Neurospora* DNA, 0.25 μg each of CTP, GTP, and UTP, [8-^{14}C]ATP (specific activity 3 X 10^5 cpm/0.1 μmole), and RNA polymerase. The reaction was allowed to proceed for 10 min.

Effect of an Activator on Transcription *In Vitro* in the Presence of Inhibitor Isolated from *N. crassa*

A protein factor isolated from red kidney beans (*Phaseolus vulgaris*) stimulates RNA synthesis in plasmolyzed *E. coli* cells (Erhenberg, personal communication). We used this activator (Fv) to check whether it can compete with the inhibitor isolated from *Neurospora*. When both the activator and the inhibitor are added to the system for RNA synthesis, there is a partial reversal of inhibition by the inhibitor (Table XII). If inhibitor is added 5 min before the activator, the total synthesis is only slightly increased (Table XIII). This indicates that the site of action of both these factors on the DNA is probably the same. The slight increase in the synthesis due to the addition of activator after the treatment with inhibitor indicates the same. Thus the activator may be of the derepressing type and the inhibitor may function as a repressor.

GENERAL DISCUSSION AND CONCLUSIONS

From the hybridization data, it is evident that gene activity is quite high at the 8-hr growth period as compared to 16 and 24 hr. A very similar observation was also made by DNA·RNA hybridization using hydroxylapatite column chromatography. It is also clear from the competition experiments that there are new species of RNA during the various stages of growth. Thus the three stages of growth showed differences in the extent and quality of active genes, indicating differential gene action in *Neurospora* during the growth period of 8-24 hr.

It is to be noted that the estimate of gene activity derived from our experiments concerns only those RNA molecules synthesized during the short

Table XIII. Effect of Activator (Fv) in the Presence of Inhibitor

Experiment	Cpm on paper		
	1	2	3
Blank	135		
Control (no inhibitor)	853	865	850
Control + Fv	853	860	860
With inhibitor	313	300	330
Inhibitor added 5 min before the addition of the Fv	396	414	448

period of labeling. However, even when the cultures were labeled for longer times, the pattern was same, except for the fact that the percent hybridization was much higher (unpublished data).

As the DNA function was affected in the growth period, we looked into the possibility of the presence of molecules that might bring about such control of RNA synthesis. We have shown that there are possibly two protein molecules that have a binding affinity for DNA and can thereby block transcription.

The binding of these proteins to DNA seems to be somewhat site specific, as they bind only to regions other than the ribosomal DNA region and the proteins are not always present but only at a specific time in the life cycle.

To check whether it acts at the same level as the DNA-binding proteins, we used an activator factor isolated from red kidney beans. This activator does not activate RNA polymerase but is supposed to stimulate RNA synthesis by derepressing regions of DNA (Erhenberg, unpublished data). We observed derepression of the DNA molecule, earlier repressed by the inhibitor isolated from $N.$ $crassa$, by the activator (Fv). Therefore, it is possible that this inhibitor acts at the same site as the activator, possibly by blocking the operator site O or promoter site P.

Thus it is concluded that there are at least two proteins in $N.$ $crassa$ that act as repressors of RNA synthesis and are present in the cytoplasm only during the peak RNA synthesis period, i.e., at 8-10 hr, but that later affect the amount of RNA synthesized at 16 and 24 hr, perhaps by remaining complexed with DNA in the nuclei. During this later period, the proteins are not present in the cytoplasm. These proteins affect only nonribosomal RNA, which might include significant amounts of mRNA. Such site- and time-specific proteins are significant as controlling elements of mRNA transcription and thereby for the physiology of the fungus as well.

REFERENCES

1. B. J. McCarthy and B. H. Hoyer. *Proc. Natl. Acad. Sci. (USA)* **52**:915-922 (1964).
2. E. H. Davidson, M. Crippa, and A. E. Mirsky. *Proc. Natl. Acad. Sci. (USA)* **60**:152-159 (1968).
3. J. Paul and R. S. Gilmour. *J. Mol. Biol.* **34**:305-316 (1968).
4. M. Chamberlin and P. Berg. *Proc. Natl. Acad. Sci. (USA)* **48**:81-94 (1962).
5. R. R. Burgess, A. A. Travers, J. J. Dunn, and E. F. K. Bautz. *Nature* **221**:43-46 (1969).
6. G. Hartman, K. O. Honikeley, F. Knusel, and J. Nuisch. *Biochim. Biophys. Acta* **145**:843-844 (1967).
7. S. H. Mizuno, H. Yamazaki, K. Nitta, and H. Umezawa. *Biochim. Biophys. Acta* **157**:322-332 (1968).
8. S. H. Mizuno, H. Yamazaki, K. Nitta, and H. Umezawa. *Biochem. Biophys. Res. Commun.* **30**:379-385 (1968).
9. R. C. Huang and J. Bonner. *Proc. Natl. Acad. Sci. (USA)* **48**:1216-1222 (1962).
10. D. L. Wilson and E. P. Geiduschek. *Proc. Natl. Acad. Sci. (USA)* **62**:514-520 (1969).

11. D. Gillespie and S. Spiegelman. *J. Mol. Biol.* **12**:829-842 (1965).

12. A. S. Bhagwat and P. R. Mahadevan. *Mol. Gen. Genet.* **109**:142-151 (1970).

13. J. Marmur. *J. Mol. Biol.* **3**:208-221 (1961).

14. K. S. Kirby. *Biochem. J.* **96**:266-269 (1965).

15. Y. Miyazawa and C. A. Thomas. *J. Mol. Biol.* **34**:305-316 (1965).

16. D. E. Kohne. *CarnegieInst. Yearbook* **67**:310-311 (1968).

17. U. Maitra and J. Hurwitz. *Proc. Natl. Acad. Sci. (USA)* **54**:815-822 (1965).

18. B. M. Alberts, F. J. Amodio, M. Jenkins, E. D. Gutmann, and F. L. Ferris. *Cold Spring Harbor Symp. Quant. Biol.* **33**:289-305 (1968).

19. R. G. Roeder and W. J. Rutter. *Proc. Natl. Acad. Sci. (USA)* **65**:657-682 (1970).

20. B. J. Davis. *Ann. N.Y. Acad. Sci.* **121**:404-427 (1964).

21. R. S. Dwivedi, S. K. Dutta, and D. P. Bloch. *J. Cell Biol.* **43**:51-58 (1969).

22. A. D. Riggs, H. Suzuki, and S. Bourgeois. *J. Mol. Biol.* **48**:67-83 (1970).

DISCUSSION

Question (Dutta): How do you know that with the hydroxylapatite method you obtained DNA·RNA hybrids and not DNA·DNA?

Answer: Hybrids obtained in the first elution were treated with pancreatic RNase. DNA·RNA hybrids treated in this manner do not adsorb to the hydroxylapatite, while this treatment does not affect the adsorption of the DNA·DNA hybrids.

Question (Dutta): What percent of rRNA did you get?

Answer: It was about 1%.

Question (Chanda): The inhibitor protein factor does not contain any DNase or RNase activity. Did you test whether the protein has any proteolytic activity? If it has proteolytic activity, it might affect RNA polymerase and thus eventually might affect RNA synthesis.

Answer: The inhibitor factor did not show any proteolytic activity. This was acertained by testing hydrolysis of casein with it. The TCA-soluble material of this reaction did not give any ninhydrin-positive reaction.

Question (Das): Have you characterized the RNA formed *in vitro* in the presence of the inhibitor? Have any competition experiments been done with *in vivo* RNA?

Answer: These experiments are in progress.

19

Transcriptional Systems in Eukaryotic Cells

Michael Goldberg, Jean-Claude Perriard, Gordon Hager, Richard B. Hallick, and William J. Rutter

Department of Biochemistry
University of California, San Francisco
San Francisco, California, U.S.A.

The problem of regulation of transcription is common to all biological systems. There are two significant complications in eukaryotes: (a) the nuclear chromosomes are structurally complex, and (b) independent genomes are segregated within the nucleus and in organelles such as mitochondria, chloroplasts, and centrioles. Current evidence suggests that there are at least two and perhaps several transcriptive systems in the nucleus and distinct transcriptive systems in the cytoplasmic organelles. A transcriptive system is defined as a DNA-dependent RNA polymerase, the set of genes that are specifically transcribed, and whatever regulatory elements influence the transcription.

Roeder and Rutter (37) reported that three forms of RNA polymerase (I, II, and III) can be detected in rat liver and sea urchin embryos. A heterogeneity in I and II was observed in the earliest studies (12,21,37). Further investigation has shown that there are two different structural forms of II (A and B) (13,21). I and II have been found invariably; III has been found in several organisms including rat (liver), *Xenopus*, sea urchin embryo, and yeast (4,37,38). The latter enzyme appears to be the most labile and is frequently not detected in crude extracts of higher organisms.

These polymerases probably have different transcriptive functions. This is particularly evident for I and II. Polymerase II is specifically inhibited by the mushroom toxin α-amanitin, while polymerases I and III are not affected

(4,20,29). Since the synthesis of most of the RNA species made in isolated nuclei is α-amanitin sensitive, most heterogeneous and mRNA species must be produced by II (4). The synthesis of ribosomal RNA, transfer RNA, and 5S RNA is not α-amanitin sensitive and thus is a function of I and/or III (16,34, 36,53). Since I is found largely, if not exclusively, in the nucleolus, which contains the ribosomal genes, it is presumed that this enzyme is responsible for the transcription of ribosomal RNA (39).

The role of polymerase III remains undefined at present. Several possibilities exist: (a) III may be a modified regulatory form of I. Phosphorylation of I, for example, might cause chromatographic behavior similar to that of III. However, we have been unable to convert I to III or III to I in tests involving crude cellular extracts or purified protein kinase and alkaline phosphatase (Paule and Rutter, unpublished observations). (b) III may transcribe tRNA and 5S genes. Indeed, Penman and colleagues have reported evidence consistent with but not conclusively demonstrating this view (34). (c) It has recently been demonstrated in both bacteria and higher organisms that DNA synthesis is not self-initiating but requires an RNA primer presumably synthesized by an RNA polymerase at a specific initiation site (22,26). III may therefore be involved in initiating DNA synthesis. This possibility is suggested by the presence of high levels of III in rapidly proliferating organisms such as sea urchin and *Xenopus* embryos, and yeast (4,38).

The nomenclature of the RNA polymerases is currently complicated. A nomenclature for the polymerases based solely on α-amanitin sensitivity has been proposed (11). This limits enzyme classification to two categories. We believe that there are at least three transcriptive systems in nuclei. For this reason, we prefer to retain our original terminology for the RNA polymerases (37). Eventually, it would be useful to associate enzyme terminology with a particular transcriptive system (the genes transcribed) rather than with any arbitrary property.

STRUCTURAL HOMOLOGIES BETWEEN EUKARYOTIC AND PROKARYOTIC POLYMERASES

If the eukaryotic polymerases resemble those from prokaryotic organisms, then we would expect similarities in both mechanism and regulation. One way to establish this similarity is to compare their subunit structures. Rat liver polymerase II has been purified independently in our laboratory (49) and by other groups (13,30). Polymerase II can be resolved into two forms which are distinguished by a different high molecular weight subunit (Table I). Our procedure gives approximately 10,000-fold purification with a high yield (25-30%). Four components which are present in stoichiometric quantities (Table I) can be resolved by gel electrophoresis in sodium dodecylsulfate. The sum of the

Table I. Apparent Structural Homologies Between Prokaryotic and Eukaryotic RNA Polymerases[a]

Subunit	E. coli core	II		I nucleolar
		A	B	
β'	$(155,000)_1$	$(190,000)_1$		$(200,000)$
β''			$(170,000)_1$	
β	$(145,000)_1$	$(150.000)_1$	$(150,000)_1$	$(125,000)$
α	$(40,000)_2$	$(35,000)_1$	$(35,000)_1$	$(60,000)$
α'		$(25,000)$	$(25,000)_1$	$(44,000)$
		$(16,000)$	$(16,000)$	$\sim(20,000)$
Molecular weight	380,000	400,000	400,000	$\sim$350-400,000
Structure	$\alpha_2\beta\beta'$	$\alpha\alpha'\beta\beta'$	$\alpha\alpha'\beta\beta'$	

[a]Molecular weights of subunits of E. coli RNA polymerase (8), rat liver nuclear II (49), and nucleolar I were estimated by sodium dodecylsulfate-acrylamide gel electrophoresis (43). Molecular weights of the native enzyme molecules were estimated from their sedimentation coefficients in glycerol-density gradients (4, 8).

molecular weights of the four components approximates the molecular weight of the native molecule. The overall structure resembles that of the prokaryotic polymerases.

Purification of polymerase I has been less successful, since recovery of activity is often low during fractionation. Two chromatographically distinguishable activities of polymerase I are present in extracts of nuclei (Goldberg, Paule, Rutter, unpublished observations). Our early attempts at purification showed that highly purified polymerase I had a subunit structure different from that of polymerase II (40).

In order to obtain higher yields and more stable enzyme, we have recently taken advantage of the observation of Roeder and Rutter (39) that I activity is enriched in the nucleolus. Polymerase-I activity was solubilized from nucleoli by sonication in a buffer of high ionic strength. Subsequent purification was similar to that employed previously for polymerase II, except that we have adapted the method of ion-filtration chromatography (24) to fractionate the nucleolar extract under high ionic strength conditions, minimizing association of the polymerases with other proteins and DNA. High-resolution chromatography on DEAE-Sephadex and centrifugation in glycerol gradients yielded a preparation which was nearly homogeneous and had a specific activity approaching that of polymerase II. Sodium dodecylsulfate gel electrophoresis (43) of RNA polymerase obtained across the glycerol gradient revealed the presence of two high molecular weight subunits corresponding in intensity to the peak of enzyme activity. We have estimated their molecular weight to be 200,000 ($\pm$10%) and

120,000 (±10%), respectively. Electrophoresis of the enzyme on acrylamide gels under conditions that maintain enzyme activity (6) yielded a single band of polymerase activity. Re-electrophoresis on sodium dodecylsulfate gels of the protein associated with this band of activity again indicated the presence of the same two high molecular weight subunits. A number of lower molecular weight components are also present, but we are uncertain of their relationship to the polymerase-I molecule.

Polymerases I and II are each composed of two high molecular weight and several lower molecular weight subunits. Since the molecular weights of corresponding subunits of I and II are different, the molecules are probably distinct entities. The overall structure is analogous to that of the *Escherichia coli* core RNA polymerase (8). We believe that the general structural similarity of prokaryotic and eukaryotic RNA polymerases implies a similarity of mechanism and regulation. This would suggest that eukaryotic RNA polymerases require factors similar to the σ factor (9).

There has been an active search for specific transcription factors for several years. The following types of factor activities have previously been described: (a) Nonspecific factors such as DNAse, which can stimulate eukaryotic polymerase activity by introducing single-strand breaks into the template DNA, presumably adding false initiation sites (11,23). Bovine serum albumin, presumably a nonspecific protein, stimulates both I and II, though to somewhat different degrees (40). (b) Factors isolated independently of the RNA polymer-

Table II. Alteration of Template Specificity After Chromatography of I on rRNA-Sepharose[a]

	Relative activity (%)	
Template	Sepharose I	rRNA-Sepharose I
Native calf thymus DNA	78	4
Denatured calf thymus DNA	100	42
Poly(dC)	93	97
Protein (% recovery)	100	60

[a]Ribosomal RNA-Sepharose was prepared by coupling rat liver rRNA to Sepharose 4B-200 after activation with CNBr (48). Columns were equilibrated and eluted with 0.05 M tris (pH 7.9), 25% glycerol (v/v), 0.005 M Mg^{2+}, 0.1 mM EDTA, 0.5 mM dithiothreitol, containing 0.1 M ammonium sulfate. The preparation of nucleolar polymerase I (insensitive form I) used in these experiments is described elsewhere (Goldberg *et al.*, in preparation). RNA synthesis was measured in the presence of 0.05 M ammonium sulfate as previously described (4). Polydeoxycytidylate was a gift of Dr. Fred J. Bollum. Proteins were determined according to Rutter (41).

ase that stimulate II activity on native but not denatured DNA. Such stimulation is highly variable (2-20 X) (27,42,45). (c) Factors that initially copurify with the polymerases. Such factors have up to a threefold stimulation of activity (14,15,18). (d) A factor we have recently isolated from highly purified polymerase I. The relationship of this factor to polymerase I bears a strong resemblance to that of σ and *E. coli* core polymerase.

Polymerase I was chromatographed on a variety of columns prepared from immobilized nucleic acids. These included DNA-cellulose (2), polyuridylate-Sepharose, and rRNA-Sepharose (48). The enzyme eluted from each of these columns was assayed on three templates, native calf thymus DNA, denatured calf thymus DNA, and polydeoxycytidylate [poly(dC)]. Chromatography on Sepharose (Table II) or poly(U)-Sepharose had no effect on template preference, while chromatography on DNA-cellulose caused a modest loss in the ability of I to transcribe native DNA. However, elution of polymerase I from rRNA-Sepharose resulted in an almost complete loss of activity on native DNA, a partial loss of activity on denatured DNA, and total recovery of activity on poly(dC) (Table II). These results suggest the possibility that a factor regulating activity on native DNA was removed during chromatography on rRNA-Sepharose. To test this possibility, column fractions were assayed for such a factor. A protein fraction (form-I factor) eluting at high ionic strength restored the ability of rRNA-Sepharose purified I (factor-sensitive form I) to transcribe native DNA.

Form-II enzyme when chromatographed on similar materials, such as DNA-cellulose or phosphocellulose, also loses its ability to transcribe native DNA (factor-sensitive form II). Activity can be restored by a protein factor (form-II factor) purified from calf thymus cytoplasm (Weinberg and Rutter, unpublished observations). Similar activities appear to be present in a number of tissues.

A summary of the effect of protein factors on both RNA polymerases is shown in Table III. Factor-I and -II activity was tested on polymerase I before and after chromatography on rRNA-Sepharose (insensitive and sensitive form I) and on polymerase II before and after purification on phosphocellulose (insensitive and sensitive form II). Form-I factor exerted a large effect on the transcription of native calf thymus DNA and a moderate effect on the transcription of denatured DNA by sensitive form I. Form-II factor had no effect on sensitive form I. Both form-II and form-I factors stimulated sensitive form-II activity on native calf thymus DNA but had little effect on denatured calf thymus DNA. Whether form-I factor contains more than one stimulatory protein is not yet known. Little or no effect of the factors on the insensitive forms of the enzymes acting on native or denatured calf thymus DNA was observed. The factors produced a variable inhibition of the activity on poly(dC) template. The characteristics of form-I factor stimulation of sensitive form-I activity are presented in greater detail in Fig. 1. The saturation by form-I factor occurred at a protein

Table III. Effect of Protein Factors on RNA Polymerases I and II[a]

	Relative activity		
	nCT DNA	dCT DNA	poly(dC)
Insensitive form I			
+form-I factor	1	1	0.3
+form-II factor	1	1	0.9
Sensitive form I			
+form-I factor	13-100	2.5	0.5
+form-II factor	1	0.9	0.2
Insensitive form II			
+form-I factor	1	1	0.6
+form-II factor	1.6	1.3	1
Sensitive form II			
+form-I factor	4.7	1.2	0.9
+form-II factor	9.2	1.7	0.8

[a]Sensitive form I was enzyme prepared by chromatography on rRNA-Sepharose. Insensitive form II was prepared by chromatography on DEAE-Sephadex. Subsequent chromatography on phosphocellulose of the DEAE preparation yielded the sensitive polymerase II (49). The minimum response of sensitive form-I polymerase to form-I factor is a thirteenfold stimulation of RNA synthesis on native calf thymus DNA. This stimulation could be much higher. It is difficult to quantitate since sensitive form I does not transcribe native DNA. nCT, Native calf thymus; dCT, denatured calf thymus; poly(dC), polydeoxycytidylate.

concentration comparable to the enzyme protein concentration in the assays. Under these conditions, the DNA concentration was tenfold higher. As noted above, the activity of polymerase I on poly(dC) decreases with increasing concentration of form-I factor. Neither albumin nor form-II factor exerts any effect on polymerase-I activity.

Enzymes containing these factors exhibit some degree of specificity for the DNA template (Table IV). I transcribes rat liver nucleolar DNA (which is enriched in ribosomal DNA) more efficiently than does II. This preference by I is not simply due to the high G+C content of ribosomal RNA since DNA from *Micrococcus lysodeikticus* (which has an even higher G+C content) is transcribed less efficiently by I than by II. Shearing of the native calf thymus DNA decreased the activities of both enzymes and reduced the I/II activity ratio from 1.73 to 1, the same value seen for denatured DNA. This suggests that shearing of native DNA may abolish template specificity, perhaps by creating artificial initiation sites.

In conclusion, we have obtained a factor from purified polymerase I (form-I factor) that confers specificity on I for transcription of native DNA. This form-I factor copurifies with I and can be specifically removed by chromatography on rRNA-Sepharose. Since the factor is maximally active at low factor/enzyme ratios, this might suggest direct interaction with the polymerase. There is an obvious similarity between the relationship of sensitive form-I to form-I factor and of *E. coli* "core" RNA polymerase to σ factor. Both enzymes have two high and several low molecular weight subunits. Both *E. coli* holoenzyme and insensitive form-I enzyme prefer their physiological templates. What remains to be established is the extent of the functional analogy between form-I factor and σ.

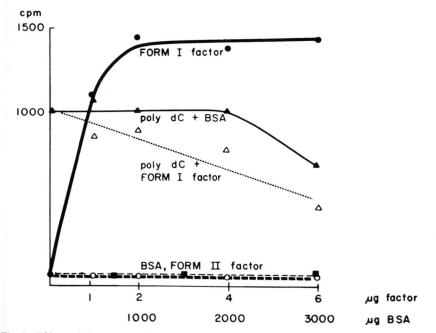

Fig. 1. Effect of form-I and form-II transcription factors on RNA synthesis by sensitive RNA polymerase I. Form-I factor was eluted at high ionic strength from the rRNA-Sepharose column (Goldberg *et al.,* in preparation). Form-II factor was a gift of F. Weinberg. RNA synthesis was measured as described in Table II. Factors or bovine serum albumin were added to sensitive form I at 4°C and preincubated for 15 min. Protein, 1-6 μg per assay, was added in the factor-containing preparations, and up to 3000 μg albumin per assay (0.06 ml) was present in the controls. Assays contained 18 μg of native calf thymus DNA or 2.4 μg poly(dC).

Table IV. Effect of DNA Template on Activity Ratio of RNA Polymerases I and II[a]

DNA	I/II
Native calf thymus DNA	1.75
Sheared native calf thymus DNA	1.0
M. lysodeikticus DNA	0.63
Rat liver nucleolar DNA	3.6
Denatured calf thymus DNA	1.05
Sheared denatured calf thymus DNA	0.93

[a]The activity ratios are the ratios of V_{max} for the different templates as determined by Hofstee plots (19). Native calf thymus DNA and *Micrococcus lysodeikticus* DNA were commercially available samples. Rat liver nucleolar DNA (prepared from purified nucleoli) was a gift of Graeme Bell. Samples of the calf thymus DNA were sheared by passage through a French pressure cell to an approximate mol wt of 150,000. Assay conditions are described in Table II. The insensitive enzymes as described in Table III were used.

MITOCHONDRIAL TRANSCRIPTION

An alternate approach to the study of transcription is to focus on those eukaryotic organelles which are known to contain their own genetic apparatus. These systems have the advantage of a relatively small and more manageable genome. Therefore, the study of mitochondrial RNA synthesis may be useful in probing general transcribing mechanisms in eukaryotic cells.

Studies on protein synthesis have emphasized that the translation system of mitochondria resembles that of bacteria, leading to the supposition that RNA synthesis is also of a prokaryotic nature. This contention is supported by reports that *in vivo* mitochondrial transcription (44) or *in vitro* RNA synthesis by mitochondrial RNA polymerase (25,35) is sensitive to rifampicin, an inhibitor of bacterial transcription. In contrast, others (17,47,50,51) have found mitochondrial transcription to be insensitive to rifampicin.

Highly purified RNA polymerases have been obtained from both *Neurospora* (25) and *Xenopus* mitochondria (51). The *Xenopus* enzyme is insensitive to rifampicin, whereas the *Neurospora* enzyme is sensitive. These enzymes are single polypeptides of molecular weight 64,000 resembling the single-subunit T7 bacteriophage polymerase (110,000) rather than the multisubunit bacterial and eukaryotic RNA polymerases (450,000-500,000). It is paradoxical that the *Neurospora* polymerase, a low molecular weight protein, interacts with rifampicin, whereas a high molecular weight subunit of the bacterial enzyme (β, mol wt 160,000) binds this inhibitor (52).

We have been studying RNA polymerase activity in mitochondria from *Saccharomyces cerevisae* and find evidence for a high molecular weight, multisubunit rifampicin-insensitive enzyme. Three activities can be resolved from extracts of purified mitochondria by chromatography on DEAE-Sephadex and DNA-cellulose. Seventy to eighty percent of this activity is contained in the first fraction eluted from DEAE-Sephadex (mito 1). The second peak of activity can be resolved into an α-amanitin-sensitive activity similar to nuclear II and an α-amanitin-insensitive activity.

Mito 1 has characteristics that distinguish it from the nuclear enzymes (Table V). It is relatively resistant to inhibition by the AF/013 derivative of rifamycin. The other activities are inhibited by rifamycin AF/013 to the same extent as the nuclear enzymes I, II, III (1). Mito 1 also transcribes mitochondrial DNA more effectively than the other mitochondrial activities. These activities may be nuclear contaminants, but a role in mitochondrial transcription cannot be excluded.

Table   V.   Properties   of   Yeast   Mitochondrial   RNA
Polymerase[a]

	Mito 1	Fraction 2	Fraction 3
Percent total activity	70-80%	15%	5%
α-Amanitin inhibition	0	95%	10%
Rifampicin inhibition	0	0	0
Rifamycin AF/013 inhibition	10%	80%	80%
Activity ratio: $\dfrac{\text{yeast mitochondrial DNA}}{\text{denatured calf thymus}}$	1.0	0.02	0.10

[a]The RNA polymerase activity was solubilized from purified mitochondria with 0.1% Brij-58 (a non-ionic detergent) and 0.3 M KC1, and resolved into three fractions as described in the text. RNA synthesis was measured as described in Table II. The following inhibitor concentrations were used: α-amanitin, 50 μM; rifampicin, 100 μg/ml; rifamycin AF/013, 5 μg/ml. Yeast mitochondrial DNA was prepared according to the procedure of Richard Kolodner (personal communication).

Mito 1 has been purified to high specific activity (one-fourth to one-third that of homogeneous nuclear II). Electrophoresis of the purified enzyme under conditions that maintain the native structure reveals a single protein band coincident with the polymerase activity. Electrophoresis in the presence of sodium dodecylsulfate and mercaptoethanol (which is known to dissociate proteins into subunits) gives rise to two prominent peptides of approximate mol wt 190,000 and 150,000. Low molecular weight subunits may also be present. The native enzyme cosediments with β-galactosidase at 16S both in crude extracts and in highly purified form, at ionic strengths varying between 0.05 M and 1.0 M KCl. This suggests a molecule with a molecular weight of approximately 500,000 and with little tendency to aggregate at low salt concentration.

The characteristics of mito 1 described above suggest that it is a mitochondrial enzyme. Its molecular weight and subunit structure resemble those of nuclear enzymes I and II, and contrasts with those reported for the *Neurospora* and *Xenopus* mitochondrial polymerases. We have found no evidence of a small enzyme in yeast mitochondria using methods similar to those employed in the isolation of the *Neurospora* and *Xenopus* enzymes.

Three possibilities for explaining the discrepancy are apparent. First, mitochondria from different organisms could contain distinct RNA polymerases. We consider this unlikely. Second, the enzyme we have isolated from yeast mitochondria could in fact be due to nuclear contamination. The facts that mitochondrial fractions are highly enriched in mito 1 and that the isolated enzyme has characteristics different from those of the nuclear polymerases argue against this possibility. Third, the low molecular weight enzymes found by others might be subunits derived from a more complex molecule. It has recently been reported that the a subunit of *E. coli* RNA polymerase can carry out the polymerization of ATP, and to a lesser extent other nucleoside triphosphates (32). Therefore, an isolated subunit may partially retain the activity of its parent molecule. In this context, we note that the specific activity of the *Neurospora* enzyme is high, while that of the *Xenopus* enzyme is very low. Thus it is conceivable that these molecules have retained to a varying degree the activity of a putative high molecular weight polymerase. One way to discriminate between these possibilities would be the isolation and characterization of transcription complexes from mitochondria.

A TRANSCRIPTION COMPLEX FROM CHLOROPLASTS

DNA-dependent RNA polymerases previously have been isolated from chloroplasts of maize seedlings (5) and wheat leaf (33). In the course of our purification of RNA polymerase, we have isolated from chloroplasts of *Euglena* a transcription complex composed of the chloroplast DNA plus the RNA polymerase and other proteins that also bind to the DNA. Because the existence of this complex suggests that a specific interaction exists between chloroplast polymerase and DNA, we have begun to investigate its properties in detail.

Chloroplasts were isolated from *Euglena gracilis* Z (31). Purified chloroplasts were lysed with the non-ionic detergent Triton X100. Further purification was achieved by differential centrifugation and gel filtration chromatography on Agarose A-5M (Fig. 2). The RNA polymerase was eluted with the bulk, if not all, of the chloroplast DNA as a sharp band in the void volume of this column. However, more than 99% of the protein and all the pigment were retained by the column. The RNA polymerase in the fractions of highest specific activity (18 nmoles UMP incorporated/10 min at 30°C) has been purified at least 600-fold from the chloroplast lysate. The specific activity is based on the transcription of endogeneous DNA, which is present at a concentration of 1 μg/ml; this concentration of DNA is about 1% of that needed to saturate the isolated nuclear

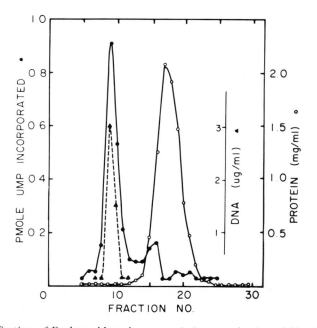

Fig. 2. Purification of Euglena chloroplast transcription complex by gel filtration chromatography on Agarose A-5M. Details of the purification procedure are described elsewhere (Hallick *et al.*, in preparation). Protein was estimated as previously described (41). DNA was determined by the diphenylamine method (10). The RNA polymerase reaction contained 0.05 M tris-Cl (pH 7.9), 0.02 M MgCl$_2$, 0.04 M (NH$_4$)$_2$SO$_4$, 0.6 mM ATP, CTP, and GTP, and 0.01 mM [5,6-^{3}H] UTP. After 10 min incubation at 30°C, reactions were stopped by pipetting 0.04 ml of the reaction mixture onto Whatman DE81 filter discs, as previously described (4).

enzymes. Addition of a tenfold excess of exogenous chloroplast DNA did not influence the reaction. These results imply that a specific complex does exist between the polymerase and the endogenous DNA.

The buoyant density of the transcription complex DNA in neutral CsCl gradients was identical to that of chloroplast DNA (1.685 g/cm^3). No nuclear DNA (1.707 g/cm^3) contamination was evident.

The only requirements for maximal RNA synthesis by the complex are the four ribonucleoside triphosphates and a divalent cation. Mg^{2+} is preferred over Mn^{2+}. As seen in Fig. 3, the complex transcribes for several hours *in vitro*. RNA synthesis is inhibited by actinomycin D, as would be expected for a DNA-dependent reaction.

It has previously been suggested that *Euglena* chloroplast RNA polymerase is "prokaryotic" because rifampicin blocks the accumulation of chloroplast rRNA *in vivo* (7). Rifampicin even at high concentrations (100 µg/ml) has no effect on the kinetics of the reaction carried out by the transcription complex. Since

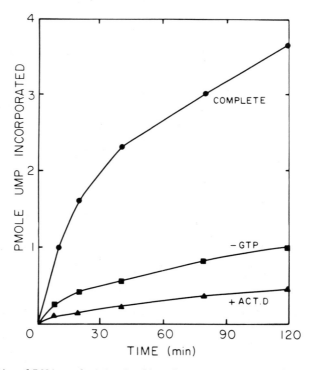

Fig. 3. Kinetics of RNA synthesis by the chloroplast transcription complex. RNA synthesis was measured *in vitro* as described in Fig. 2. ●, Complete reaction mixture; ▲, complete reaction mixture plus 50 µg/ml actinomycin D; ■, reaction mixture minus GTP.

rifampicin is an inhibitor of initiation of transcription, it is possible that the complex is not initiating *in vitro,* but only completing RNA strands. Alternatively, the enzyme present in this complex is not rifampicin sensitive.

Since the endogenous DNA template is transcribed, it is possible that the chloroplast genome has been isolated relatively intact. The RNA sequences synthesized *in vitro* may be the same as those made *in vivo.* If the product of the transcription complex is a symmetrical transcript of both strands (as has been reported for the *in vivo* transcription of mitochondrial DNA in HeLa cells; ref. 3), one would expect the base composition of this *in vitro* RNA to be the same as that of chloroplast DNA, 25% G+C. However, the base composition is different from that of chloroplast DNA, suggesting that the DNA in this complex is not symmetrically transcribed.

In collaboration with Dr. O. C. Richards, we have begun to characterize the *in vitro* RNA transcript by hybridization with isolated heavy, light, and satellite single-stranded DNA from *Euglena* chloroplasts. In a reaction carried out with DNA excess, 60% of the RNA hybridized to the light single-strand population, 53% to the heavy, and 13% to the satellite DNA (based on S1 nuclease digestion as a measure of hybridization; refs. 28 and 46). Therefore, the RNA product is complementary to the chloroplast DNA.

In conclusion, we have obtained a highly purified complex of chloroplast DNA and its attendant RNA polymerase. This material has the properties of a transcription complex: (a) it transcribes at very low levels of DNA; (b) it is indifferent to exogenous DNA; (c) the RNA product is complementary to the organelle DNA but is not a simple symmetrical copy of it.

ACKNOWLEDGMENTS

The authors thank Graeme Bell for buoyant density analysis of DNA samples, Michael Glowalla for his assistance in the purification of RNA polymerase from yeast mitochondria, and Henry Salmona for his help in the isolation of rat liver polymerases. This work was supported by USPHS, NIH grants HD 04617 and GM 49794; NSF grant No. 35256; American Cancer Society grant PF-794; Giannini Foundation; and the Swiss National Foundation.

REFERENCES

1. R. Adman, L. D. Schultz, and B. D. Hall. Transcription in yeast: Separation and properties of multiple RNA polymerases. *Proc. Natl. Acad. Sci. (USA)* **69**:1702 (1972).
2. B. Alberts and G. Herrick. DNA-cellulose chromatography. *Meth. Enzymol.* **21**:198 (1971).
3. Y. Aloni and G. Attardi. Symmetrical *in vivo* transcription of mitochondrial DNA in HeLa cells. *Proc. Natl. Acad. Sci. (USA)* **68**:1757 (1971).
4. S. P. Blatti, C. J. Ingles, T. J. Lindell, P. W. Morris, R. F. Weaver, F. Weinberg, and W. J.

Rutter. Structure and regulatory properties of eukaryotic RNA polymerase. *Cold Spring Harbor Symp. Quant. Biol.* **35**:649 (1970).

5. W. Bottomley, H. J. Smith, and L. Bogorad. RNA polymerase of maize: Partial purification and properties of the chloroplast enzyme. *Proc. Natl. Acad. Sci. (USA)* **68**:2412 (1971).

6. I. R. Brown. Polyacrylamide gel electrophoresis of DNA polymerase from Ehrlich ascites tumor cells and recovery of active enzyme. *Biochim. Biophys. Acta* **191**:731 (1969).

7. R. D. Brown, D. Bastia, and R. Haselkorn. Effect of rifampicin on transcription in chloroplasts of *Euglena*. In *Lepetit Colloquium on RNA Polymerase and Transcription*, North-Holland, Amsterdam, p. 309 (1969).

8. R. R. Burgess. Separation and characterization of the subunits of ribonucleic acid polymerase. *J. Biol. Chem.* **244**:6168 (1969).

9. R. R. Burgess, A. A. Travers, J. J. Dunn, and E. K. F. Bautz. Factor stimulating transcription by RNA polymerase. *Nature* **221**:43 (1969).

10. K. Burton. A study of the conditions and mechanism of the diphenylamine reaction for the colorimetric estimation of DNA. *Biochem. J.* **62**:315 (1956).

11. P. Chambon, F. Gissinger, J. L. Mandel, C. Kedinger, M. Gniazdowski, and M. Meihlac. Purification and properties of calf thymus DNA-dependent RNA polymerases A and B. *Cold Spring Harbor Symp. Quant. Biol.* **35**:693 (1970).

12. C. J. Chesterton and P. H. W. Butterworth. A new form of mammalian DNA-dependent RNA polymerase and its relationship to the known forms of the enzyme. *FEBS Letters* **12**:301 (1971).

13. C. J. Chesteron and P. H. W. Butterworth. Purification of the rat liver form B DNA-dependent RNA polymerases. *FEBS Letters* **15**:181 (1971).

14. M. E. Dahmus and S. Lee. Multiple forms of RNA polymerase from Novikoff ascites cells and their response to a purified stimulation factor. *Fed. Proc.* **31**:428 (1972).

15. E. DiMauro, C. P. Hollenberg, and B. D. Hall. Transcription in yeast: A factor that stimulates yeast RNA polymerase. *Proc. Natl. Acad. Sci. (USA)* **69**:2818 (1972).

16. E. Egyhazi, B. D'Monte, and J. E. Edstrom. Effects of alpha-amanitin on *in vitro* labeling of RNA from defined nuclear components in salivary gland cells from *Chironomus tentans*. *J. Cell Biol.* **53**:523 (1972).

17. F. Herzfeld. The insensitivity of RNA synthesis to rifampicin in *Neurospora* mitochondria. *Z. Physiol. Chem.* **351**:658 (1970).

18. T. Higashinakagawa, T. Onishi, and M. Muramatsu. A factor stimulating the transcription by nucleolar RNA polymerase in the nucleolus of rat liver. *Biochem. Biophys. Res. Commun.* **48**:937 (1972).

19. B. H. J. Hofstee. On the evaluation of the constants Vm and Km in enzyme reactions. *Science* **116**:329 (1952).

20. C. Kedinger, M. Gniazdowski, J. L. Mandel, F. Gissinger, and P. Chambon. Alpha-amanitin: A specific inhibitor of one of the two DNA-dependent RNA polymerase activities from calf thymus. *Biochem. Biophys. Res. Commun.* **38**:165 (1970).

21. C. Kedinger, P. Nuret, and P. Chambon. Structural evidence for two alpha-amanitin sensitive RNA polymerases in calf thymus. *FEBS Letters* **15**:169 (1971).

22. W. Keller. RNA-primed DNA synthesis *in vitro*. *Proc. Natl. Acad. Sci. (USA)* **69**:1560 (1972).

23. W. Keller and R. Goor. Mammalian RNA polymerase: Structural and functional properties. *Cold Spring Harbor Symp. Quant. Biol.* **35**:671 (1970).

24. L. H. Kirkegaard, T. J. A. Johnson, and R. M. Bock. Ion filtration chromatography: A powerful new technique for enzyme purification applied to *E. coli* alkaline phosphatase. *Anal. Biochem.* **50**:122 (1972).

25. H. Küntzel and K. P. Schäfer. Mitochondrial RNA polymerase from *Neurospora crassa*. *Nature New Biol.* **231**:265 (1971).

26. K. G. Lark. Evidence for the direct involvement of RNA in the initiation of DNA replication in *E. coli* 15T⁻ *J. Mol. Biol.* **64**:47 (1972).

27. D. Lentfer and A. G. Lezius. Mouse myeloma polymerase B: Template specificities and the role of a transcription-stimulating factor. *Europ. J. Biochem.* **30**:278 (1972).

28. J. Leong, A. Garapin, N. Jackson, L. Fanshier, W. Levinson, and J. M. Bishop. Virus-specific ribonucleic acid in cells producing Rous sarcoma virus: Detection and characterization. *J. Virol.* **9**:891 (1972).

29. T. J. Lindell, F. Weinberg, P. W. Morris, R. G. Roeder, and W. J. Rutter. Specific inhibition of nuclear RNA polymerase II by alpha-amanitin. *Science* **170**:447 (1970).

30. J. L. Mandel and P. Chambon. Purification of RNA polymerase B activity from rat liver. *FEBS Letters* **15**:175 (1971).

31. J. E. Manning, D. R. Wolstenholme, R. S. Ryan, J. A. Hunter, and O. C. Richards. Circular chloroplast DNA from *Euglena gracilis*. *Proc. Natl. Acad. Sci. (USA)* **68**:1169 (1971).

32. S. Ohasa and A. Tsugita. Poly A synthesizing activity in a constitutive subunit of RNA polymerase. *Nature New Biol.* **240**:35 (1972).

33. G. M. Polya and A. T. Jagendorf. Wheat leaf RNA polymerases. I. Partial purification and characterization of nuclear, chloroplast and soluble DNA-dependent enzymes. *Arch. Biochem. Biophys.* **146**:635 (1971).

34. R. Price and S. Penman. A distinct RNA polymerase activity synthesizing 5.5S, 5S and 4S RNA in nuclei from adenovirus 2 - infected HeLa cells. *J. Mol. Biol.* **70**:435 (1972).

35. B. D. Reid and P. Parsons. Partial purification of mitochondrial RNA polymerase from rat liver. *Proc. Natl. Acad. Sci. (USA)* **68**:2830 (1971).

36. R. H. Reeder and R. G. Roeder. Ribosomal RNA synthesis in isolated nuclei. *J. Mol. Biol.* **67**:433 (1972).

37. R. G. Roeder and W. J. Rutter. Multiple forms of DNA-dependent RNA polymerase in eukaryotic organisms. *Nature* **224**:234 (1969).

38. R. G. Roeder, R. H. Reeder, and D. D. Brown. Multiple forms of RNA polymerase in *Xenopus laevis:* Their relationship to RNA synthesis *in vivo* and their fidelity of transcription *in vitro*. *Cold Spring Harbor Symp. Quant. Biol.* **35**:729 (1970).

39. R. G. Roeder and W. J. Rutter. Specific nucleolar and nucleoplasmic RNA polymerases. *Proc. Natl. Acad. Sci. (USA)* **65**:675 (1970).

40. W. J. Rutter, P. W. Morris, M. Goldberg, M. Paule, and R. Morris. The role of RNA polymerases in transcriptive specificity in eukaryotic organisms. In J. K. Pollak and J. Wilson Lee (eds.), *The Biochemistry of Gene Expression in Higher Organisms,* Australia and New Zealand Book Company, Sydney, Australia, p. 89 (1973).

41. W. J. Rutter. Protein determination in embryos. In F. H. Wilt and N. K. Wessels (eds.), *Methods in Developmental Biology,* Thomas Y. Crowell New York, p. 671 (1967).

42. K. H. Seifart, P. P. Juhasz, and B. J. Benecke. A protein factor from rat liver tissue enhancing the transcription of native templates by homologous RNA polymerase B. *Europ. J. Biochem.* **33**:181 (1973).

43. A. L. Shapiro, E. Vinuela, and J. V. Maizel. Molecular weight estimation of polypeptide chains by electrophoresis in SDS-polyacrylamide gels. *Biochem. Biophys. Res. Commun.* **28**:815 (1967).

44. Z. G. Shmerling. The effect of rifamycin on RNA synthesis in the rat liver mitochondria. *Biochem. Biophys. Res. Commun.* **37**:965 (1969).

45. H. Stein and P. Hausen. A factor from calf thymus stimulating DNA-dependent RNA polymerase isolated from this tissue. *Europ. J. Biochem.* **14**:270 (1970).

46. W. D. Sutton. A crude nuclease preparation suitable for use in DNA reassociation experiments. *Biochim. Biophys. Acta* **240**:522 (1971).
47. M. J. Tsai, G. Michaelis, and R. S. Criddle. DNA-dependent RNA polymerase from yeast mitochondria. *Proc. Natl. Acad. Sci. (USA)* **68**:473 (1971).
48. A. F. Wagner, R. L. Bugianesi, and T. Y. Shen. Preparation of Sepharose-bound poly(rI:rC). *Biochem. Biophys. Res. Commun.* **45**:185 (1971).
49. R. F. Weaver, S. P. Blatti, and W. J. Rutter. Molecular structures of DNA-dependent RNA polymerases (II) from calf thymus and rat liver. *Proc. Natl. Acad. Sci. (USA)* **68**:2994 (1971).
50. E. Wintersberger and U. Wintersberger. Rifamycin insensitivity of RNA synthesis in yeast. *FEBS Letters* **6**:58 (1970).
51. G. Wu and I. B. Dawid. Purification and properties of mitochondrial deoxyribonucleic acid dependent ribonucleic acid polymerase from ovaries of *Xenopus laevis*. *Biochemistry* **11**:3589 (1972).
52. W. Zillig, K. Zechel, D. Rabussay, M. Schachner, V. S. Sethi, P. Palm, A. Heil, and W. Seifart. On the role of different subunits of DNA-dependent RNA polymerase from *E. coli* in the transcription process. *Cold Spring Harbor Symp. Quant. Biol.* **35**:47 (1970).
53. E. A. Zylber and S. Penman. Products of RNA polymerases in HeLa cell nuclei. *Proc. Natl. Acad. Sci. (USA)* **68**:2861 (1971).

DISCUSSION

Question (Burma): How do the different forms of polymerases including the mitochondrial enzymes differ antigenically? Is there any cross-reaction between the different types?
Answer: There are no published studies on this point.

Question (Pradhan): Does factor II reverse α-amanitin inhibition?
Answer: No.

Question (Pradhan): Is it possible that factors I and II are chromosomal proteins?
Answer: Yes. However, factor I copurifies with the enzyme over several thousandfold. Thus it may interact with the enzyme as well. RNA polymerase might be classified as a chromosomal protein.

Question (Gallo): In your study of the relative inhibition of nuclear I RNA polymerase and the mitochondrial I by AF/013 did either enzyme preparation contain detergent? If so, were the amounts exactly the same? The reason for the question is that these detergents result in micelle formation which removes the rifamycin derivative from interaction with enzymes.
Answer: No detergents were present in the assay.

Question (Ganguly, Das, and Mazumder): We are very much interested to know much more about your so-called heat-stable and heat-unstable factors.
Answer: So are we.

20

Transcription of Double-Stranded Viral and Cellular DNAs by Purified Mammalian DNA-Dependent RNA Polymerases

P. Chambon, J. L. Mandel, F. Gissinger, C. Kedinger, M. Gross-Bellard, and P. Hossenlopp

Institut de Chimie Biologique
Unité de Recherche sur le Cancer
de l'INSERM et Centre de Neurochimie du CNRS
Faculté de Médecine
Strasbourg, France

The multiplicity and different intranuclear localizations of DNA-dependent RNA polymerases have suggested that gene expression in animal cells is regulated, at least in part, by distinct RNA polymerases with different template specificities (1). One of the most direct ways to support this hypothesis would be to show *in vitro* that the various purified enzymes specifically transcribe different parts of the deproteinized chromosomal DNA. A first step in such a study is to ask whether the purified enzymes alone can in fact initiate RNA synthesis on an intact double-stranded DNA or whether the presence of additional initiation factor(s), similar to the *Escherichia coli* σ factor (2,3), is required. Previous studies involving normal calf thymus DNA preparations and the initiation inhibitor AF/013 (4-7) have suggested that purified AI and B enzymes initiate at different sites on calf thymus DNA and that the B enzymes could in fact initiate on "true" double-stranded regions of the DNA, while AI enzyme could lack an initiation factor. It is nevertheless clear that the possible specificity of the animal enzymes cannot be unequivocally demonstrated using these ordinary preparations of DNAs, since all of them contain a high number of single-stranded nicks ("high" compared to the expected number of true promoter sites), acting as efficient nonspecific initiation sites (8,9). On the other hand, using intact phage DNAs, we have shown (9,10) that the purified calf thymus enzymes can bind to phage DNAs but do not initiate RNA synthesis and behave, in many respects, like the bacterial core enzyme, which requires the σ initiation factor to initiate RNA synthesis on phage DNAs (11). Since the phage DNAs are obviously nonphysiological templates for the animal RNA polymerases, two interpretations could be proposed to explain these results: either that some general initiation factor(s) is lost during the purification of the calf thymus RNA polymerases or that the animal enzymes are unable to recognize the initiation signals present in the DNA of these too remote organisms. Studies of the transcriptability of intact DNA of animal viruses (SV40 and adenovirus), which do not possess their own polymerase and therefore are transcribed, at least early after the infection, by one of the cellular DNA-dependent RNA polymerases, should help to discriminate between these two alternatives. Analysis of the transcriptability of the high molecular weight chromosomal DNA, free of single-stranded nicks, which was recently prepared by Gross-Bellard *et al.* (12), should also be informatory. We have performed both types of studies and we have also characterized the RNA transcripts synthesized by AI and B enzymes on SV40 DNA form I,[1] in the hope of revealing that the two types of enzyme exhibit different template specificities and also to investigate whether the animal RNA polymerases exhibit the two main features of the prokaryotic transcription, namely, selectivity and asymmetry (2,3). We discuss here the results of these studies, which lead us to conclude that the purified mammalian RNA polymerases initiate RNA synthesis only very poorly, if at all, on unnicked "regular" double-stranded DNAs.

TRANSCRIPTION OF A VIRAL SUPERCOILED CIRCULAR DNA

SV40 DNA form I (FI) is a supercoiled double-stranded circular DNA with a molecular weight of about 3.3×10^6. Study of its *in vitro* transcription by animal DNA dependent RNA polymerases appealed to us for several reasons: (a) its circular structure resolves the problem of nonspecific initiation at single-stranded nicks or at ends of DNA molecules; (b) *in vivo,* early viral mRNA is complementary to about 30% of the sequences of one of the DNA strands, while late after infection additional mRNA appears that is complementary to the remaining 70% of the other DNA strand, suggesting that *in vivo* transcription could be selective and asymmetrical (13-19); (c) *in vitro* transcription of SV40 DNA-FI by *E. coli* holoenzyme is asymmetrical and primarily from the DNA strand that is transcribed early *in vivo* (16,18-20).

[1] Abbreviations: SV40 DNA form I (FI), supercoiled circular DNA of simian virus 40; SV40 DNA form II (FII), open circular DNA of simian virus 40; SV40 DNA form III (FIII), linear DNA of simian virus 40.

Table I shows that SV40 DNA-FI is readily transcribed by calf thymus AI and B RNA polymerases at low ionic strength in the presence of Mn^{2+}. The most surprising finding was the very poor transcriptability of SV40 DNA-FI by enzyme AI in the presence of Mg^{2+}. This result markedly contrasts with the classical observation that enzyme AI is equally stimulated by Mn^{2+} or Mg^{2+} when the template is calf thymus DNA (Table I and refs. 1, 21). It is also interesting to note that SV40 DNA-FII (open double-stranded circular form) and even more so SV40 DNA-FIII (double-stranded linear form) are very poor templates for both AI and B enzymes and that SV40 DNA-FI is efficiently transcribed by *E. coli* core enzyme, as previously reported by Sugden and Sambrook (22).

The size of the RNAs synthesized by calf thymus polymerases AI and B on SV40 DNA-FI was analyzed by sedimentation through formaldehyde-sucrose gradients. As shown in Fig. 1a, most of the RNA made in 30 min by enzyme AI is much larger than 28S rRNA, like the RNA made by *E. coli* holoenzyme on the same template (Fig. 1b and refs. 23, 24). RNA polymerase AI can therefore pass over its own initiation site on SV40 DNA-FI and synthesize RNA that has at least twice the length of a DNA strand. On the other hand, the RNA made by calf thymus B enzymes has a definite maximum size (Fig. 2) that is always less than a complete transcript of the viral genome, irrespective of the divalent cation in the incubation medium (Fig. 2a,b). As reported elsewhere (25), this result was not due to the presence of traces of RNase in the B enzyme preparation. Furthermore, measurement of the incorporation of $[\gamma\text{-}^{32}P]$ ATP and $[\gamma\text{-}^{32}P]$ GTP and calculation of the average chain lengths of the RNAs synthesized by AI and B enzymes on SV40 DNA-FI have confirmed the much larger size of the RNA transcripts made by enzyme AI (25). These determinations indicate also

Table I. Transcription of Allomorphic Forms of SV40 DNA[a]

Enzyme	Divalent cation	Salt (mM)	DNA (0.20 µg)			
			SV40-FI (pmoles)	SV40-FII (pmoles)	SV40-FIII (pmoles)	N-CT (pmoles)
CT-AI	Mn^{2+}	—	32.4	13.0	7.2	45.7
		AS= 16	24.1	12.5	—	41.1
	Mg^{2+}	—	5.6	9.6	5.5	31.6
CT-B	Mn^{2+}	AS= 25	27.3	11.7	4.8	18.7
	Mg^{2+}	AS= 16	4.1	4.1	1.1	10.0
E. coli holoenzyme	Mg^{2+}	KCl= 120	110.9	—	53.3	47.7
E. coli core enzyme	Mg^{2+}	KCl= 120	21.4	—	19.1	31.3

[a]RNA synthesis was determined as previously described (52) and is expressed in pmoles $[^3H]$UTP incorporated in 10 min at 37°C. Mn^{2+} (3 mM), Mg^{2+} (8 mM), ammonium sulfate (AS), and KCl were added to the incubation medium as indicated in the table. CT-AI, purified calf thymus AI enzyme; CT-B, purified calf thymus B enzymes; N-CT, native calf thymus DNA (52). For details, see Mandel and Chambon (53).

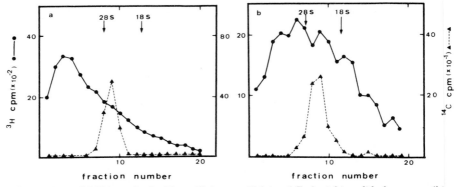

Fig. 1. Size of RNA synthesized by calf thymus AI (a) and Escherichia coli holoenzyme (b) on SV40 DNA form I. Reproduced with permission from *FEBS Letters* **29**:109 (1973).

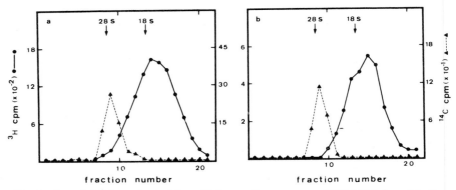

Fig. 2. Size of RNA synthesized by calf thymus B enzymes on SV40 DNA form I in the presence of Mn²⁺ (a) or Mg²⁺ (b). Reproduced with permission from *FEBS Letters* **29**:109 (1973).

that AI and B enzymes have multiple initiation sites on SV40 DNA-FI, since both ATP and GTP were found at the 5′ end of the synthesized RNA chains.

The possible asymmetry of the transcription catalyzed by calf thymus enzymes AI and B on SV40 DNA-FI was analyzed by self-annealing assay of the synthesized RNAs. As shown in Table II, the transcription is largely symmetrical with both enzymes, irrespective of the incubation conditions and of the SV40 DNA form. In contrast, the *E. coli* holoenzyme transcription is essentially asymmetrical, as previously found by Westphal (20). On the other hand, it is interesting to note that *E. coli* core enzyme does not transcribe preferentially one of the DNA strands, a result in keeping with the symmetrical transcription of phage DNAs by this enzyme (2,3). Since the size of the RNA synthesized by enzyme AI is larger than the SV40 genome size, these results demonstrate that

Table II. Symmetrical Transcription of SV40 DNA by AI and B RNA Polymerases[a]

Enzyme	Incubation conditions	SV40 DNA template	Ribonuclease resistance after self-annealing (%)
CT-AI	Mn^{2+}, no salt	FI	76.9
CT-B	Mn^{2+}, AS 25 mM	FI	62.4
	Mg^{2+}, AS 16 mM	FI	56.5
	Mn^{2+}, AS 25 mM	FIII	66.6
RL-B	Mn^{2+}, AS 25 mM	FI	69.5
	Mg^{2+}, AS 16 mM	FI	50.7
E. coli holoenzyme	Mg^{2+}, KCl 120 mM	FI	20.0
	Mn^{2+}, KCl 120 mM	FI	21.0
	Mg^{2+}, KCl 120 mM	FIII	27.6
	Mg^{2+}, KCl 120 mM	Denatured FI	67.3
E. coli core enzyme	Mn^{2+}, no salt	FI	66.9

[a]RNAs were synthesized and self-annealed as described elsewhere (25). Mn^{2+} (3 mM), MG^{2+} (8 mM), ammonium sulfate (AS), and KCl were added to the incubation medium as indicated in the table. CT-AI, purified calf thymus AI enzyme; CT-B, purified calf thymus B enzymes; RL-B, rat liver B enzymes. For details, see Mandel and Chambon (25).

Table III. Hybridization of RNAs Synthesized *in Vitro* by Calf Thymus AI Enzyme and *E. coli* Holoenzyme with RNA Made *in Vitro* by Calf Thymus B Enzymes on SV40 DNA-FI[a]

Labeled RNAs present during the hybridization period and enzymes used for their synthesis		RNAase resistance of [^{3}H]RNA after hybridization
[^{3}H]RNA	[^{32}P]RNA	(%)
CT-AI	—	23.6
CT-AI	CT-AI	84.2
CT-AI	CT-B	74.9
E. coli holoenzyme	—	11.2
E. coli holoenzyme	CT-AI	76.6
E. coli holoenzyme	CT-B	68.6

[a]Concentrations of [^{3}H]RNA and [^{32}P]RNA were 3.3×10^{-3} μg/ml and 4×10^{-2} μg/ml, respectively. Hybridization was performed at 68°C for 3 hr. CT-AI, purified calf thymus AI enzyme; CT-B, purified calf thymus B enzymes. For details, see Mandel and Chambon (25).

enzyme AI transcribes the two strands of SV40 DNA-FI over their entire length. In the case of the B enzymes, the smaller size of the RNA transcripts suggests that, although symmetrical, the *in vitro* transcription of SV40 DNA-FI could nevertheless exhibit some selectivity, only a part of the genome being transcribed. This alternative is clearly not the case, since most of the AI or *E. coli* transcripts can be hybridized with the RNA synthesized by the B enzymes (Table III). In these experiments, the concentration of the AI and *E. coli* transcripts was low enough to prevent their self-annealing. One should therefore conclude that the maximum definite size of the RNA synthesized by the B enzymes on SV40 DNA-FI does not reflect the selective transcription of some part of the genome. Other results, not shown (25), suggest that this maximum size is related to an inhibition of chain elongation by the RNA product.

Taken together, these results demonstrate that the *in vitro* transcription of SV40 DNA by the two types of calf thymus RNA polymerase does not exhibit the two main features of the *in vivo* and *in vitro* prokaryotic transcription, which, to be faithful, should be asymmetrical and selective. Similar results were obtained with the rat liver B enzymes, whose purification did not involve a phosphocellulose chromatography step in order to prevent the loss of a possible animal σ-like factor (25,26). Our results are at variance with previous reports showing that SV40 DNA-FI was asymmetrically transcribed *in vitro* by the KB cell (27) or rat liver (28) RNA polymerases, and primarily from the DNA strand that is also transcribed *in vitro* by *E. coli* enzyme (27). However, more recent results are in keeping with our observations, since they indicate that RNAs synthesized *in vitro* by cellular DNA-dependent RNA polymerases on either SV40 DNA-FI (Sambrook, personal communication) or polyoma DNA-FI (Monjardino, personal communication) are largely symmetrical. In this respect, it is important to stress that the lack of selectivity and asymmetry of the *in vitro* transcription of SV40 DNA-FI by either type of animal DNA dependent RNA polymerases does not necessarily mean that the *in vitro* situation does not reflect at all the *in vivo* process, since it was recently shown that the viral cytoplasmic mRNAs are probably derived from much larger nuclear precursors (15,29-32) and that *in vivo* transcription could be at least in part symmetrical (33).

The ability of both AI and B RNA polymerases to transcribe a double-stranded circular DNA suggests that these enzymes can initiate on an intact native double-stranded DNA and that no additional initiation factors are required. In fact, it was recently shown that supercoiled circular DNAs are not perfectly double-stranded and contain, due to conformational constraints, small denatured-like regions (34-37). In this respect, it is noteworthy that the *E. coli* core enzyme, which very poorly initiates RNA synthesis on linear unnicked double-stranded phage DNAs, transcribes efficiently SV40 DNA-FI as well as other supercoiled circular DNAs (38). If one assumes that the purified animal

RNA polymerases are in fact unable to initiate on a regular double-stranded DNA, this peculiar structure of SV40 DNA-FI would explain why it is much better transcribed than the linear form III and also why Mn^{2+} is much more efficient than Mg^{2+} in stimulating its transcription, since it is known that Mn^{2+} has a destabilizing effect on double-stranded DNA (39,40).

TRANSCRIPTION OF VIRAL AND CELLULAR LINEAR DOUBLE-STRANDED DNAs

As discussed above, the ability of the purified animal enzymes to transcribe supercoiled double-stranded SV40 DNA-FI does not prove that, in fact, they are not lacking some factor(s) that would be required to initiate RNA synthesis on regular double-stranded DNAs.

We first chose another viral DNA—adenovirus-2 DNA—to answer this question, since (a) it has a well-defined unnicked linear double-stranded structure and its molecular weight (23×10^6) is high enough to minimize the importance of the initiation which could occur at the ends of the DNA molecules; (b) it was recently shown that the adenovirus genome is transcribed *in vivo* both by an amanitin-sensitive (B type) RNA polymerase (41-43) and by an amanitin-resistant (A type) enzyme (41,44). Results presented in Table IV show that native adenovirus-2 DNA is very poorly, if at all, transcribed by purified calf thymus AI and B RNA polymerases, irrespective of the divalent cation present in the incubation medium. It is transcribed neither by a partially purified calf thymus B enzyme preparation (fraction DCB) nor by rat liver B RNA polymerases, the purification of which avoids the use of a phosphocellulose chromatography step. As expected, native adenovirus DNA is also very poorly transcribed by *E. coli* core enzyme. Transcription is blocked at the initiation step, since denatured adenovirus-2 DNA (Table IV) and adenovirus DNA nicked with pancreatic DNAase (results not shown) are readily transcribed by the animal enzymes.

These results indicate either that the animal enzymes lack a general initiation factor required for initiation on any regular double-stranded DNA or that transcription of an animal viral DNA requires some additional factor(s), which could be of cellular or viral origin. In an attempt to distinguish between these two possibilities, we prepared and used as template a high molecular weight unnicked cellular DNA (12). This DNA preparation, obtained from CV1 cells, has an average mol wt of 2×10^8 and does not contain any detectable single-stranded nicks. As shown in Table V, this DNA is also very poorly transcribed by the purified calf thymus AI and B enzymes. Determination of the incorporation of γ-^{32}P-labeled ATP and GTP, as well as measurement of pyrophosphate exchange, revealed that initiation is in fact blocked on such a

Table IV. Transcription of Adenovirus-2 DNA[a]

Enzyme	Salt (mM)	Divalent cation	DNA (0.5 μg)	[α-^{32}P] ATP incorporated (pmoles) (10 min, 37°C)
CT-AI	AS = 25	Mn^{2+}	N-Ad2	0.7
			D-Ad2	28.8
			N-CT	36.2
		Mg^{2+}	N-Ad2	1.2
			N-CT	29.3
CT-B (PC2)	AS = 25	Mn^{2+}	N-Ad2	2.3
			D-Ad2	133
			N-CT	42
		Mg^{2+}	N-Ad2	0.1
			N-CT	29.6
CT-B (DCB)	AS = 25	Mn^{2+}	N-Ad2	3.5
			N-CT	19.6
		Mg^{2+}	N-Ad2	1.5
			N-CT	11.2
RL-B	AS = 25	Mn^{2+}	N-Ad2	2.3
			N-CT	30
		Mg^{2+}	N-Ad2	0.0
			N-CT	15.6
E. coli holoenzyme	KCl = 120	Mg^{2+}	N-Ad2	52
			N-CT	104
E. coli core enzyme	KCl = 120	Mg^{2+}	N-Ad2	5.6
			N-CT	38.4

[a]Calf thymus AI enzyme (CT-AI) was 0.35 μg of fraction GG (54), calf thymus B enzymes (CT-B) were either 0.70 μg of fraction PC2 (55) or 20 μg of fraction DCB (52), rat liver B enzymes (RL-B) were 0.6 μg of the glycerol-gradient fraction (26). *E. coli* holoenzyme (0.40 μg) and *E. coli* core enzyme (0.30 μg) were prepared as described in the footnote to Table V. RNA synthesis was determined as previously described (52). Mn^{2+} and Mg^{2+} were 4 and 8 mM, respectively. Ammonium sulfate (AS) or KCl was added to the incubation mixture as indicated in the table. N-Ad2, Intact native adenovirus-2 DNA; D-Ad2, denatured adenovirus-2 DNA; N-CT, native calf thymus DNA (52).

template. The ready transcription of this DNA, when denatured or nicked with DNAase, confirmed that the blockage is at the initiation step (results not shown). It is interesting that *E. coli* core enzyme also transcribes this high molecular weight eukaryotic DNA very poorly and that its stimulation by the σ factor is on the order of that obtained on intact linear phage DNAs (38,45).

Table V. Transcription of High Molecular Weight DNA from CV1 Cells[a]

Enzyme	Salt (mM)	Divalent cation	DNA (0.5 µg)	$[\alpha\text{-}^{32}\text{P}]$ UTP incorporated (pmoles) (10 min, 37°C)
CT-AI	AS = 25	Mn^{2+}	CV1	19.3
			N-CT	95.7
		Mg^{2+}	CV1	9.4
			N-CT	79.5
CT-B	AS = 25	Mn^{2+}	CV1	7.35
			N-CT	91.4
		Mg^{2+}	CV1	1.4
			N-CT	46.6
E. coli holoenzyme	KCl = 120	Mg^{2+}	CV1	77.7
			N-CT	78.0
E. coli core enzyme	KCl = 120	Mg^{2+}	CV1	14.0
			N-CT	111.3
E. coli core enzyme + σ factor	KCl = 120	Mg^{2+}	CV1	117.5
			N-CT	140.6

[a]Calf thymus AI enzyme (CT-AI) was 0.7 µg fraction GG (54), and calf thymus B enzymes (CT-B) were 1.0 µg fraction PC2 (55). E. coli holoenzyme (0.30 µg) was prepared according to Berg et al. (56) and further purified on a glycerol gradient. E. coli core enzyme (0.70 µg) and σ factor (0.20 µg) were separated as described by Burgess et al. (45), but phosphocellulose chromatography was repeated twice. RNA synthesis was determined as previously described (52). Mn^{2+} and Mg^{2+} were 4 and 8 mM, respectively. Ammonium sulfate (AS) or KCl was added to the incubation mixture as indicated in the table. CV1, DNA from CV1 cells (an established line of African green monkey kidney cells) prepared as described elsewhere (12); N-CT, native calf thymus DNA (52).

CONCLUSION

Our results demonstrate that purified calf thymus AI and B RNA polymerases, as well as the purified rat liver B enzymes, are unable to efficiently transcribe an intact linear double-stranded DNA of viral or cellular origin; in fact, RNA synthesis was never higher than that achieved with E. coli core enzyme, which is known to initiate very poorly, if at all, on linear unnicked double-stranded DNAs (2,3). Several hypotheses, some of them not necessarily mutually exclusive, could account for these observations: (a) a general initiation factor, similar to the E. coli σ factor, is lost during the purification and the purified animal enzymes resemble the E. coli core enzyme; (b) the animal enzymes are highly species specific and transcribe only their homologous DNA, like the phage or mitochondrial RNA polymerases (3,46), which would explain the failure of calf thymus or rat liver enzymes to transcribe CV1 DNA; (c) the very limited RNA synthesis on cellular DNA is not meaningless (especially if it turned out that some elongation factor(s) could stimulate it) and corresponds to initiations at a small number of specific sites, which are laboriously located by the enzymes, which would also imply that, unlike the bacterial enzymes, the animal RNA polymerases are highly specific; (d) the animal RNA polymerases are intrinsically unable to initiate RNA synthesis on a naked intact double-stranded DNA. In this hypothesis, initiation would occur only when the secondary structure of DNA is altered. This could be achieved either (i) by the introduction of single-stranded nicks (47), (ii) by binding of some regulatory factors (protein or RNA; refs. 48-50), or (iii) by the supercoiling of the DNA in the chromatin, which would result in loops of single-stranded DNA (51). In this respect, it is interesting that RNA synthesis is readily initiated by animal enzymes on supercoiled DNA form I of SV40 or PM2 phage (10). Studies aimed at distinguishing between these various hypotheses are in progress.

ACKNOWLEDGMENTS

We thank Dr. Doerfler (Köln) for a generous gift of adenovirus-2 DNA. The technical assistance of Mrs. M. Acker, Mrs. K. Dott, Mrs. C. Hauss, and Mr. G. Dretzen is gratefully acknowledged. F. Gissinger is Attaché de Recherche CNRS, and P. Hossenlopp is Boursier de la Ligue Nationale Française contre le Cancer. This investigation was supported by grants from the Centre National de la Recherche Scientifique (ATP differenciation), the Institut National pour la Santé et la Recherche Médicale, and the Commissariat à l'Energie Atomique.

REFERENCES

1. Transcription of Genetic Material. *Cold Spring Harbor Symp. Quant. Biol.* **35**:641-737 (1970).
2. R. R. Burgess. *Ann. Rev. Biochem.* **40**:711 (1971).
3. E. K. F. Bautz. In J. W. Davidson and W. E. Cohn (eds.), *Progress in Nucleic Acid Research and Molecular Biology,* Vol. 12, Academic Press, New York, pp. 129–160 (1972).
4. P. Chambon, M. Meilhac, S. Walter, C. Kedinger, J. L. Mandel, and F. Gissinger. In A. Hollaender (ed.), *Gene Expression and Its Regulation,* Plenum Press, New York, pp. 75–90 (1973).
5. P. Chambon, F. Gissinger, C. Kedinger, J. L. Mandel, M. Meilhac, and P. Nuret. *Acta Endocrinol. Suppl.* **168**:222 (1972).
6. M. Meilhac, Z. Tysper, and P. Chambon. *Europ. J. Biochem.* **28**:291 (1972).
7. M. Meilhac and P. Chambon. *Europ. J. Biochem.,* **35**:454 (1973).
8. V. Vogt. *Nature* **223**:854 (1969).

9. M. Gniazdowski, J. L. Mandel, F. Gissinger, C. Kedinger, and P. Chambon. *Biochem. Biophys. Res. Commun.* **38**:165 (1970).
10. P. Chambon, F. Gissinger, J. L. Mandel, C. Kedinger, M. Gniazdowski, and M. Meilhac. *Cold Spring Harbor Symp. Quant. Biol.* **35**:693 (1970).
11. A. A. Travers and R. R. Burgess. *Nature* **222**:537 (1969).
12. M. Gross-Bellard, P. Oudet, and P. Chambon. *Europ. J. Biochem.,* **36**:32 (1973).
13. Y. Aloni, E. Winocour, and L. Sachs. *J. Mol. Biol.* **31**:415 (1968).
14. K. Oda and R. Dulbecco. *Proc. Natl. Acad. Sci. (USA)* **60**:525 (1968).
15. W. Tonegawa, G. Walter, A. Bernardini, and R. Dulbecco. *Cold Spring Harbor Symp. Quant. Biol.* **35**:823 (1970).
16. G. Khoury, J. C. Byrne, and M. A. Martin. *Proc. Natl. Acad. Sci. (USA)* **69**:1925 (1972).
17. G. Khoury and M. A. Martin. *Nature New. Biol.* **238**:4 (1972).
18. D. M. Lindstrom and R. Dulbecco. *Proc. Natl. Acad. Sci. (USA)* **69**:1517 (1972).
19. J. Sambrook, P. A. Sharp, and W. Keller. *J. Mol. Biol.* **70**:57 (1972).
20. H. Westphal. *J. Mol. Biol.* **50**:407 (1970).
21. P. Chambon, F. Gissinger, C. Kedinger, J. L. Mandel, and M. Meilhac. In H. Busch (ed.), *The Cell Nucleus,* Academic Press, New York, in press (1973).
22. B. Sugden and J. Sambrook. *Cold Spring Harbor Symp. Quant. Biol.* **35**:663 (1970).
23. H. Westphal and E. D. Kiehn. *Cold Spring Harbor Symp. Quant. Biol.* **35**:819 (1970).
24. A. H. Fried and F. Sokol. *J. Gen. Virol.* **17**:69 (1972).
25. J. L. Mandel and P. Chambon. *Europ. J. Biochem.,* in press (1973b).
26. J. L. Mandel and P. Chambon. *FEBS Letters* **15**:175 (1971).
27. W. Keller and R. Goor. *Cold Spring Harbor Symp. Quant. Biol.* **35**:671 (1970).
28. M. Herzberg and E. Winocour. *J. Virol.* **6**:667 (1970).
29. R. Jaenisch. *Nature New Biol.* **235**:46 (1972).
30. R. A. Weinberg, S. O. Warnaar, and E. Winocour. *J. Virol.* **10**:193 (1972).
31. F. Sokol and R. I. Carp. *J. Gen. Virol.* **11**:177 (1971).
32. S. Rozenblattt and E. Winocour. *Virology* **50**:558 (1972).
33. Y. Aloni. *Proc. Natl. Acad. Sci. (USA)* **69**:2404 (1972).
34. M. F. Maestre and J. C. Wang. *Biopolymers* **10**:1021 (1971).
35. W. W. Dean and J. Lebowitz. *Nature* **231**:5 (1971).
36. H. Delius, M. J. Mantell, and B. Alberts. *J. Mol. Biol.* **67**:341 (1972).
37. P. Hossenlopp, P. Oudet, and P. Chambon. *Europ. J. Biochem.,* in press (1973).
38. M. Sugiura, T. Okamoto, and M. Takanami. *Nature* **225**:598 (1970).
39. J. A. Anderson, G. P. P. Kuntz, H. H. Evans, and T. J. Swift. *Biochemistry* **10**:4368 (1971).
40. G. Luck and C. Zimmer. *Europ. J. Biochem.* **29**:528 (1972).
41. R. Price and S. Penman. *J. Virol.* **9**:621 (1972).
42. R. D. Wallace and J. Kates. *J. Virol.* **9**:627 (1972).
43. N. Ledinko. *Nature* **233**:247 (1971).
44. R. Price and S. Penman. *J. Mol. Biol.* **67**:433 (1972).
45. R. R. Burgess, A. A. Travers, J. J. Dunn, and E. K. F. Bautz. *Nature* **221**:43 (1969).
46. H. Kuntzel and K. P. Schafer. *Nature New Biol.* **231**:265 (1971).
47. A. Cascino, S. Riva, and E. P. Geiduscheik. *Cold Spring Harbor Symp. Quant. Biol.* **35**:213 (1970).
48. R. J. Britten and E. H. Davidson. *Science* **165**:349 (1969).
49. S. Bram. *Biochimie* **54**:1005 (1972).
50. J. Paul. *Nature New Biol.* **238**:444 (1972).
51. F. Crick. *Nature* **234**:25 (1971).

52. C. Kedinger, M. Gissinger, M. Gniazdowski, J. L. Mandel, and P. Chambon. *Europ. J. Biochem.* **28:**269 (1972).
53. J. L. Mandel and P. Chambon. *Europ. J. Biochem.,* in press (1973a).
54. F. Gissinger and P. Chambon. *Europ. J. Biochem.* **28:**277 (1972).
55. C. Kedinger and P. Chambon. *Europ. J. Biochem.* **28:**283 (1972).
56. D. Berg, K. Barrett, and M. Chamberlin. In L. Grossman and K. Moldave (eds.), *Methods in Enzymology,* Vol. XXI, Academic Press, New York p. 506 (1971).

21

Factors Affecting the Selection of a Template for the Characterization of Multiple DNA-Dependent RNA Polymerases of Mammalian Tissues

Peter H. W. Butterworth and Sarah Jane Flint

Department of Biochemistry, University College London
London, England, U.K.

and

C. James Chesterton

Department of Biochemistry, King's College London
London, England, U.K.

The first step in the expression of genetic information in any cell is the production of an RNA transcript from the DNA by the DNA-dependent RNA polymerase. Factors that regulate the expression of certain genes or classes of genes might be expected to act by some direct effect on the transcription apparatus. The general picture that has emerged from a study of gene-expression control in prokaryotes tends to support this thesis. Our understanding of the phenomenon of "polymerase-mediated control" has developed from investigations of bacteriophage infection of *Escherichia coli*. It is now generally accepted that host *E. coli* RNA polymerase transcribes at least a part of the phage genome (the "early" regions), whereas a modified host RNA polymerase (in the case of T4) or even a new phage-specified polymerase (as in the case of T7) transcribes the "late" regions (1,2). These observations suggest that the host *E. coli* RNA polymerase, the modified T4 polymerase, and the new phage-specified polymerase recognize different nucleotide sequences and thus bind to and transcribe from different initial binding sites (promoter sites) on phage DNA. Thus at least one "positive" control mechanism resides in the ability of different polymerase species to recognize different promoter sites.

In the last few years, our knowledge concerning the machinery of RNA synthesis in eukaryotes has increased greatly. The major stimulus to research in this area was the publication by Roeder and Rutter (3) of a system for the solubilization of the rat liver DNA-dependent RNA polymerase activity and its resolution into two species (termed forms A and B or I and II). Forms A and B are conveniently distinguished by the inhibition of form B by a-amanitin (4). Since this initial discovery of multiple eukaryotic RNA polymerases, the number of polymerase forms has continued to increase. It now appears that there are at least three form-A polymerases: forms AI and AII, which are restricted to the nucleolus (5-7), and form AIII, which is thought to be nucleoplasmic (5). Form-B polymerase is exclusively nucleoplasmic, and at least two forms (BI and BII) have been recognized (8).

The presence of multiple DNA-dependent RNA polymerases in the cells of higher organisms may be taken to suggest that there is a role for the polymerases in the control of gene expression analogous to that described above for the prokaryotes; that is, the different polymerase species may have different initial binding-site ("promoter-site"?) specificities, thus transcribing different classes of genes.

The characterization of the different eukaryotic RNA polymerases is still in a primitive state. They have been characterized by their different elution properties from ion-exchange celluloses, the different conditions of ionic strength and divalent metal ion concentration required to give optimal activity *in vitro,* their ability to transcribe native and/or denatured DNA, their sensitivity to the toadstool toxin a-amanitin, their intracellular localization, and, to a certain extent, their subunit structure. Much of the evidence concerning template specificity of these enzymes is vague, negative, or indirect. As the form-A polymerases (excluding AIII) are restricted to the nucleolus (5,6), which is the locus of the ribosomal cistrons, this polymerase is thought to be responsible for the synthesis of ribosomal RNA: the best evidence for this comes from an analysis of stage-4 oocytes of *Xenopus laevis,* where 95% of RNA synthesis is of ribosomal RNA. As RNA synthesis in these cells is not inhibited by a-amanitin, the involvement of form-A polymerase is implied (9). On the other hand, form-B RNA polymerases are nucleoplasmic and are therefore thought to be responsible for the synthesis of most forms of RNA excluding ribosomal RNA.

The major problem facing those interested in the template specificity of each of the multiple RNA polymerases of eukaryotic cells is the choice and preparation of a suitable DNA template for these studies. Much of our knowledge concerning the specificities of prokaryotic RNA polymerases has been derived from studies using simple bacteriophage DNAs, elegant genetic analysis, and meaningful RNA·DNA hybridization studies of the *in vitro* synthesized products. However, any approach to the study of differential template specificities of the eukaryotic RNA polymerases is hampered by the gross complexity of the eukaryotic genome, and the hopes that animal viral templates might prove as useful as bacteriophage DNAs have yet to be realized. Two possibilities therefore are open to us: either the nucleoprotein complex "chromatin" can be used as a template for these studies, or attempts may be made to deproteinize the chromatin to yield "native" DNA.

CHROMATIN

Studies using rat liver chromatin and purified rat liver DNA-dependent RNA polymerases in our laboratories (10) yielded several important findings:

a. Chromatin preparations contain endogenous form-B RNA polymerase. This activity was not inhibited by rifampicin AF/013 and is thus thought to be involved only in the elongation of RNA chains.
b. The lack of any α-amanitin-resistant activity is taken to mean that nucleolar chromatin, which is known to contain form-A polymerase (5,6,11), is absent from these preparations.
c. Chromatin is transcribed by added, purified form-B polymerase (BI + BII), whereas added form-AI polymerase does not transcribe this template.

These observations suggest that there are discrete differences in the template specificities of these two groups of polymerase. Using competition studies, it was also clearly demonstrated that form-B rat liver polymerases and a bacterial RNA polymerase (derived from *Micrococcus lysodeikticus*) bind to and transcribe from different sites on the chromatin DNA.

There is little doubt that chromatin might be an "ideal" template for studies on the specificities of the different form-B polymerases that have yet to be resolved preparatively from rat liver nuclei. However, the further extension of this work may be severely restricted by our lack of understanding concerning the structure of "chromatin." It is also clear that nucleolar chromatin might be the template of choice for the form-A polymerases, and we are currently investigating this possibility.

NATIVE DNA

It seems to be inevitable that, at least for the present, studies of the template specificities of the mammalian RNA polymerase must resort to the use of protein-free ("native") DNA. The DNA isolated from eukaryotic nuclei is of high but heterogeneous molecular weight, and the isolation procedures unavoidably result in a certain amount of shearing of the DNA and the insertion of a number of single-stranded breaks ("nicks"). It is known that certain types of "nicks" act as pseudo-promoters for some RNA polymerases (12,13).

Before being able to study template specificity, it is important to ascertain first the effect of changes in the integrity of the DNA on the activity of the various classes of mammalian RNA polymerase. The results that emerge turn out to be extremely complex, and at least two opposing effects are evident. Several parameters are discussed below.

Treatment of Rat Liver DNA with Pancreatic Deoxyribonuclease

Figure 1 shows that treatment by low concentrations of pancreatic deoxyribonuclease (generating increasing numbers of "nicks") activates the template toward the form-A polymerase, whereas the activity of the form-B polymerase changes little. Higher concentrations of nuclease appear to reduce the activity of both forms of the enzyme. [It should be pointed out that there is an intriguing similarity between these results and those of Dausse *et al.* (13) and Hinkle *et al.* (14) using *E. coli* "core" and "holo" RNA polymerase.]

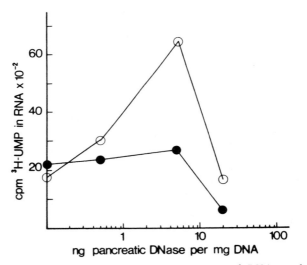

Fig. 1. Effect of pancreatic deoxyribonuclease treatment of DNA on the activity of form-AI and form-B rat liver RNA polymerases. Partially purified, nuclease-free form-AI RNA polymerase was prepared as described by Butterworth *et al.* (10); the purification of form-B RNA polymerase and the assays for RNA synthesis were carried out as previously described (7). Nuclease treatment, using pancreatic deoxyribonuclease (Sigma), followed the procedure of Aposhian and Kornberg (17). The numbers of "nicks" on the DNA were assayed using the end-labeling technique with polynucleotide kinase (15). The numbers of "nicks"/100 μg DNA were as follows: untreated DNA, 44; DNA treated with 0.5 ng nuclease/mg DNA, 742; DNA treated with 5.0 ng nuclease/mg DNA, 1074; the DNA treated with 20 ng nuclease was not assayed for "nick" content. ○, Form-AI polymerase activity; ●, form-B polymerase activity.

Is form-A activity totally dependent on "nicks" in the DNA? There is no absolute answer to this question, as we have never prepared DNA containing no "nicks." It has been found repeatedly that DNA having very low numbers of "nicks" (about ten per 100 μg DNA, which corresponds to approximately one "nick" per double strand in high molecular weight DNA) is a good template for form-A RNA polymerase, but attempts to demonstrate a direct relationship between the numbers of "nicks" and form-A polymerase activity have been unsuccessful.

Part of the reason for this failure is that nuclease treatment reduces the molecular weight of the DNA. The molecular weight of DNA may be measured conveniently by the "end-labeling" technique of Weiss *et al.* (15). This technique gives the average molecular weight of DNA species in a mixture. A DNA preparation having an average molecular weight of 1.05×10^7 was treated with two concentrations of pancreatic deoxyribonuclease under the same conditions. Using 0.5 ng nuclease/mg DNA, the average molecular weight was reduced to 1.74×10^6; after a similar treatment with 5.0 ng nuclease/mg DNA, the average molecular weight was reduced to 1.10×10^6. Therefore, nuclease treatment introduces a further parameter, one of the DNA size *or* the number of DNA "ends." These results prompted us to investigate further the effect of DNA size on template activity for the mammalian RNA polymerases.

Sepharose Fractionation of DNA

In the simplest case, we fractionated on Sepharose 4B DNA that had not been nuclease treated. The DNA was heterogeneous, and fractions were bulked over three ranges of molecular weight (Fig. 2). Each bulked fraction was assayed for its template properties. Fifteen percent of the DNA was not recovered from the column and is thought to be of low molecular weight. The data are summarized in Table I. It can be seen that the activity of the form-B polymerase did not change markedly on fractionation of the DNA or with decreasing molecular weight of the DNA. However, the activity of the form-A polymerase increased on fractionation of the DNA, and this is thought to be due to the removal of low molecular weight DNA by the gel filtration procedure. The activity of the form-A polymerase decreased as the molecular weight of the DNA decreased. Unfortunately, a definitive interpretation of these data is difficult because of the variation in the number of "nicks" in the separate fractions, the lowest molecular weight fraction containing vastly more "nicks" than the others. For a true study of the effect of DNA molecular weight on template activity, a large number of DNA preparations were fractionated on Sepharose, and the template activity of DNA fractions having different molecular weights but about the same low numbers of "nicks" (about 20 "nicks"/100 μg DNA) was studied with form-A and -B rat liver RNA polymerase. Figure 3 shows that for both

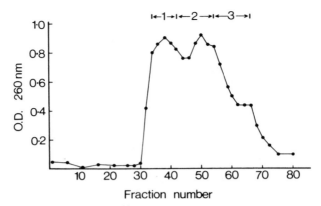

Fig. 2. Fractionation of DNA on Sepharose 4B. DNA was prepared by a minor modification of the technique of Paul and Gilmour (18). DNA at 500 μg/ml was applied to a column of Sepharose 4B (Pharmacia, Sweden) equilibrated with 0.01 *M* tris-Cl (*p*H 8.0), 0.1 m*M* EDTA, and 0.1 *M* KCl. Fractions were bulked and concentrated using polyethylene glycol 6000.

Table I. Effect of Fractionation of Bulk DNA on the Activity of Form-AI and Form-B RNA Polymerases

DNA fraction	Average mol wt[a]	"Nicks"/100 μg DNA[a]	RNA polymerase activity[b]	
			Form AI	Form B
Bulk DNA before fractionation	1.05×10^7	44.0	1786	2239
Sepharose fraction 1	1.85×10^7	6.5	4059	1720
Sepharose fraction 2	6.5×10^6	28.2	3455	1854
Sepharose fraction 3	3.2×10^6	319.0	2718	1954

[a]Average molecular weights and numbers of "nicks" were assayed by the end-labeling technique using polynucleotide kinase (15).

[b]Cpm [^{3}H]UMP incorporated into acid-precipitable RNA according to the technique of Chesterton and Butterworth (7).

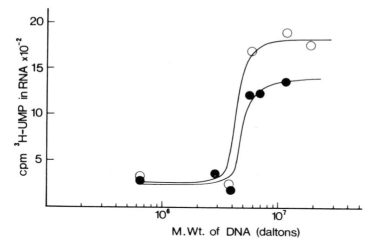

Fig. 3. Effect of DNA molecular weight on the activity of form-A and form-B RNA polymerases. Several preparations of DNA were fractionated on columns of Sepharose 4B. Using the end-labeling technique (15), the molecular weight and "nick" content of the fractions were compared, and, for the data presented in this figure, the major variable is the DNA molecular weight, each DNA having a low "nick" content (see text). Assays for template activity were carried out as described in the caption of Fig. 1. ○, Form-AI polymerase activity; ●, form-B polymerase activity.

enzymes there is a sharp decrease in polymerase activity as the DNA molecular weight drops from 5 to 3×10^6. This could be due to one of several effects. We favor the notion that the polymerases form abortive complexes at "ends," because DNA having molecular weights in the region of 3×10^6 but containing large numbers of "nicks" (about 300 "nicks"/100 μg DNA double strand) is a good template for either form-A or form-B polymerase.

Sonication

As the isolation of DNA containing no single-stranded breaks does not seem feasible, the effect of sonication of DNA was studied to ascertain whether this treatment would cleave the DNA at "nicks." Preliminary experiments indicate that this technique has considerable potential. Careful examination of Fig. 4 reveals that after very brief sonication (approximately 2 sec) there is a considerable reduction in the number of single-stranded breaks, resulting in a decrease in form-A polymerase activity. It is interesting that the subsequent increase in numbers of "nicks" is not accompanied by an increase in form-A polymerase activity and that form-B polymerase activity only slowly declines with increasing sonication time. Both of these phenomena are probably a result of the production of double-stranded "ends" (see below).

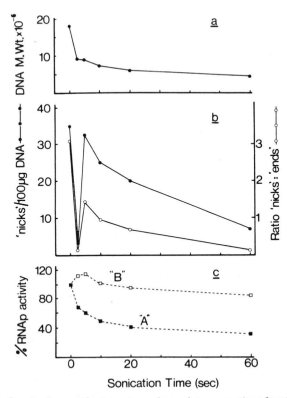

Fig. 4. Effect of sonication on the integrity and template properties of rat liver DNA. DNA was sonicated for varying periods of time (sec), and aliquots were taken and assayed for (a) average molecular weight of DNA species (15); (b) "nicks"/100 μg DNA (•) and the ratio of "nicks" to "ends" (○) (15); (c) template activity for form-AI polymerase (■) and for form-B polymerase (□). See caption of Fig. 1 for details of assay procedure.

However, this is a difficult technique to apply as a routine procedure: the duration of the brief burst of sonication required to reduce the numbers of "nicks" is critical and is highly dependent on DNA concentration and size.

The slight inhibition of form-B and the significant inhibition of form-A polymerase activity by 60 sec of sonication (Fig. 4) must be due to a reduction in the size of the DNA, thereby generating double-stranded "ends" (diplotomic cleavage) (16). If it is assumed that polymerases form abortive complexes at these "ends," removal of the low molecular weight DNA species (e.g., by molecular filtration) should relieve the inhibition. Again, this is found to be the case, as is shown in Table II.

Table II. Fractionation of DNA Sonicated for 60 sec[a]

DNA fraction	Average mol wt	RNA polymerase activity[b]	
		Form AI	Form B
Bulk DNA after sonication	—	1804	2097
Sepharose fraction 1	5.4×10^6	3722	2501
Sepharose fraction 2	4.8×10^6	2967	2147
Sepharose fraction 3	2.9×10^6	(641)	(400)

[a]DNA was sonicated for 60 sec in 0.01 M tris-Cl (pH 8.0) and 0.1 mM EDTA and was fractionated on Sepharose 4B as shown in Fig. 2.

[b]Cpm [^{3}H]UMP incorporated into acid-precipitable RNA according to the technique of Chesterton and Butterworth (7). Assays were carried out at a DNA concentration of 10 μg/0.25 ml assay except for Sepharose fraction 3 where 5 μg/0.25 ml assay was used.

CONCLUSIONS

On the basis of the data presented here, it is probably reasonable to predict that there are hierarchies of binding sites for polymerases on DNA: true initial binding sites (or "promoters") and single-stranded breaks (at least of the type inserted by pancreatic deoxyribonuclease), both of which produce productive complexes, and "ends" (probably double-stranded) which produce abortive complexes. It would be predicted that the polymerases have the highest affinity for their "promoters." An interesting but tentative interpretation of the data presented here is that the form-A polymerase (assuming its function to be the expression of the ribosomal cistrons) has few "promoters" in bulk DNA; therefore, its activity changes as the degree of modification of the DNA template increases. On the other hand, if the form-B polymerases are responsible for the transcription of all extranucleolar DNA, it would be anticipated that there would be relatively large numbers of "promoters" for this enzyme for which the enzyme would have a high affinity. Therefore, the activity of this polymerase is less likely to be affected by changes in the integrity of the DNA, and, so long as assays are carried out at limiting enzyme concentration, the effect of factors such as "nicks" in the DNA on the activity of form-B polymerase may be minimal.

The numbers of "ends" in the DNA can be controlled by careful fractionation procedures, but some knowledge of the numbers of single-strand breaks in the DNA would seem to be a prerequisite for the design of critical experiments to define the absolute template specificities of the multiple eukaryotic DNA-dependent RNA polymerases.

ACKNOWLEDGMENTS

We are grateful for the excellent technical assistance of Miss Karen Pollock and Mr. Brian Jenkins. This work was supported by grants from the Science Research Council (B/SR/7803 and B/SR/7804) and the Wellcome Foundation.

REFERENCES

1. A. Travers. *Nature New Biol.* **229**:69 (1971).
2. E. K. F. Bautz. In *Progress in Nucleic Acid Research and Molecular Biology,* Vol. 12, Academic Press, New York, p. 129 (1972).
3. R. G. Roeder and W. J. Rutter. *Nature (Lond.)* **224**:234 (1969).
4. C. Kedinger, M. Gniazdowski, J. L. Mandel, Jr., F. Gissinger, and P. Chambon. *Biochem. Biophys. Res. Commun.* **38**:165 (1970).
5. R. G. Roeder and W. J. Rutter. *Proc. Natl. Acad. Sci. (USA)* **65**:675 (1970).
6. C. J. Chesterton and P. H. W. Butterworth. *FEBS Letters* **12**:301 (1971).
7. C. J. Chesterton and P. H. W. Butterworth. *Europ. J. Biochem.* **19**:232 (1971).
8. C. Kedinger, P. Nuret, and P. Chambon. *FEBS Letters* **15**:169 (1971).
9. G. P. Tocchini-Valentini and M. Crippa. *Nature (Lond.)* **228**:993 (1970).
10. P. H. W. Butterworth, R. F. Cox, and C. J. Chesterton. *Europ. J. Biochem.* **23**:229 (1971).
11. I. Grummt and R. Lindigkeit. *Europ. J. Biochem.* **36**:244 (1973).
12. V. Vogt. *Nature (Lond.)* **223**:854 (1969).
13. J.-P. Dausse, A. Sentenac, and P. Fromageot. *Europ. J. Biochem.* **31**:394 (1972).
14. D. C. Hinkle, J. Ring, and M. J. Chamberlin. *J. Mol. Biol.* **70**:197 (1972).
15. B. Weiss, T. R. Live, and C. C. Richardson. *J. Biol. Chem.* **243**:4530 (1968).
16. C. C. Richardson. *J. Mol. Biol.* **15**:49 (1966).
17. H. V. Aposhian and A. Kornberg. *J. Biol. Chem.* **237**:519 (1962).
18. J. Paul and R. S. Gilmour. *J. Mol. Biol.* **34**:305 (1968).

22

RNA Polymerases and Controlling Factors from Plant Cell Nuclei

B. B. Biswas, H. Mondal, A. Ganguly, Asis Das, and R. K. Mandal

Bose Institute
Calcutta, India

Transcriptional regulation in higher organisms occurs by activation or inactivation of entire chromosomes, large chromosomal segments, and possibly smaller units. The phenomenon of puffing (1), where fairly large sections of chromosomes are activated together, may indicate the expression of the functionally related clusters. That such clusters of genes actually occur in higher organisms has been shown (2). Crick's (3) hypothesis that the function of most of the DNA is to regulate the activity of the rest of the DNA seems to originate from several lines of evidences. Britten and Davidson (4) suggested that the control is exerted by the extra DNA carried by higher organisms, especially by the repetitive DNA, and they pointed out the necessity of a sensor gene and integrator genes besides the regulator and structural genes. Georgiev *et al.* (5) have recently invoked similar types of multielemental control systems in eukaryotes. Thus inasmuch as different investigators have hypothesized a number of regulatory elements, regulation of the transcription process in the eukaryotes must be studied in detail.

The RNA polymerase of higher organisms has been resolved into two or three species, and the requirements of these species seem to be different. What can be generalized is that there are at least two or three forms of RNA polymerase present in the nuclei of eukaryotic cells. Moreover, it has been pointed out that one is associated with the nucleolus, responsible for ribosomal RNA synthesis, and the other with the nucleoplasm, responsible for mRNA or non-ribosomal RNA synthesis (6,7). In fact, very little is known about initiation or termination factors in eukaryotic cells (8-10).

Our intention was to find out whether RNA polymerases and the factors are associated with the chromatin. Since chromatin contains DNA, RNA, histone, and nonhistone proteins, it is pertinent to ask whether the protein parts have any role in RNA synthesis. Histone has now been classified as a general repressor for RNA polymerase (11-13). This inhibition of RNA polymerase can, however, be counteracted nonspecifically by many substances (14). Nonhistone protein has some role in derepression (15); also, this protein is heterogeneous (16). RNA polymerases (8) and several enzymes (16) have also been detected in the nonhistone fraction of the chromatin. Is it possible that RNA synthesis in eukaryotes is modulated during the division cycle by the production of nonhistone proteins of different composition and conformation? We have found that initiation and termination factors as well as RNA polymerases are present in the nonhistone fraction of chromatin (17,18).

In this chapter, we shall discuss the properties of three RNA polymerases isolated from the chromatin of coconut endosperm cell nuclei (17,18) as well as other proteins from the nuclei that could modulate the activity of these polymerases.

Table I. Enzyme Purification Summary[a]

600 green coconuts (2-3 months old)
      ↓ scraping
200 g endosperm tissue
      ↓ homogenization, washing
5 g chromatin
      ↓ 2 M NaCl extraction
500 mg soluble chromatin
      ↓ dialysis, centrifugation
143 mg nonhistone protein
      ↓ CM-cellulose chromatography
140 mg CM-cellulose unabsorbed protein
      ↓ ammonium sulfate fractionation
27.5 mg 30-55% ammonium sulfate fraction
      ↓ DEAE-cellulose chromatography

i.   2 mg R_I $\xrightarrow{\text{QAE-Sephadex chromatography}}$ 0.2 mg R_I
ii. 5 mg R_{II} $\xrightarrow{\text{Biogel A gel filtration}}$ 0.8 mg R_{II}
iii. 1 mg R_{III} $\xrightarrow{\text{Biogel P300 gel filtration}}$ 0.3 mg R_{III}
iv. 2 mg F_B $\xrightarrow{\text{QAE-Sephadex chromatography}}$ 0.15 mg F_B

[a]Details of the purification procedure will be published elsewhere.

RNA POLYMERASES

It was reported earlier from this laboratory that the RNA polymerase activity of the chromosomal nonhistone protein can be resolved into two species by DEAE-cellulose chromatography, the first activity being sensitive to the action of rifampicin. When the second activity peak was passed through a QAE-Sephadex column, the RNA polymerase was again resolved into two species. The polymerase eluted at 0.08 M KCl was designated RNA polymerase II and was subsequently purified extensively by Biogel A gel-filtration chromatography. The activity of the polymerase eluted at 0.12 M KCl was designated RNA polymerase III and purified further by Biogel P300 gel-filtration chromatography. A summary of the purification of the RNA polymerases is given in Table I. All three RNA polymerases exhibited single bands on polyacrylamide gel electrophoresis with different pHs, gel concentrations, and stains (Fig. 1).

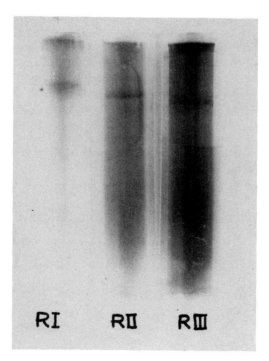

Fig. 1. Polyacrylamide gel electrophoresis of purified RNA polymerases. The enzyme fractions after the last purification steps were analyzed at pH 8.3 on polyacrylamide gels containing 5% acrylamide and 0.133% methylene bisacrylamide, as described by Davis (26). One-hundred micrograms of the enzyme preparations was applied, and electrophoresis was performed at 4 ma/tube for 2 hr. Gels were soaked in 7.5% acetic acid and stained with Coomassie blue.

The purified polymerases were then tested for their structural similarity or dissimilarity by electrophoresis on polyacrylamide gels in the presence of sodium dodecylsulfate. A schematic representation of the electropherograms is given in Fig. 2. The polymerases showed similarity in that all contained four different polypeptides and the core enzyme was composed of six subunits as estimated by densitometric tracing. When we comparatively analyzed the molecular weights of these subunits, we concluded that subunit a, with a molecular weight of 180,000, was conserved in all the enzymes. Subunit b was changed in RNA polymerase III, whereas subunit d was changed in RNA polymerase I. Subunit c was different in all cases (Table II).

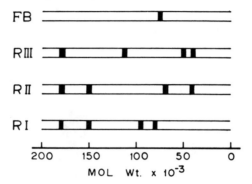

Fig. 2. *Schematic representation of dodecylsulfate-polyacrylamide gel electrophoretic patterns of RNA polymerases and factor B.* The analysis was performed in 5% acrylamide in the presence of 0.1% sodium dodecylsulfate, at 8 ma/tube for 2 hr, as described by Weber and Osborn (27).

Table II. Molecular Weights of the Subunits of RNA Polymerase

	Subunit				Mol wt of the enzyme $\times 10^{-3}$
	a	b	c	d	
R_I					
Mol wt $\times 10^{-3}$	180	150	95	80	735
Mol ratio	1	2	1	2	
R_{II}					
Mol wt $\times 10^{-3}$	180	150	69	42	633
Mol ratio	1	2	1	2	
R_{III}					
Mol wt $\times 10^{-3}$	180	112	50	40	534
Mol ratio	1	2	1	2	

All three polymerases are stimulated by fraction B (as in the case of RNA polymerase I) (18), which has been purified extensively by QAE-Sephadex column chromatography. Contrary to our previous report, we have found that all the purified enzymes are inhibited by rifampicin to different degrees (Table III). RNA polymerase I is inhibited completely at a concentration of 2 μg/ml of rifampicin. But 8 μg/ml and 4 μg/ml of rifampicin are required to inhibit RNA polymerase II and RNA polymerase III, respectively. We have also found that we can make all these polymerases resistant to rifampicin by making a complex of enzyme and factor B and that the enzyme-factor complex can be inhibited by gradually increasing the concentration of rifampicin, as reported earlier in the case of RNA polymerase I (18). Thus core enzyme is sensitive while holoenzyme is resistant to rifampicin. RNA polymerase I has been found to be sensitive to a-amanitin, while polymerases II and III are comparatively resistant (18).

In Vitro Products of RNA Polymerases

We have already reported that RNA polymerase I synthesizes a heterogeneous species of RNA (10–20S) (18). When we analyzed this RNA by DNA·RNA competition-hybridization experiments, it was found that the RNA species are nonribosomal. RNA polymerase II makes an RNA species *in vitro* that competes 90–92% with coconut ribosomal RNA (Fig. 3a), and this RNA, after polyacrylamide gel electrophoresis, shows the presence of different rRNA species. The product of RNA polymerase III is complex in nature, since about 20% of this

Table III. **Stimulation by Factor B and Inhibition by Rifampicin of Coconut RNA Polymerases**

Reaction system	[^{3}H] UMP incorporated[a]	
	pmoles/mg enzyme	Percent inhibition by rifampicin (2 μg/ml)
1. R$_I$ + Coco DNA	4	
2. 1 + factor B	208	
3. 1 + Rif + factor B	3	100
4. R$_{II}$ + Coco DNA	7	
5. 4 + factor B	513	
6. 4 + Rif + factor B	213	58
7. R$_{III}$ + Coco DNA	11	
8. 7 + factor B	704	
9. 7 + Rif + factor B	111	86

[a]50 μg RNA polymerase, 5 μg factor B (all purified fractions), and 10 μg DNA were used. The assay method was as described earlier (17).

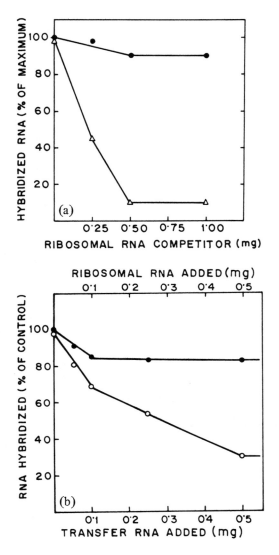

Fig. 3. Characterization of in vitro synthesized RNA products by DNA·RNA hybridization. Ribosomal RNA was isolated by hot phenol plus dodecylsulfate from coconut ribosomes. ^{3}H-Labeled RNAs were synthesized *in vitro* by three enzymes separately in the presence of factor B and tritium-labeled nucleoside triphosphates and were isolated by hot phenol plus dodecylsulfate (18). Hybridization was performed following the method of Gillespie and Spiegelman (28). (a) *In vitro* products of R_I and R_{II} were competed with ribosomal RNA; 20 μg denatured DNA and 50 μg [3H] RNA were used. •, R_I product; △, R_{II} product. (b) *In vitro* products of R_{III} were competed with rRNA and tRNA (isolated from coconut cytoplasm by DEAE-cellulose column chromatography); 10 μg denatured DNA and 30 μg [3H] RNA were used. •, rRNA; ○, tRNA.

RNA can be competed for by coconut rRNA and 70% of the RNA by coconut tRNA (Fig. 3b).

From the results we have discussed so far, it is evident that one can isolate from the chromosomal nonhistone proteins three RNA polymerases that not only differ greatly in their subunit structure but also synthesize *in vitro* mainly three distinct types of RNA species.

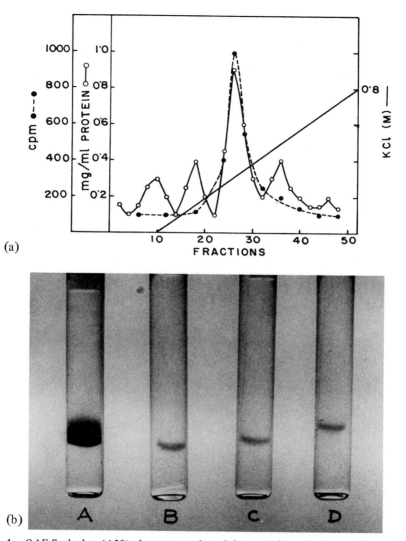

Fig. 4a. QAE-Sephadex (A50) chromatography of factor B from chromatin. The protein preparation in 0.01 M tris-Cl buffer (pH 8.0) containing 1 mM mercaptoethanol, 0.1 mM EDTA, and 5% v/v glycerol was passed through a QAE-Sephadex column, precycled, and equilibrated with the same buffer. The column was washed and then eluted with a 0-0.8 M KCl linear gradient in the abovementioned buffer. Fractions of 2 ml were collected. Aliquots containing 5 μg of protein were assayed with 50 μg of QAE enzyme (R$_I$) as described earlier (17). •, Factor-B activity, ○, protein (mg/ml); ——, KCl (M).

Fig. 4b. Polyacrylamide gel electrophoresis of purified factor B. The procedure was the same as described in Fig. 1. (A) QAE factor B, 50 μg at 7% gel; (B) QAE factor B, 10 μg at 7% gel; (C) at 7.5% gel; (D) at 8% gel.

Factor B as Initiation Factor

By DEAE-cellulose column chromatography, we isolated a protein fraction (F_B) (17) which is needed to synthesize RNA by all three species of RNA polymerase. Factor B was further purified to homogeneity by QAE-Sephadex column chromatography (Fig. 4a), as has been tested by polyacrylamide electrophoresis (Fig. 4b). That factor B acts as an initiation factor is indicated by the following evidence (18):

a. In the absence of factor B, RNA polymerases show only minimal activity with coconut DNA as the template.

b. Factor B can bind with RNA polymerases, and the enzyme-F_B complex then binds to DNA, but factor B alone cannot bind to DNA.

c. It promotes the incorporation of $[\beta,\gamma\text{-}^{32}P_2]$ ATP into RNA, and this stimulation reaches a plateau rather quickly, while the incorporation of $[^{14}C]$ ATP in the interior of the RNA chain continues.

d. It is active with native homologous DNA as the template, but not with denatured or λ DNA.

e. RNA molecules synthesized in its presence are of higher sedimentation value (10-20S) than that synthesized in its absence (4S).

f. It can completely counteract the inhibitory effect of rifampicin, which is known to inhibit RNA synthesis at the initiation step.

Indoleacetic Acid Stimulation of RNA Synthesis by RNA Polymerase I *In Vitro*

Several laboratories have reported that indoleacetic acid can stimulate RNA synthesis in plant cells. We have performed experiments with isolated coconut cells and nuclei that confirm this (Table IV). Until the present, the effect of indoleacetate has been shown *in vivo* or in a isolated system, but its actual effect on the RNA polymerase reaction *per se* has not been demonstrated. It was thus interesting to see the effect of indoleacetate on the purified RNA polymerases isolated from the plant cell nuclei. It has been noted that this substance cannot stimulate RNA synthesis by RNA polymerase alone, needing for stimulation the presence of another nuclear protein (Table V). This aspect has already been discussed (19).

This protein was tested for indoleacetate binding capacity by equilibrium dialysis. It was found that this protein can bind $[^{14}C]$ indoleacetate (19). This binding was confirmed by polyacrylamide gel electrophoresis, as shown in Fig. 5. Thus this protein might be analogous to the auxin acceptor protein reported earlier (20).

Table IV. Effect of Indoleacetate on RNA Synthesis by Isolated Coconut Cells and Nuclei[a]

System	pmoles [^{14}C] uridine incorporated/ mg RNA
Cell suspension	
1. Control	363
2. Indoleacetate (10^{-6} M) treated	1112
Nuclear suspension	
1. Control	666
2. Indoleacetate (10^{-6} M) treated	1050

[a]Isolated cell and nucleus (17) were incubated in 1 ml mixture containing 0.25 M glucose, 0.001 M MgCl$_2$, 0.01 M tris-Cl (pH 7), 0.4 μmole [^{14}C] uridine (3 $\times$ 10^6 cpm/μmole), and 0.1 ml of 0.2% alcohol in the control or 0.1 ml of 10^{-5} M indoleacetate in the system, at 37°C for 30 min. RNAs were isolated by hot phenol, precipitated by alcohol, and dissolved in acetate buffer (pH 5.2). RNA was measured by UV absorption, and incorporation was determined by measuring radioactivity in liquid scintilation counter in dioxan base.

Table V. Factor Essential for Indoleacetate to Stimulate RNA Polymerase I[a]

Reaction system	[^{3}H] UTP incorporated (cpm)
R$_I$ + factor B + Coco DNA	336
R$_I$ + factor B (without DNA)	56
R$_I$ + factor B + Coco DNA + indoleacetate	328
Nucleoplasm only	72
Nucleoplasm + indoleacetate	68
R$_I$ + factor B + Coco DNA + nucleoplasm	412
R$_I$ + factor B + Coco DNA + nucleoplasm + indoleacetate	727

[a]10 μg enzyme, 1 μg factor B, 10 μg DNA, 10 μg nucleoplasm, and 10^{-6} M indoleacetate were used. The assay procedure was as usual.

The next question was, how does the acceptor protein mediate the reaction? When RNA polymerase I and F$_B$ were allowed to react with the acceptor protein complex and DNA and the mixture was layered on a linear sucrose gradient, it was found that the acceptor protein does not bind to enzyme-F$_B$ complex but that it does bind to DNA. We then measured the binding of the acceptor protein complex with DNA on cellulose nitrate filters. It was found that the DNA· [^{14}C] indoleacetate·acceptor complex was retained on the filter paper (19).

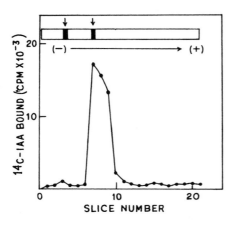

Fig. 5. *Lack of binding of acceptor protein with RNA polymerase I and factor B.* Five micrograms of acceptor protein, 10^{-6} M [2-^{14}C]indoleacetate (specific activity 8 × 10^5 cpm/nmole), 10 μg RNA polymerase I, and 1 μg factor B were incubated for 15 min at 37°C in buffer (pH 8). The aliquot of the incubation mixture was electrophoresed on 5% polyacrylamide gel as in Fig. 2. The gels were sliced and dissolved in H_2O_2 and counted with dioxan-based liquifluor (30). The band nearer the cathode indicated the RNA polymerase - factor B complex, and the distal band indicated the indoleacetate - acceptor protein complex.

New Species of RNA Synthesis Mediated by Indoleacetate and Acceptor Protein

The stimulation of RNA synthesis in the presence of indoleacetate and acceptor protein might be due to more efficient synthesis of the same types of RNA than that in the absence of the acceptor, or to the synthesis of additional new species of RNA. These possibilities were tested by DNA·RNA hybridization. Various amounts of labeled RNA synthesized in the absence of indoleacetate and acceptor were hybridized with denatured coconut DNA to obtain a saturation level. At this point, different amounts of RNA synthesized in the presence of the acceptor were added in order to see whether any additional RNA was hybridized (Fig. 6). The extent of hybridization was doubled in the latter case, which indicates that RNA synthesized in the presence of indoleacetate hybridizes at additional sites of DNA that are not complementary to RNA made in its absence (19).

Effect of Indoleacetate on rRNA Synthesis by RNA Polymerase II

Because, as discussed above, indoleacetate can influence nonribosomal RNA synthesis by RNA polymerase I, it was thought worthwhile to test whether it can also influence rRNA synthesis by RNA polymerase II. It has been found that indoleacetate stimulates RNA synthesis by RNA polymerase II by about 1.5-to twofold. When RNA polymerase II was inhibited by rifampicin and indoleacetate and acceptor protein were added, an enhancement of RNA synthesis was still noted (Fig. 7).

We wanted to find the type of RNA species synthesized by RNA polymerase II in the presence of indoleacetate by DNA·RNA competition hybridization. We

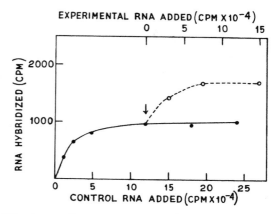

Fig. 6. Hybridization of in vitro synthesized RNA with DNA. [³H]RNA was synthesized by RNA polymerase I and factor B in either the presence (experimental) or the absence (control) of acceptor protein and indoleacetate. The liquid hybridization technique of Attardi *et al.* (29) was used. Various amounts of labeled RNA (2.4 × 10³ cpm/μg in case of control and 2 × 10³ cpm/μg in case of experimental RNA) were incubated with 5 μg of heat-denatured coconut DNA in 2 ml of 2× SSC buffer (0.15 *M* NaCl, 0.015 *M* tri-sodium citrate) at 70°C for 10 hr. After slow cooling to room temperature, the mixture was treated with 10 μg of pancreatic RNase (freed from DNase by heating at 80°C for 15 min). After incubation with RNase for 15 min at 21°C, the mixture was passed through Millipore HAWP filters. The filters were washed with 100 ml of 2× SSC and counted with 10 ml of dioxan-based liquifluor and 1 ml of water, in which the filters completely dissolved giving a uniform phase. ●, Hybridization of varying amounts of control RNA synthesized in the absence of indoleacetate. ○, Hybridization of varying amounts of experimental RNA synthesized in the presence of indoleacetate when added on top of a saturating amount (12 × 10⁴ cpm) of control RNA.

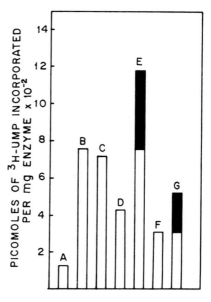

Fig. 7. Effect of indoleacetate and acceptor protein on RNA synthesis by RNA polymerase II. (A) Coconut DNA (10 μg) + RNA polymerase II (50 μg); (B) A + factor B (5 μg); (C) B + indoleacetate (10⁻⁶ *M*); (D) B + acceptor protein (10 μg); (E) B + indoleacetate + acceptor protein; (F) A + rifampicin (4 μg/ml) + factor B; (G) F + indoleacetate + acceptor protein. Assay conditions were similar to those described earlier (17).

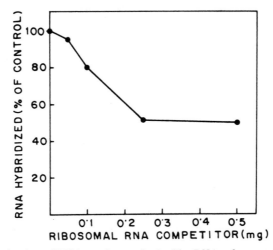

Fig. 8. *Characterization of RNA species synthesized by RNA polymerase II in the presence of indoleacetate and acceptor protein by DNA·RNA competition hybridization.* ^{3}H-Labeled RNA was isolated from a reaction mixture containing coconut DNA, RNA polymerase II (200 μg), factor B (20 μg), rifampicin (6 μg/ml), indoleacetate (10^{-6} M), and acceptor protein (40 μg) by hot phenol. Fifty micrograms of [3H] RNA was hybridized with 10 μg of denatured DNA in the presence of different amounts of coconut ribosomal RNA.

found that about 40% of the RNA synthesized under the experimental conditions was nonribosomal (Fig. 8). We conclude that RNA polymerase II, which synthesizes only ribosomal RNA (90%), can synthesize nonribosomal RNA under certain conditions. (Characterization of the new species of nonribosomal RNA is in progress.)

CONCLUSION

Three distinct RNA polymerases from the nonhistone proteins of chromatin of coconut endosperm cell nuclei have been isolated and purified. However, RNA polymerases may not be entirely bound to the chromatin. There might be an equilibrium between the bound and the free forms, since RNA polymerase and the factors present in the chromatin would have to be separated from the chromatin followed by reassociation in order to recycle the process *in vivo.* From the polyacrylamide gel electrophoretic pattern, it is apparent that these species have been extensively purified. The molecular weights of these polymerases are recorded as 730,000, 635,000 and 530,000, respectively. The subunit nature of these enzymes is well documented as compared to the species isolated from animal sources. In no case are lower molecular weight subunits discernible (21). However, the reconstitution of these enzymes from subunits has not yet been achieved.

Besides these RNA polymerases, two nonhistone proteins have been isolated that could modulate RNA polymerase activity; one has been purified to homogeneity (mol wt 76,000), has a single subunit, and acts as an initiation factor (18). The other one, though not extensively purified, has a definite role in the release and/or termination of RNA chains (18). All three species of RNA polymerase require the same initiation factor (factor B).

The product, analyzed by polyacrylamide gel electrophoresis as well as by the DNA·RNA competition-hybridization technique, has been found to be different and characteristic of the particular enzyme. RNA polymerase I synthesizes nonribosomal RNA, whereas polymerase II synthesizes ribosomal RNA; the product of polymerase III seems to be partly ribosomal and partly of a tRNA type when total homologous native DNA is used as template.

Another protein fraction has been isolated from the nucleoplasm of the same source that can accept indoleacetic acid, a plant growth hormone. That the acceptor protein complex interacts with DNA but not with RNA polymerase or initiation factor (factor B) *per se* and that an additional species of RNA is synthesized in case of polymerase I have been documented. The same complex can also increase the synthesis of rRNA by polymerase II, but the RNA synthesized in the presence of the acceptor protein seems to be nonribosomal. That this nonribosomal RNA might act as an activator RNA, as suggested in the model of Britten and Davidson (4), is an interesting possibility. It seems that there might be a number of nonhistone proteins in the chromatin that can modulate the transcription. Results from several laboratories are consistent with the concept of these proteins as regulators of gene expression in eukaryotic cells (22-25). All these evidences suggest that there are certain positive controlling elements in the chromatin that can modulate the transcription. Some of these controlling elements have been identified in the present study. The initiation complex seems to be a ternary complex or complex of higher order, but the exact mechanism by which this type of control is operative in the chromosome is yet to be understood.

ACKNOWLEDGMENTS

The technical assistance of Mr. Subhas Deb Roy is acknowledged with thanks. This research was supported by a USDA PL-480 grant (No. FG-In-321) and an equipment grant from the Department of Atomic Energy, Government of India.

REFERENCES

1. S. Beerman. *Genetics* **54**:569 (1966).
2. M. Lezzi. *Internat. Rev. Cytol.* **29**:127 (1970).
3. F. Crick. *Nature* **234**:25 (1971).

4. R. J. Britten and E. H. Davidson. *Science* **165**:349 (1969).
5. G. P. Georgiev, A. P. Ryskov, C. Coutelle, V. L. Manitieva, and E. R. Avakyan. *Biochim. Biophys. Acta* **259**:259 (1972).
6. C. C. Widnell and J. R. Tata. *Biochim. Biophys. Acta* **123**:478 (1966).
7. R. G. Roeder and W. J. Rutter. *Nature* **224**:234 (1969).
8. H. Mondal, R. K. Mandal, and B. B. Biswas. *Biochem. Biophys. Res. Commun.* **40**:1194 (1970).
9. H. Stein and P. Hausen. *Europ. J. Biochem.* **14**:270 (1970).
10. E. D. Mauro, C. P. Hollenberg, and B. D. Hall. *Proc. Natl. Acad. Sci. (USA)* **69**:2818 (1972).
11. J. Bonner. *The Molecular Biology of Development,* Oxford University Press, Oxford (1965).
12. J. A. V. Butler, E. W. Johns, and D. M. P. Phillips. *Progr. Biophys. Mol. Biol.* **18**:209 (1968).
13. G. P. Georgiev. *Ann. Rev. Genet.* **3**:155 (1969).
14. J. H. Frenster. *Nature* **206**:680 (1965).
15. J. Paul and R. S. Gilmour. *J. Mol. Biol.* **34**:305 (1968).
16. S. C. R. Elgin, S. C. Froehner, J. E. Smart, and J. Bonner. In E. J. DuPraw (ed.), *Advances in Cell Molecular Biology,* Vol. 1, Academic Press, New York, p. 1 (1971).
17. H. Mondal, R. K. Mandal, and B. B. Biswas. *Europ. J. Biochem.* **25**:463 (1972).
18. H. Mondal, A. Ganguly, A. Das, R. K. Mandal, and B. B. Biswas. *Europ. J. Biochem.* **28**:143 (1972).
19. H. Mondal, R. K. Mandal, and B. B. Biswas. *Nature New Biol.* **240**:111 (1972).
20. A. G. Mathysse and C. Phillips. *Proc. Natl. Acad. Sci. (USA)* **63**:897 (1969).
21. F. Gissinger and P. Chambon. *Europ. J. Biochem.* **28**:277 (1972).
22. R. Stellwagen and R. Cole. *Ann. Rev. Biochem.* **38**:951 (1969).
23. R. S. Gilmour and J. Paul. *FEBS Letters* **9**:242 (1970).
24. T. C. Spelsberg and L. Hnilica. *Biochem. J.* **120**:435 (1970).
25. C. Ten, C. Teng, and V. J. Allfrey. *J. Biol. Chem.* **246**:3597 (1971).
26. B. J. Davis. *Ann. N.Y. Acad. Sci.* **121**:404 (1964).
27. K. Weber and M. Osborn. *J. Biol. Chem.* **244**:4406 (1969).
28. D. Gillespie and S. Spiegelman. *J. Mol. Biol.* **12**:829 (1965).
29. G. Attardi, P. C. Huang, and S. Kabat. *Proc. Natl. Acad. Sci. (USA)* **54**:185 (1965).
30. J. B. Boyd and H. K. Mitchell. *Anal. Biochem.* **14**:441 (1966).

DISCUSSION

Question (Chakravorty): In the experiment where you showed the retention of [^{3}H]DNA on Millipore filters, what percent of the input DNA can be retained on the Millipore filter with the help of acceptor protein? Moreover, your indoleacetate-binding protein is not pure. Did you run any control experiment with other types of DNA to check whether your acceptor protein contains any basic protein causing nonspecific binding to the Millipore filter?

Answer: Under the experimental conditions, 36–40% of the DNA is retained. With *E. coli* DNA there is nonspecific binding, but this can be washed from the Millipore filter by treating with 0.3 *M* KCl. Under identical conditions in the case of coconut DNA, at least 30% of DNA is retained.

Question (Gurnani): Did acceptor protein bind to DNA in the absence of indoleacetate? Did indoleacetate bind to DNA in the absence of the acceptor protein?

Answer: Acceptor protein alone binds to DNA and inhibits RNA synthesis by RNA polymerase I. Indoleacetate *per se* can bind to DNA, but this binding at physiological concentration is very labile.

Question (Burma): What is the ratio of binding between the protein and indoleacetate? Apparently the protein has to be obtained in pure form to do this, but can you give us some rough idea?

Answer: From our experiment where the indoleacetate-acceptor complex is isolated by gel electrophoresis or by Biogel and taking the molecular weight of the protein as 100,000, the ratio of protein and indoleacetate comes to roughly 2.5:1.

Question (Salahuddin): What ionic strength did you use in your binding experiments by equilibrium dialysis? If the ionic strength is very low, the distribution of indoleacetic acid will be greatly influenced by Gibbs-Donan equilibrium.

Answer: The concentration of protein was less than 10^{-4} M and the salt concentration in the buffer 10^{-1} M. The distribution of indoleacetate is not affected by Donan equilibrium under these conditions.

Question (Sarkar): Do you know which subunit is responsible for rifampicin sensitivity? Could you detect any conformational change in the indoleacetate-protein complex?

Answer: No. Since the protein is not absolutely pure, such an attempt has not been made.

Question (Das): The initiation factor leads to the production of longer RNA. Thus it means that the factor also stabilizes the complex or that the synthesis in the absence of the factor is random and physilogically useless. Have you done any experiment, competition hybridization or other, to differentiate between these possibilities?

Answer: Since RNA of lower molecular weight is only synthesized in the absence of initiation factor, we think that RNA synthesis might be random and biologically nonfunctional. We have not done any hybridization experiments with this RNA.

Question (Pradhan): Have you checked the effect of indoleacetate on Mg^{2+}-dependent and $Mn^{2+}/(NH_4)_2SO_4$-dependent RNA polymerase activities in intact nuclei? Could you tell us how much of RNA polymerase is solubilized from coconut nuclei?

Answer: From our previous experiments, we know that both nonribosomal and ribosomal RNA synthesis are increased *in vivo* with indoleacetate. Sixty percent of the total RNA polymerase activity of the nuclei could be isolated from the preparation of our chromatin.

23

Restriction of RNA Synthesis by RNA Polymerase from Avian Erythrocyte Nuclei

R. K. Mandal, Hemanta K. Mazumder, and B. B. Biswas

Bose Institute
Calcutta, India

The biochemistry of cell division and its regulation are intricate problems of molecular biology today. Generally speaking, all animal cells go through a period (G_1) following mitosis during which no DNA synthesis takes place. This is true for rapidly dividing cells as well as for those in the process of transformation from a nondividing to a dividing state. However, the period is one of intense activity so far as RNA synthesis is concerned, and this RNA synthesis is necessary for subsequent entry of the cells into the S phase. In some cells such as brain cells and nucleated erythrocytes of avian and amphibian species, this period is prolonged indefinitely into a state G_0. But while brain cells make RNA and protein all the time, nucleated erythrocytes are extreme examples where the function of the nucleus is permanently shut off. From this consideration, we wanted to look for the factor or factors responsible for inhibiting the transcriptional activity of DNA in avian erythrocyte nuclei.

It is well known that all the precursor cells of avian erythrocytes are very active in RNA synthesis, but the rate falls practically to zero in the mature nucleated erythrocyte (7,14). There is a concomitant increase, in the chromatin, of an erythrocyte-specific, serine-rich histone called "F2C fraction." Though circumstantial evidence indicates that the F2C histone may be responsible for the repression of transcriptional activity of erythrocyte nuclei, it is by no means persuasive (1,3). There might be other reasons for this nonfunctioning of DNA. First, the DNA template itself may be irreversibly damaged, e.g., partially denatured, cross-linked, or degraded. Second, key enzymes such as DNA poly-merase, RNA polymerase, or their regulatory factors, if any, may be absent.

BEHAVIOR OF CHICKEN ERYTHROCYTE DNA ON HYDROXYLAPATITE COLUMNS

To test the first possibility, we isolated DNA from mature chicken erythro-cytes by a modification of Marmur's method (9) and examined it by hydroxyl-apatite column chromatography (12). Figure 1 shows the elution profile of a mixture of ^{32}P-labeled native *Escherichia coli* DNA and native chicken erythro-cyte DNA. Chicken erythrocyte DNA was eluted a fraction or two after *E. coli* DNA. This slight difference was always reproducible in a number of chromato-graphic runs. The elution pattern of a mixture of heat-denatured ^{32}P-labeled *E. coli* DNA and heat-denatured chicken erythrocyte DNA is shown in Fig. 2. It can be seen that both were eluted exactly at the same position. Also, the heat-denatured chicken erythrocyte DNA applied to the column was quantita-tively recovered in one peak, indicating that it contained no cross-linked frac-tion. Otherwise, that fraction of DNA would have been resistant to denaturation and eluted after the denatured DNA peak. Thus hydroxylapatite column chro-

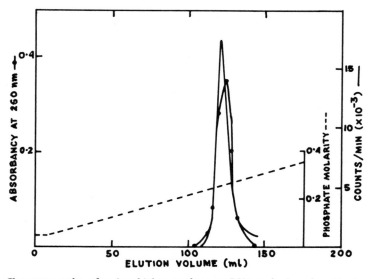

Fig. 1. *Chromatography of native chicken erythrocyte DNA on hydroxylapatite.* A mixture of 4.0 A_{260} units of chicken erythrocyte DNA and 0.8 A_{260} unit of ^{32}P-labeled *E. coli* DNA (containing 70,000 cpm) was put on a 1.2- by 3.5-cm hydroxylapatite column. DNA was eluted with a linear gradient of 0.05-0.4 *M* sodium phosphate (*p*H 6.8). Fractions of 4 ml were collected at a flow rate of 1 ml/3 min.

matography revealed no significant abnormality in the chicken erythrocyte DNA. Regarding the possibility of fragmentation or degradation of DNA in chicken erythrocytes, the indication obtained was negative. The higher viscosity and sedimentation rate (results not presented) indicated that chicken erythrocyte DNA is larger than DNA isolated from calf thymus or chicken liver. Possibly due to the low level of nuclease activity in chicken erythrocytes, the chance of DNA degradation during its isolation was much less than with chicken liver or calf thymus.

PRESENCE OF RNA POLYMERASE IN CHICKEN ERYTHROCYTE CHROMATIN

The presence of DNA and RNA polymerases in chicken erythrocytes was next checked. Previously, Mondal *et al.* (10) in our laboratory had isolated and purified RNA polymerases and some controlling factors from chromatinic acidic proteins of plant cell nuclei. The same procedure with some modification was applied to isolate chromosomal acidic proteins from chicken erythrocytes and young chicken liver. The composition of crude chromatin (including the nucleolochromosomal apparatus) is shown in Table I. For comparison, the compo-

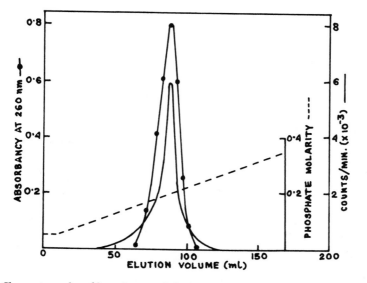

Fig. 2. Chromatography of heat-denatured chicken erythrocyte DNA on hydroxylapatite. A mixture of 4.0 A_{260} units of heat-denatured chicken erythrocyte DNA and 0.5 A_{260} unit of heat-denatured ^{32}P-labeled *E. coli* DNA (50,000 cpm) was chromatographed under the conditions described in the caption of Fig. 1.

Table I.   Composition of Chromatin[a]

Chromatin source	DNA	RNA	Histone	Nonhistone
Pea bud[b]	1.00	0.12	1.05	0.50
Coconut endosperm[c]	1.00	0.50	1.00	0.50
Chicken liver[d]	1.00	0.11	0.80	1.50
Chicken erythrocyte[d]	1.00	0.01	0.84	0.38
Chicken liver[e]	1.00	0.28	1.10	0.60
Chicken erythrocyte[e]	1.00	0.03	1.00	0.29

[a]The amounts of RNA, histone, and nonhistones are expressed with
respect to DNA taken as 1.
[b]Bonner et al. (4).
[c]Mondal et al. (10).
[d]Dingman and Sporn (6).
[e]Present study.

sitions of purified chromatin from some other sources are also presented.
Needless to say, the composition will vary considerably with the method of
isolation. We only point out that in chicken erythrocyte chromatin the relative
amount of RNA was one-tenth and of nonhistone chromosomal proteins one-
half that of chicken liver chromatin, both isolated by the same method in the
present study.

The total chromosomal acidic protein from chicken erythrocytes was assayed for RNA and DNA polymerases by the incorporation of [^{3}H] UTP and
[^{3}H] dATP, respectively. The results presented in Table II indicate the presence
of RNA polymerase and the absence of DNA polymerase activity.

The existence of multiple RNA polymerases in eukaryotic cells is now
accepted (Chambon et al., Chapter 20, this volume, and refs. 5,10,13). Also, in
chicken erythrocytes both the amount of total chromosomal nonhistone proteins
and RNA-synthesizing capacity decrease with progressive maturation (2). However, no attempt to isolate RNA polymerases from mature chicken erythrocytes
has come to our notice. We therefore fractionated total chromosomal acidic
proteins from chicken erythrocytes on DEAE-cellulose columns and tested the
fractions for RNA polymerase activity. The results are presented in Fig. 3. Three
RNA polymerases, R_I, R_{II}, and R_{III}, were detected. By analogy with plant chromatin fractions, we tested the protein fraction eluted at higher salt concentration
for any stimulatory activity. From the results presented in Table III, it can be seen
that all the three RNA polymerases from chicken erythrocytes had only minimal

Table II. Assay of RNA and DNA Polymerases in Chromosomal Acidic Proteins from Chicken Erythrocyte Nuclei[a]

System	[³H]dATP incorporation in DNA (cpm)	[³H]UTP incorporation in RNA (cpm)
Blank	200	
Complete	182	
Blank		150
Complete		425
Omit NTP[b]		195

[a]The complete incubation mixture in a final volume of 0.25 ml contained tris-Cl buffer (pH 8.0), 10 μmoles; $MgCl_2$, 2.5 μmoles; EDTA, 0.025 μmole; mercaptoethanol, 1.5 μmoles; calf thymus DNA, 20 μg; a mixture of dCTP, dGTP, dTTP, and [³H]dATP, 50 nmoles each (specific activity of [³H]dATP = 13 cpm/pmole), in the case of DNA synthesis, or a mixture of ATP, CTP, GTP, and [³H]UTP, 50 nmoles each (specific activity of [³H]UTP = 12 cpm/pmole), in the case of RNA synthesis; and chromatin acidic protein, 100 μg. Incubation was for 30 min at 37°C. Reaction was stopped by 10% trichloroacetic acid, and the precipitate was collected and washed on Millipore filters and counted in toluene liquifluor in a Beckman LS100 scintillation counter.
[b]NTP, unlabeled nucleoside triphosphate mixture.

activity in the absence of any added factors. The addition of protein fraction B from chicken erythrocytes had no stimulatory effect. But the addition of coconut initiation factor B (11) stimulated the activity of all three RNA polymerases. In contrast, RNA polymerases isolated from young chicken liver chromosomal acidic proteins by the same method (Fig. 4) had about ten times higher specific activity, and they were not stimulated by either chicken liver fractions or coconut factor B (Table III). This indicates that chicken liver RNA polymerases have the stimulatory factor associated with them.

The active chicken liver RNA polymerase was used to test the template activity of chicken erythrocyte DNA. Results presented in Table IV showed that chicken erythrocyte DNA is as active a template as calf thymus DNA. These results indicate that chicken erythrocyte nuclei contain both template DNA and RNA polymerases but may be deficient in regulatory factor(s). This may well explain the low RNA-synthesizing capacity of mature chicken erythrocytes. This

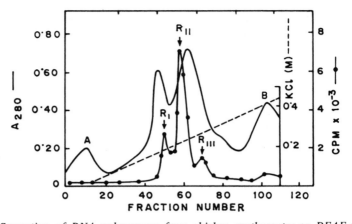

Fig. 3. Separation of RNA polymerases from chicken erythrocytes on DEAE-cellulose. Nuclei isolated from washed chicken erythrocytes by brief hypotonic shock were disrupted in low-salt buffer. From the crude chromatin, nonhistone proteins were isolated by the method of Mondal et al. (10). Twenty-two milligrams of 30-55% ammonium sulfate saturated fraction of the nonhistone protein was placed on a DEAE-cellulose column (1.2 by 25 cm) and eluted with a KCl gradient in 0.01 M tris (pH 8), 5 mM mercaptoethanol, 0.1 mM EDTA, 5% glycerol. Fractions collected at a flow rate of 1 ml/5 min were assayed for RNA polymerase activity by the ^{32}PP$_i$ exchange method (8).

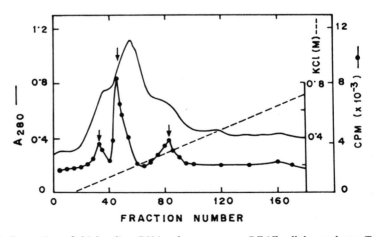

Fig. 4. Separation of chicken liver RNA polymerases on a DEAE-cellulose column. Twenty-five milligrams of 30-55% ammonium sulfate saturated fraction of chicken liver chromatin nonhistone proteins was chromatographed on a DEAE-cellulose column. Other conditions were the same as in Fig. 3.

Table III. RNA Polymerases from Chicken Erythrocyte and Liver Chromatin Nonhistone Proteins[a]

Enzyme system	[^{3}H] UTP incorporation (pmoles/mg/30 min) in fractions from	
	Chicken erythrocytes	Chicken liver
30-55% AS	75	210
R_I	400	4000
R_I + Coco B	1500	4000
R_{II}	800	5600
R_{II} + Coco B	1200	5600
R_{III}	340	600
R_{III} + Coco B	1380	600

[a]Assay mixture was the same as in Table II. Fifty micrograms of enzyme protein and 5 μg of fraction B were used where indicated.

Table IV. Template Activity of Chicken Erythrocyte DNA with Chicken Liver RNA Polymerase II[a]

System	[^{3}H] UTP incorporation (cpm)
Blank	243
Complete	1666
Complete - CT DNA[b]	361
Complete - CT DNA + CEN DNA[b]	1420

[a]The assay system was the same as in Table II; 40 μg of chicken liver RNA polymerase II (from DEAE-cellulose column) was used per incubation.

[b]CT, calf thymus; CEN, chicken erythrocyte nuclei.

study does not, however, preclude the existence of alternative mechanisms of transcription shutoff. For example, there may be positive inhibition of RNA synthesis by some inhibitors. Studies on this point are in progress.

Finally, we wish to point out here the changes brought about in the elution behavior of RNA polymerases from DEAE-cellulose. In the nomenclature of the present study (and also of Biswas et al., Chapter 22, this volume), R_I is the non-nucleolar RNA polymerase sensitive to a-amanitin and R_{II} is nucleolar RNA polymerase insensitive to a-amanitin. R_{III} is also insensitive to the drug. In studies of others, the nucleolar RNA polymerase is eluted first from DEAE-cellulose. We studied this problem in depth and found that this altered elution was due to a high initial salt (1 M) treatment of chromatin. Chicken liver nuclei were incubated in low-salt buffer according to Chesterton and Butterworth (6), and the nucleolar a-amanitin-insensitive RNA polymerase which eluted at 0.12-0.14 M salt was solubilized. When this enzyme was treated in vitro with 1 M

NaCl, dialyzed, and again put into a DEAE-cellulose column, it eluted at 0.2-0.24 M salt but still remained insensitive to a-amanitin. This change in elution behavior may be due to some irreversible change in conformation of the enzyme and/or loss of some proteins not necessary for the enzyme activity.

ACKNOWLEDGMENT

This research was supported by a grant from the Department of Atomic Energy, Government of India.

REFERENCES

1. R. Appels and J. R. E. Wells. *J. Mol. Biol.* **70**:425 (1972).
2. R. Appels and A. F. Williams. *Biochim. Biophys. Acta* **217**:531 (1970).
3. M. A. Billet and J. Hindley. *Europ. J. Biochem.* **28**:451 (1972).
4. J. Bonner, M. E. Dahmus, D. Fambrough, R. C. C. Huang, K. Marushige, and D. Y. H. Tuan. *Science* **161**:529 (1968).
5. C. J. Chesterton and P. H. W. Butterworth. *Europ. J. Biochem.* **19**:232 (1971).
6. C. W. Dingman and M. B. Sporn. *J. Biol. Chem.* **239**:3483 (1964).
7. D. Kabat and G. Attardi. *Biochim. Biophys. Acta* **138**:382 (1967).
8. J. Krakow and E. J. Fronk. *J. Biol. Chem.* **244**:5988 (1969).
9. J. Marmur. *J. Mol. Biol.* **3**:208 (1961).
10. H. Mondal, R. K. Mandal, and B. B. Biswas. *Europ. J. Biochem.* **25**:463 (1972).
11. H. Mondal, A. Ganguly, A. Das, R. K. Mandal, and B. B. Biswas. *Europ. J. Biochem.* **28**:143 (1972).
12. Y. Miyazawa and C. A. Thomas. *J. Mol. Biol.* **11**:223 (1965).
13. R. G. Roeder and W. J. Rutter. *Nature* **224**:234 (1969).
14. A. F. Williams. *J. Cell Sci.* **10**:27 (1971).

DISCUSSION

Comment (Rutter): We have found that many times the enzymes fractionate differently on columns due to complexes with protein and/or DNA. This can be eliminated by ion-elution fractionation according to Bock. Then they will fractionate normally.

Question (Burma): Has it not been shown by cell fusion techniques that hemoglobin can be produced in erythrocytes by fusing these cells with HeLa cells with the help of Sendai virus?

Answer: Yes. In this case, some factor(s) from the HeLa cells activates the erythrocyte nuclei, which synthesize RNA followed by protein. But this activation process has not yet been studied at the isolated RNA polymerase level.

Question (Sarkar): Did you attempt to titrate your RNA polymerase with factor to decide whether your enzyme contains a limiting amount of the factor?

Answer: At low concentrations of factor B, RNA polymerase activity increases with the amount of factor B added. But as our DEAE-cellulose fractions of RNA polymerases are rather crude, a stoichiometric titration cannot be done.

24

On the Regulation of Pre-mRNA Biosynthesis and Transport

E. M. Lukanidin, O. P. Samarina, A. P. Ryskov, and G. P. Georgiev

Institute of Molecular Biology
Academy of Sciences of the U.S.S.R.
Moscow, U.S.S.R.

In this chapter, I shall present some new data on the structure of nuclear pre-mRNA (precursor of mRNA, also called dRNA and HnRNA) and on the properties of nuclear ribonucleoprotein particles containing pre-mRNA. These problems are closely related to an understanding of the regulation of mRNA synthesis and transport.

DOUBLE-HELICAL REGIONS (HAIRPIN-LIKE STRUCTURES) IN THE NUCLEAR PRE-mRNA

According to the hypothetical model describing the organization of the transcriptional unit in eukaryotes (5), it consists of two parts—acceptor and structural zones. The structural zone consists of one or a few structural genes. The acceptor zone does not carry any structural information. The latter contains the acceptor sites in DNA that interact with regulatory proteins and consequently may control the folding of DNA as well as the movement of RNA polymerase along the transcriptional unit.

Some of the acceptor sites may be reiterated, making it possible to switch different transcriptions on or off by one regulatory agent.

Experiments on the hybridization properties of the 5'-end and 3'-end sequences gave evidence in favor of the localization of mRNA near the 3' end of the giant pre-mRNA molecule. This is in good agreement with the model (6). Poly(A) studies also confirmed the 3'-end localization of mRNA in pre-mRNA (25). On the other hand, 5' ends were found to be synthesized on the reiterated DNA sequences, and the corresponding sequences were not observed in the cytoplasm (ref. 6 and some unpublished data). These results are in good agreement with the above-mentioned model.

There remains the question of what the structure of the acceptor zone is. To analyze this problem, we tried to look for some specific base sequences in pre-mRNA typical of pseudo-mRNA (ps-mRNA) or of the part of pre-mRNA that is not transferred to the cytoplasm. One example of such sequences are the double-stranded (ds) hairpin-like structures in pre-mRNA. Nuclear ds-RNA was first described by Harel and Montagnier (8). Ryskov *et al.* (25) and then Jelinek and Darnell (10) found that the ds-RNA is a part of nuclear pre-mRNA and probably has a hairpin-like structure.

Ds-RNA was isolated from Ehrlich carcinoma nuclear pre-mRNA by means of RNase treatment at rather high ionic strength followed by gel filtration through Sephadex G75 (Fig. 1). The RNase-resistant material was further purified from poly(A) according to the membrane filter technique of Lee *et al.* (12), which selectively removes the poly(A).

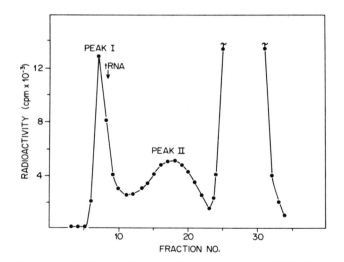

Fig. 1. Fractionation of RNase-stable material of nuclear pre-mRNA through Sephadex G75. Pre-mRNA fractions were mixed with a stock solution of pancreatic and T1 RNases (final concentrations were 50 μg/ml and 100 μg/ml, respectively). The solution was incubated for 1 hr at $37°$C. The reaction was stopped by addition of 200 μg/ml Pronase. The solution in 2× NaCl-citrate was loaded onto a Sephadex G75 column, equilibrated with 0.2 *M* sodium acetate. The elution was accomplished with sodium acetate, and 3-5 ml fractions were collected.

Peak I obtained after the fractionation of light nuclear pre-mRNA (10-20S) consists almost exclusively of poly(A). However, in heavy nuclear pre-mRNA (greater than 35S), this peak contains only traces of poly(A) and the main part of it represents ds-RNA (see below). The base composition of this material is symmetrical, with a G+C content of 45-50%.

Peak II does not contain poly(A). Its base composition is also symmetrical and is characterized by a high G+C content (approximately 75%). The double-stranded nature of these materials was confirmed by hydroxylapatite chromatography and thermoelution. The hairpin-like structure of ds-RNA was suggested on the basis of snap-back experiments. The melting of RNA with rapid cooling did not remove the double-stranded material. This means that the complementary strands in RNA are close to one another and are easily reconstituted after melting.

After RNase treatment, melting leads to separation of two strands; this suggests cleavage of the loop of the hairpins by RNase.

The size of ds-RNA was determined either by means of thin-layer gel chromatography or by determining the amount of orthophosphate liberated by phosphatase.

The ds-RNA of the first peak contains 100 or more base pairs; the ds-RNA of the second peak contains an average of 10-20 base pairs. Long hairpins are present almost exclusively in giant pre-mRNA but are absent from light pre-mRNA, cytoplasmic mRNA, and rRNA precursors. Short hairpins are also present in light pre-mRNA.

The important thing is that RNA hairpins are transcripts from the highly reiterated DNA base sequences. The isolated double-stranded material after melting (followed by strand separation) hybridizes very efficiently with DNA. The half-hybridization of RNA takes place at a DNA-driven $C_0 t$ value equal to about 10. Similar hybridization curves were observed with material of both peak I and peak II (Fig. 2A).

To determine the complexity of the long hairpins, renaturation experiments were developed. Renaturation takes place in a rather narrow interval of $C_0 t$ values—between 0.01 and 1 mole/sec. $C_0 t_{1/2}$ equals about 0.05–0.1. These calculations show that the long hairpins of the Ehrlich carcinoma cells are represented by 250-500 kinds of sequences (Fig. 2B).

We then looked for the existence of corresponding structures in the denatured DNA of mouse. It was found that sheared denatured DNA after annealing even at a $C_0 t$ value as low as $10^{-6} - 10^{-7}$ contains about 2% of sequences resistant to DNase S1, which attacks single-strand regions only. These DNAse-resistant sequences were isolated by hydroxylapatite chromatography. In contrast to ds-RNA, it was impossible to melt them irreversibly—this probably depends on the survival of the hairpin loop during DNase S1 treatment. To avoid this difficulty, double-stranded material prepared from denatured DNA was melted

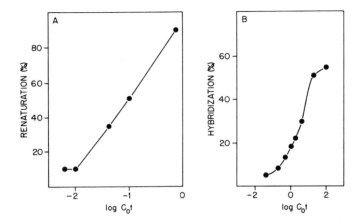

Fig. 2. Hybridization and renaturation of double-stranded regions (long hairpins) isolated from Ehrlich carcinoma pre-mRNA. (A) RNase-resistant material of pre-mRNA was purified by means of Sephadex G75 chromatography (as in Fig. 1). Peak I [long hairpins + poly(A)] was collected, filtered through a nitrocellulose membrane (12) to remove poly(A), extensively deproteinized by dodecylsulfate-phenol-chloroform treatment (to remove RNase), and precipitated with ethanol in the presence of *E. coli* tRNA, which was used as a nonlabeled carrier. The material was then dissolved in a small volume of water (10 µg of double-stranded RNA/ml), denatured by heating in a boiling-water bath for 15 min, and cooled rapidly. One-tenth volume of 20× NaCl-citrate was added, and the samples (1-10 µg/ml) were incubated at 65°C for the time necessary to obtain the appropriate C_0t value (not more than for 8 hr to avoid RNA degradation). After annealing, the sample was diluted with 2× NaCl-citrate to 50 µl and 1:10 (w/w) of RNase was added; the mixture was incubated for 15 min at 37°C, placed on fiberglass filters (Whatman GF/C), dried, washed with 5% trichloroacetic acid and ethanol, and then counted in an SL30 (Intertechnique) spectrometer using a toluene scintillator. Nonannealed samples contained 10-15% RNase-resistant material. (B) The fractions of RNase-stable material were dissolved in water, heated for 10 min in a boiling-water bath, and then cooled rapidly. One-tenth volume of 20× NaCl-citrate was added, and the samples containing 1-2 µg of a material having a specific activity of 10,000 cpm/µg were annealed to immobilize DNA at 65°C or in some experiments at 50°C. DNA was added in excess. Hybridization was made with DNA immobilized on nitrocellulose filters according to Gillespie and Spiegelman (7).

in the presence of CH_2O. The free CH_2O was rapidly removed by gel filtration through Sephadex G25 in the cold, and the DNA sample was immediately treated with DNase S1. More than 90% of the material was destroyed. After very short annealing in 2× NaCl-citrate,[1] DNA again becomes DNase resistant. This demonstrates the presence of hairpin-like structures in the isolated DNA. In native DNA, the hairpins are represented by two inverted repetitive sequences.

The last question was whether or not the RNA hairpins were transcripts of the inverted repetitions discovered in DNA. To answer this question, the hairpins

[1]NaCl-citrate is 0.15 *M* NaCl containing 0.015 *M* Na$_3$ citrate (pH 7.1).

Table I. Hybridization of pre-mRNA Hairpins with DNA Hairpins[a]

Experiment No.	Hybridization conditions					Radioactivity				
	DNA[b] hairpins (μg)	RNA[b] hairpins (μg)	Volume in 6x NaCl-citrate[c] (ml)	Time (hr)	Hybridized	Nonhybridized		RNA, hybridized to DNA (%)	RNA, renatured (%)
						Total	RNase-stable		
1	0.70	0.030	0.050	2	390	1000	570	28	41
2	0.30	0.025	0.020	2	350	740	460	32	42
3	No DNA	0.03	0.050	2	5	1500	—	0.3	—
4	Total DNA, 70.0	0.13	2.0	0.8	400	6300	—	6	—

[a]The double-stranded material from pre-mRNA was isolated as described in Fig. 2A. The hairpins from denatured DNA were isolated according to Church et al. (2). The cells were labeled by injection of [methyl-³H]thymidine (1.5 mCi per mouse each time) on the fourth and fifth days after inoculation of cells. The animals were killed on the seventh day. [³H]Thymidine-labeled DNA of Ehrlich ascites carcinoma cells was isolated by the detergent-phenol-chloroform method, sheared by sonication, denatured, reannealed at $C_0t \sim 10^{-5}$, and treated with DNase S1 (29) to destroy the single-stranded regions. Double-stranded DNase-resistant material was concentrated and purified by hydroxylapatite chromatography. It was then mixed with nonlabeled, sheared E. coli DNA, reprecipitated with ethanol, and denatured by heating in the presence of 3.7% formaldehyde. The solution was diluted with 6X NaCl-citrate to a DNA concentration of 0.5 μg/ml and poured through a hydroxylapatite-membrane filter several times. The filter was washed with 5 ml of 6X NaCl-citrate, and dried at room temperature for 2 hr, and then in a vacuum at 80°C for 2 hr. It was incubated in 6X NaCl-citrate at 65°C and in Denhardt's mixture (3). The amount of DNA fixed was measured by counting ³H. RNA was added in 6X NaCl-citrate and annealed at 65°C. The conditions of annealing are presented in the table. After annealing, the filter was washed several times with 6X NaCl-citrate, treated with RNase (50 μg/ml), again washed with 6X NaCl-citrate and then with ethanol, and counted. The supernatant was separated into two parts to determine the total and RNase-stable acid-insoluble radioactivity. All radioactivity measurements for ³²P and ³H were made in an SL40 Intertechnique spectrometer using a toluene scintillator.

[b]Specific activity of DNA was about 10,000 cpm/μg (³H) and that of RNA was about 50,000 cpm/μg (³²P). DNA-driven C_0t value was about 0.1, and RNA-driven C_0t value was about 0.05.

[c]NaCl-citrate = 0.15 M NaCl plus 0.015 M Na₃ citrate (pH 7.1).

from DNA were melted in the presence of formaldehyde, diluted with 6X NaCl-citrate, and immobilized immediately on membrane filters according to Gillespie and Spiegelman (7). Denatured ds-RNA was hybridized to these filters under conditions of DNA excess. The DNA-driven C_0t was of the same order as, or slightly higher than, the RNA-driven C_0t (when the data were corrected for the immobilization of DNA). It was found that RNA hybridization with DNA was only slightly less than RNA renaturation (Table I) (26). This indicates that DNA inverted repetitions serve as templates for the synthesis of RNA hairpins. Calculations show that the genome contains approximately 600 types of hairpins, each of which is repeated about 500 times on the average. These sequences (long hairpins) are very specific for giant pre-mRNA and are probably present in almost all pre-mRNA molecules. We suggest that they may correspond to acceptor sites that interact with regulatory or/and structural proteins of chromosomes. Work is in progress to test this possibility.

ON THE MECHANISM AND REGULATION OF mRNA TRANSPORT

Structure of Nuclear Complexes Containing Pre-mRNA

In recent years, data have been obtained that confirm the following structural organization of nuclear particles containing pre-mRNA:

According to the model, giant pre-mRNA combines with a number of specific protein macroglobular particles and is distributed on the surface of these particles. These protein particles are called "informofers." Each informofer is combined with an RNA chain of mass = 200,000 daltons, forming 30S nuclear ribonucleoprotein (RNP) particles (27).

Each informofer consists of a number (25-50) of identical protein subunits with molecular weights of about 40,000, which we call "informatin."

The important fact that confirms the existence of the informofer as a protein entity is the survival of the informofer after complete removal of RNA with 2 M NaCl (Fig. 3) (14). The easy reconstitution of RNP after removal of the dissociating agent and the sensitivity of the RNA in the particles to RNase treatment suggest the localization of pre-mRNA mainly on the surface of informofers.

Several papers have recently appeared that demonstrate the high heterogeneity of proteins isolated from pre-mRNP using dodecylsulfate-polyacrylamide gel electrophoresis (4,19). We have verified these findings and were also able to observe the additional slow-moving bands with higher concentrations of protein (Fig. 4). The total amount of the protein in these bands was not more than 10% of the total protein; 90% of the material was informatin. When the protein was treated with strong denaturation agents such as trichloroacetic acid, the amount

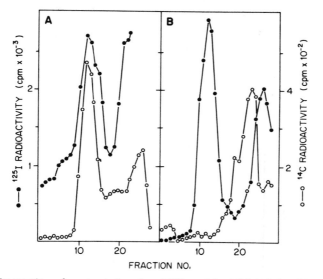

Fig. 3. Sedimentation of nontreated nuclear RNP particles (A) labeled in RNA and protein and free informofers (B). (A) Nuclei were isolated from livers of rats 45 min after injection of [^{14}C]orotic acid. RNP particles were extracted from nuclei at pH 8.0 as described previously (27), partly purified by gel filtration through Sephadex G200, and labeled with ^{125}I according to Bale *et al.* (1). The material was subsequently centrifuged through a 15-30% sucrose gradient for 14 hr at 24,000 rpm in an SW25 rotor (Spinco L2). (B) RNP particles were collected from the 30S zone in Fig. 3A and dialyzed against 2 *M* NaCl. The mixture was then layered onto a 15–30% sucrose gradient in 2 *M* NaCl and centrifuged for 14 hr at 24,000 rpm in an SW25 rotor (Spinco L2). ●, ^{125}I radioactivity; ○, ^{14}C radioactivity.

of heavy material (probably irreversible aggregates) increased. Our interpretation of this result is that informofers consist of informatin only and that the 30S RNP particles may also contain some additional proteins engaged in pre-mRNA processing. Neissing and Sekeris (18,20) found specific RNase and polyadenylate synthetase in nuclear 30S particles. It is possible that, depending on conditions, the amount of these functional proteins may vary significantly.

Binding of Informofers to Different Parts of Pre-mRNA

It was indicated above that pre-mRNA contains sequences of mRNA (at the 3′ end) and ps-mRNA as well as some "service" sequences such as poly(A) added post-transcriptionally. To understand the regulation of mRNA transport, the question of what sequences are combined with informofers must be answered. Previous competition-hybridization experiments showed that both mRNA and ps-mRNA sequences are present in 30S particles (16). The binding of ps-mRNA

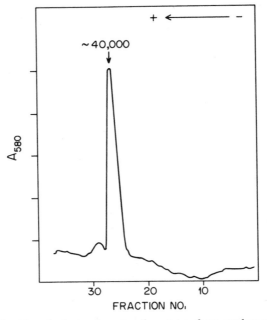

Fig. 4. Polyacrylamide gel electrophoresis of proteins from nuclear particles. Particles isolated from rat liver nuclei as in Fig. 3A were treated with RNase, and the protein was isolated as previously described (27). The proteins were submitted to polyacrylamide gel electrophoresis in 7.5% gels (*p*H 7.1) containing sodium dodecylsulfate as described by Weber *et al.* (30).

with informofers is clear, as this RNA comprises most of the pre-mRNA. The question about mRNA is less clear, and it was additionally explored in experiments with virus-specific mRNA, which is synthesized in the nuclei of human cells infected by adenovirus.

The adenovirus-infected cells were labeled, and nuclear RNP particles were isolated, fixed with formaldehyde, and analyzed on CsCl gradients. The RNA from the peak with a buoyant density of 1.4 g/cm^3 was hybridized with adenovirus DNA. It was found that the percent of RNA hybridized with viral DNA is the same in total nuclear pre-mRNA, in 30S particles, in polyparticles, and in the particles purified by CsCl-density gradient. In separate experiments, it was found that the particles obtained from the infected cells contain informofers. Thus the adenovirus-specific RNA is combined with informofers (31).

We then looked for the presence of poly(A) in 30S particles. The RNP particles were isolated from rat liver or Ehrlich ascites carcinoma cells labeled with ^{32}P. RNA was isolated from 30S particles, hydrolyzed with RNase, and chromatographed on Sephadex G75. The RNase-resistant material was collected, and its base composition was determined. Unexpectedly, we found almost no poly(A) in 30S particles, although the total RNA of the nuclear extract contained about 1% of poly(A). Thus in contrast to the other parts of pre-mRNA, poly(A) seems not to be bound to informofers. The 4S peak from the gradient that originated mainly from degraded RNA was also free of poly(A). On the other hand, the material isolated from the intermediate zone (14-15S) contained all the poly(A) (Fig. 5). Poly(A) thus appears to be bound to the special particles, which differ from informofers. It is interesting that nuclear poly(A)-containing particles have the same S value as the cytoplasmic ones (11). It appears that poly(A) is added to mRNA, which is bound to informofers. If we prevented RNase degradation by using an RNase inhibitor during the isolation of RNP particles, the poly(A) could be observed in the informofers.

Comparison of Informofers with Cytoplasmic mRNP Particles

To understand the mechanism of mRNA transport, it must be known whether or not the informofer is transported with mRNA to the cytoplasm. In cytoplasm, two kinds of mRNP have been described: free mRNP or informo-

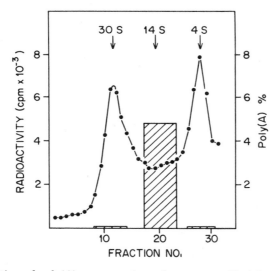

Fig. 5. *Distribution of poly(A) sequences in nuclear extracts.* Nuclei were isolated from Ehrlich ascites cells after 2 hr of labeling with [^{32} P] orthophosphate. RNP particles were extracted from the nuclei and ultracentrifuged in a sucrose gradient as described in Fig. 3A. RNA from different zones of the sucrose gradient was analyzed for the presence of poly(A) sequences. For this, RNase-stable material was isolated from RNase hydrolysates of RNA and its base composition was determined. Poly(A) content was calculated from these data. •, ^{32} P radioactivity; bar, percentage of poly(A).

somes (28) and polysome-bound mRNP (9,23). Free informosomes have not yet
been isolated in the pure state, and this excludes the direct comparison of their
protein with informatin. However, the polysomal mRNP from reticulocytes was
obtained in a more or less pure state and found to consist of two main protein
components, both of which were different from informatin when analyzed by
polyacrylamide gel electrophoresis (13). Similar results have been obtained by
others (17,22).

To check the conclusion in another way, an immunological technique was
developed (15). Antiserum was obtained after injection of hens with 30S
particles from rat liver. We could not use the gel precipitation test for direct
comparison of the immunological differences between these two kinds of mRNP

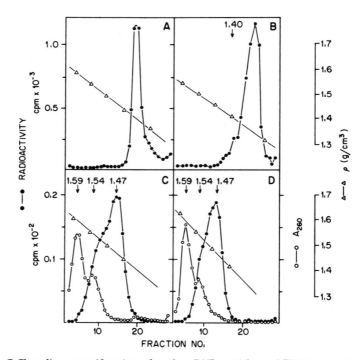

Fig. 6. CsCl-gradient centrifugation of nuclear RNP particles and EDTA-treated polysomes
before and after treatment with globulin from immunized hens. Nuclear particles were
pooled from sucrose gradients (Fig. 3A). Fifteen micrograms was incubated for 7 hr at $0°C$
with 1 mg of globulin from immunized hens, fixed with formaldehyde, and analyzed by
CsCl-gradient centrifugation. (A) Particles treated with globulin from non-immunized hens.
(B) Particles treated with globulin from immunized hens. Polysomes were isolated from
livers of rats 30 min after injection of 1 mCi of [H^3] orotic acid. The polysomes (250 μg)
were treated with EDTA and divided into two parts, one of which (C) was used as a control,
whereas the other part (D) was treated with 1 μg of globulin from immunized hens.

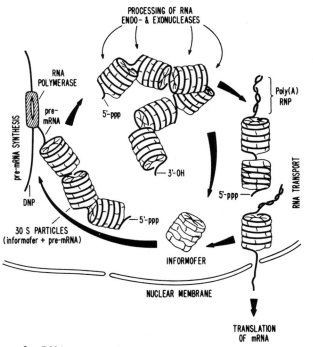

Fig. 7. Scheme of mRNA transport in mammalian cells. DNP, Deoxyribonucleoprotein; RNP, ribonucleoprotein.

because the small amount of polysomal mRNA binding protein would preclude its detection even if it were identical to informatin.

For this reason, CsCl-gradient analysis of the antigen-antibody complexes was used. Nuclear RNP particles pre-incubated with antiserum were banded in CsCl with a buoyant density of $\rho = 1.35$ g/cm^3 (Fig. 6B), demonstrating that additional protein was bound. In the control experiments, when 30S particles were incubated with the nonimmunized globulin their buoyant density was not changed, being 1.4 g/cm^3 (Fig. 6A).

These data demonstrate that under the experimental conditions 30S particles were able to combine with antibody, and so it was possible to use this technique to compare immunological differences between nuclear and polysomal mRNP.

Rat liver polysomes were treated with EDTA, and the mRNP was liberated as heterogeneous material with a buoyant density of about 1.47 g/cm^3 (Fig. 6C). This material was treated with antiglobulin, and the mixture was fixed and analyzed on a CsCl-density gradient. It was found that the buoyant density of the polysomal mRNP was not changed (Fig. 6D), thus demonstrating that antibody to 30S nuclear particles did not interact with polysomal mRNP.

These experiments show the immunological differences between polysomal and nuclear mRNP and support the idea that informofers do not cross the nuclear membrane during mRNA transport.

All these data allowed us to suggest the following hypothetical scheme for the "informofer cycle" (Fig. 7):

The informofers detach the pre-mRNA from chromosomal templates. The RNA is distributed on the surface of the informofer and is attacked by the processing enzymes, whereby ps-mRNA is degraded and some of the informofers are released. (We do not know whether, *in vivo*, informofers are released as intact particles or are degraded to subunits.) Subsequently, the mRNA sequences, complexed with informofers, are transferred to the nuclear membrane, where only the mRNA is injected into the cytoplasm. The informofers remain in the nucleus and again combine with newly synthesized pre-mRNA.

REFERENCES

1. W. F. Bale, R. W. Helminkamp, T. P. Davis, M. I. Izzo, R. L. Goodland, M. A. Contreras, and I. L. Spar. High specific activity labelling of protein with ^{131}I by the iodine monochloride method. *Proc. Soc. Exptl. Biol. Med.* **122**:407 (1966).
2. R. B. Church and G. B. Georgiev. Double-stranded regions in denatured DNA from mouse cells. *Mol. Biol.* **1**: 21 (1973).
3. D. T. Denhardt. A membrane-filter technique for the detection of complementary DNA. *Biochem. Biophys. Res. Commun.* **23**:641 (1966).
4. I. Faiferman, M. G. Hamilton, and A. O. Pogo. Nucleoplasmic ribonucleoprotein particles of rat liver. II. Physical properties and action of dissociating agents. *Biochim. Biophys. Acta* **232**:685 (1971).
5. G. P. Georgiev. On the structural organization of operon and the regulation of RNA synthesis in animal cells. *J. Theoret. Biol.* **25**:473 (1969).
6. G. P. Georgiev, A. P. Ryskov, C. Coutelle, V. L. Mantieva, and E. R. Avakyan. On the structure of transcriptional unit in mammalian cells. *Biochim. Biophys. Acta* **259**:259 (1972).
7. D. Gillespie and S. Spiegelman. A quantitative assay for DNA-RNA hybrids with DNA immobilized on a membrane. *J. Mol. Biol.* **12**:829 (1965).
8. L. Harel and L. Montagnier. Double-stranded RNA from rat liver homologous with the cellular genome. *Nature New Biol.* **229**:106 (1971).
9. E. C. Henshaw. Messenger RNA in rat liver polyribosomes: Evidence that it exists as ribonucleoprotein particles. *J. Mol. Biol.* **36**:401 (1968).
10. W. Jelinek and J. E. Darnell. Double-stranded regions in heterogeneous nuclear RNA from HeLa cells. *Proc. Natl. Acad. Sci. (USA)* **69**:2537 (1972).
11. S. Kwan and G. Brawerman. A particle associated with the polyadenylate segment in mammalian messenger RNA. *Proc. Natl. Acad. Sci. (USA)* **69**:3247 (1972).
12. S. Y. Lee, J. Mendecki, and G. Brawerman. A polynucleotide segment rich in adenylic acid in the rapidly-labeled polyribosomal RNA component of mouse sarcoma 180 ascites cells. *Proc. Natl. Acad. Sci. (USA)* **68**:1331 (1971).
13. E. M. Lukanidin, G. P. Georgiev, and R. Williamson. A comparative study of the protein components of nuclear and polysomal messenger ribonucleoprotein. *FEBS Letters* **19**:152 (1971).
14. E. M. Lukanidin, E. S. Zalmanzon, L. Komaromi, O. P. Samarina, and G. P. Georgiev. Structure and function of informofers. *Nature New Biol.* **238**:193 (1972).

15. E. M. Lukanidin, S. Olsnes, and A. Pihl. Immunological difference between informofers and the protein bound to mRNA in polysomes from rat liver. *Nature New Biol.* **240**:90 (1972).
16. V. L. Mantieva, E. R. Avakyan, and G. P. Georgiev. The nuclear ribonucleoprotein containing informational RNA. 4. Types of the nuclear dRNA bound with the informofers. *Mol. Biol. (USSR)* **3**:545 (1969).
17. C. Morel, S. Kayibanda, and K. Scherrer. Proteins associated with globin messenger RNA in avian erythroblasts: Isolation and comparison with the proteins bound to nuclear messenger-like RNA. *FEBS Letters* **18**:84 (1971).
18. J. Neissing and C. E. Sekeris. Cleavage of high-molecular-weight DNA-like RNA by a nuclease present in 30S ribonucleoprotein particles of rat liver nuclei. *Biochim. Biophys. Acta* **209**:484 (1970).
19. J. Neissing and C. E. Sekeris. The protein moiety of nuclear RNP particles containing DNA-like RNA. Presence of heterogeneous and high molecular-weight polypeptide chains. *FEBS Letters* **18**:39 (1971).
20. J. Neissing and C. E. Sekeris. A homoribopolynucleotide synthetase in rat liver nuclei associated with ribonucleoprotein particles containing DNA-like RNA. *FEBS Letters* **22**:83 (1972).
21. S. Olsnes. Characterization of protein bound to rapidly-labelled RNA in polyribosomes from rat liver. *Europ. J. Biochem.* **15**:464 (1970).
22. S. Olsnes. Further studies on the protein bound to the messenger RNA in mammalian polysomes. *Europ. J. Biochem.* **23**:557 (1971).
23. R. P. Perry and D. E. Kelley. Messenger RNA-protein complexes and newly synthesized ribosomal subunits: Analysis of free particles and components of polyribosomes. *J. Mol. Biol.* **35**:37 (1968).
24. A. P. Ryskov, R. B. Church, G. Bajszar, and G. P. Georgiev. Inverted repetitions in mammalian DNA transcribed into nucleus-restricted hairpin-like structures of pre-mRNA. *Mol. Biol.* **1**: 119 (1973).
    specific exclusively for giant dRNA. *Biochim. Biophys. Acta* **262**:568 (1972).
26. A. P. Ryskov, G. F. Saunders, V. R. Farashyan, and G. P. Georgiev. Double-helical regions in nuclear precursor of mRNA (pre-mRNA). *Biochim. Biophys. Acta* **312**: 152 (1973).
27. O. P. Samarina, E. M. Lukanidin, J. Molnar, and G. P. Georgiev. Structural organization of nuclear complexes containing DNA-like RNA. *J. Mol. Biol.* **33**:251 (1968).
28. A. S. Spirin. Informosomes. *Europ. J. Biochem.* **10**:20 (1969).
29. W. D. Sutton. A crude nuclease preparation suitable for use in DNA reassociation experiments. *Biochim. Biophys. Acta* **240**:522 (1971).
30. K. Weber and M. Osborn. The reliability of molecular weight determinations by dodecylsulfate-polyacrylamide gel electrophoresis. *J. Biol. Chem.* **244**:4406 (1969).
31. E. S. Zalmanzon, E. M. Lukanidin, L. Komaromi, and L. N. Mikhailove. Nuclear ribonucleoproteins containing informational RNA. XI. Nuclear particles containing virus-specific RNA in adenovirus-infected FL cells. *Mol. Biol. (USSR),* in press (1973).

25

The Poly(A) Sequences in Messenger RNA and Heterogeneous Nuclear RNA

Hiroshi Nakazato and Mary Edmonds

Department of Biochemistry
Faculty of Arts and Science
University of Pittsburgh
Pittsburgh, Pennsylvania, U.S.A.

The poly(A) sequences covalently bound both to the heterogeneous RNA (HnRNA) of the nucleus and to the polysome-bound messenger RNA (mRNA) of many eukaryotes (1-3) have provided chemical evidence for the precursor-product relationship long predicted to link these two species of RNA. In addition to permitting new studies of the biogenesis of mRNA in eukaryotes, the poly(A) sequences have provided the basis for techniques for the isolation and purification of both of these classes of heterogeneous RNA molecules. These techniques have allowed us to examine the location and the size of the poly(A) sequences within RNA molecules and to estimate both the number of poly(A) sequences per molecule and the fraction of mRNA and HnRNA molecules that contain poly(A) sequences. Some HnRNA molecules that contain poly(A) sequences have been compared with those that do not.

POLY(A) SEQUENCES IN MESSENGER RNA

Prior to the detection of a covalently bound poly(A) sequence, the mRNA fraction of eukaryotes had to be defined in operational terms, such as rapidly labeled, polysome-bound RNA synthesized in the presence of low levels of actinomycin D. The absence of poly(A) from ribosomal RNA and its presence in many, if not most, of the mRNA fractions bound to polysomes provided the basis for a simple assay based on the hybridization of poly(A)-containing RNA molecules to deoxythmidylate oligomers covalently bound to cellulose [oligo-(dT)-cellulose].

Properties of mRNA of HeLa Cells and Yeast

The sedimentation profile of the polysome-bound rapidly labeled RNA of HeLa cells is seen in Fig. 1A. The fraction of this RNA bound to oligo(dT)-cellulose (Fig. 1C) is free of ribosomal RNA and transfer RNA as well as RNA fragments. A close examination of the sedimentation characteristics of the unbound RNA (Fig. 1B) suggests that RNA molecules which are neither ribosomal nor transfer RNA are present. These molecules, which represent about

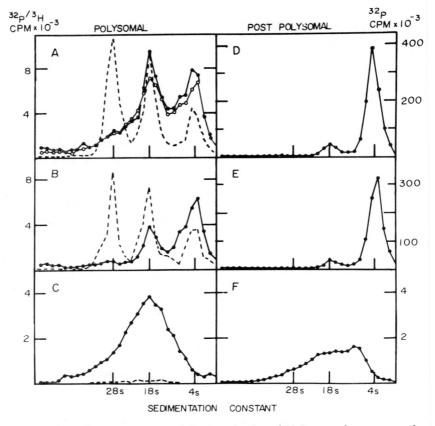

Fig. 1. Sedimentation properties of RNA molecules of HeLa cytoplasm recovered on oligo(dT)-cellulose. For details, see Nakazato and Edmonds (10).

20% of the unbound fraction, may, in fact, be mRNA molecules lacking poly(A) sequences.

The postpolysome region of a cytoplasmic gradient also contains RNA molecules with poly(A) sequences that resemble the polysome-bound mRNA fractions in both their poly(A) content (Table I) and their sedimentation properties (Fig. 1F). The poly(A) sequences from the two fractions are also the same length (Fig. 3). Until these nonpolysome-bound RNAs are shown to function as mRNAs, they should be designated as "messenger-like" RNA.

The sedimentation properties of pulse-labeled polysome-bound RNA from yeast are shown in Fig. 2. The poly(A)-containing RNA fraction that was bound to oligo(dT)-cellulose (Fig. 2C) spans a range in accord with the best estimates for the average size of yeast mRNA determined by other methods (N. S. Peterson and C. S. McLaughlin, unpublished data). The unbound RNA (Fig. 2B) shows the two characteristic ribosomal RNA species of yeast; however, in

Table I. Isolation of Messenger RNA on Oligo(dt)-Cellulose

	Total cpm			
	Original	Unbound	Bound	Percent bound
HeLa cells (10)				
Polysomal RNA				
[^{32}P] RNA, 40-min label	96,000	48,000	38,300	40.0
[^{32}P] Poly(A)	6,860	216	6,170	90.0
Percent poly(A)	7.1	0.45	16.1	
Postpolysomal RNA				
[^{32}P] RNA, 40-min label	1,213,000	1,108,000	37,600	3.1
[^{32}P] Poly(A)	6,200	885	5,770	92.0
Percent poly(A)	0.51	0.08	15.2	
Yeast (4)				
Polysomal [^{3}H] RNA,				
10-min label	–	283,000	96,700	25.0
[^{3}H] Poly(A)	–	1,390	13,000	90.0
Percent poly(A)	–	0.5	13.4	
Polio virus				
[^{32}P] RNA (virion)	215,000	42,000	188,000	87.5
[^{32}P] Poly(A)	1,630	–	1,880	–
Percent poly(A)	0.76	–	1.0	

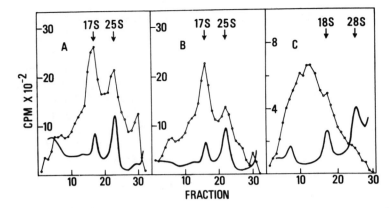

Fig. 2. Sedimentation analysis of the RNA components from yeast polysomes. From McLaughlin *et al.* (4).

contrast to the bulk RNA shown in the absorbance profile, a part of the labeled RNA is neither ribosomal nor transfer RNA. As was the case in HeLa cells, this evidence suggests that some mRNA molecules in yeast may lack poly(A) sequences. Although degradation is difficult to exclude as the source of this RNA lacking poly(A), the fact that the bulk of ribosomal RNA showed no degradation is evidence against it.

The poly(A) contents of these RNA fractions from HeLa cells and yeast are summarized in Table I. In all cases, at least 90% of the total poly(A) of unfractionated RNA was recovered in the RNA bound to oligo(dT)-cellulose, indicating that almost all poly(A) sequences in these RNAs are available for hybridization in this assay. This was also true of the purified virion RNA of poliovirus, where about 90% of purified virion RNA was retained by oligo(dT)-cellulose. The fact that a single endonucleolytic random cleavage of an RNA molecule would be expected to reduce the amount of RNA bound about 50% on the average shows that the assay can be a sensitive indicator of RNA degradation.

LENGTH OF POLY(A) SEQUENCES

Size of Poly(A) Sequences Estimated from Electrophoretic Mobilities

Poly(A) Sequences of HeLa mRNA and HnRNA

The relative homogeneity and striking similarity in size of poly(A) sequences of mRNA and of HnRNA, which originally led us to propose a model for the generation of mRNA from the HnRNA (1), on closer examination have shown the average poly(A) sequence of HnRNA to be slightly longer than that obtained from mRNA of the same cells. This discrepancy in size has been demonstrated

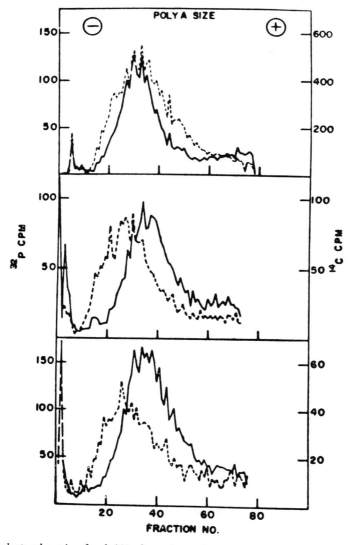

Fig. 3. Coelectrophoresis of poly(A)s from the nucleus and cytoplasm. HeLa cells were labeled for 60 min with $^{32}PO_4$ in one experiment and for 90 min in another with [^{14}C]adenosine. Nuclear RNA isolated from each experiment was separated into molecules sedimenting faster as well as slower than 45S. Cytoplasm from each experiment was fractionated into polyribosomes and more slowly sedimenting components (monosomes, subunits, etc.) prior to isolating RNA from each. The poly(A) from each RNA was electrophoresed as described (1) except for a twofold increase in duration during which the small tRNA markers moved out of the gel. For details of these procedures, see Edmonds *et al.* (1). [^{32}P]Poly(A) from >45S HnRNA is shown in the dotted line in all three panels. Top panel: [^{14}C]Poly(A) from <45S HnRNA. Center: [^{14}C]Poly(A) from polysomal RNA. Bottom: [^{14}C]Poly(A) from postpolysomal RNA.

by coelectrophoresis of poly(A) sequences from nuclear and cytoplasmic RNAs from cells labeled either for 60 min with $^{32}PO_4$ or for 90 min with [^{14}C] adenosine. Figure 3 shows electrophoretic patterns of the ^{32}P-labeled nuclear poly(A)s coelectrophoresed with ^{14}C-labeled cytoplasmic poly(A)s. Any effect on the lengths of these sequences resulting from dissimilar labeling of RNA molecules, produced in these experiments by different labeled precursors, was ruled out when results identical to Fig. 3 were obtained by coelectrophoresis of nuclear poly(A) from [^{14}C] adenosine-labeled cells and cytoplasmic poly(A) from ^{32}P-labeled cells.

It is seen that poly(A) sequences from all size classes of HnRNA are similar in size (Fig. 3, top) but are longer than poly(A) sequences from polyribosomes (Fig. 3, center) and from the RNA from more slowly sedimenting cytoplasmic components as well (Fig. 3, bottom). The lengths of poly(A) sequences from polysomal and postpolysomal RNA (see Table I) were indistinguishable (Fig. 3, center and bottom).

Poly(A) Sequences in Lower Eukaryotes and Animal Viruses

The poly(A) sequence of yeast mRNA is only about one-third the length of that of HeLa mRNA (4) (Fig. 4). The poly(A) of the mRNA of the slime mold, *Dictyosteleum discoides,* another representative of the lower eukaryotes, has recently been reported to be about 100 nucleotides in length (5).

Two animal RNA viruses, poliovirus and eastern equine encephalitis virus, also contain poly(A) sequences considerably shorter (6) than those found in the mRNA from the host cell cytoplasm where each virus is replicated (Fig. 5).

A Short Poly(A) Sequence in HnRNA

A short poly(A) sequence is regularly seen in electropherograms of nuclear poly(A) sequences such as that from the >45S HnRNA shown in Fig. 6A. This sequence, which is estimated to be about 20 nucleotides although only about 10% of total poly(A) of the nucleus, represents an approximately equivalent number of moles. The obvious questions raised by the existence of two classes of poly(A) sequences in HnRNA is considered elsewhere in this chapter.

Lengths of Poly(A) Sequences Estimated from End-Group Analysis

The evidence to be presented shortly, showing that most of the poly(A) sequences are found at the 3' end of both mRNA and HnRNA of HeLa cells and in yeast mRNA as well, permits an independent estimate of average length of poly(A) by end-group analysis. Hydroxyl groups should be found at the 3' ends of poly(A) sequences released from RNA by RNase A or RNase T1 only if they

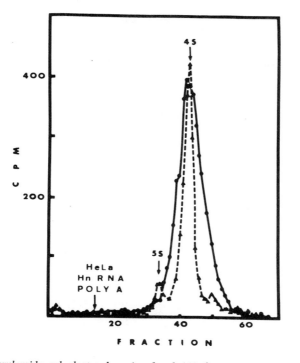

Fig. 4. Polyacrylamide gel electrophoresis of poly(A) from yeast messenger RNA. For details, see McLaughlin *et al.* (4).

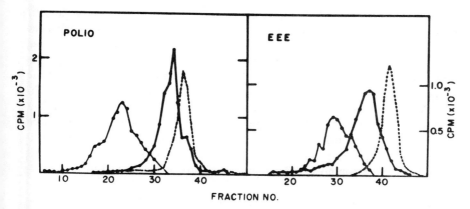

Fig. 5. Polyacrylamide gel electrophoresis of poly(A) from poliovirus RNA and eastern equine encephalitis (EEE) and from chick cell and HeLa RNA. For details, see Armstrong *et al.* (6).

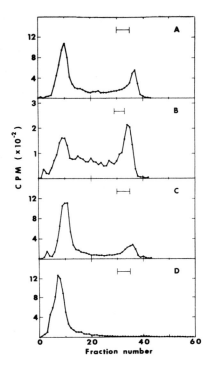

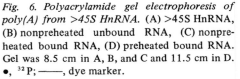

Fig. 6. Polyacrylamide gel electrophoresis of poly(A) from >45S HnRNA. (A) >45S HnRNA, (B) nonpreheated unbound RNA, (C) nonpreheated bound RNA, (D) preheated bound RNA. Gel was 8.5 cm in A, B, and C and 11.5 cm in D. ●, ^{32}P; ——, dye marker.

occupy the 3′ terminus. The ratio of label in hydroxyl groups in a single nucleoside recovered from an alkaline hydrolysate of the poly(A) sequence relative to that in the AMP recovered can give an estimate of average length. Table II summarizes data for electrophoretically purified poly(A) sequences from HeLa and yeast mRNA labeled with adenosine. The variability in the three experiments shown for HeLa mRNA may not necessarily reflect experimental deviations but may be a true difference in the average length of the sequences in mRNA from different labeling experiments (H. Nakazato, unpublished experiments). These data for HeLa cells are in close agreement with data already published for the poly(A) sequence of sarcoma 180 mRNA (7), but since even lower levels of radioactivity were recovered in adenosine in these experiments (7) the possible contamination of the poly(A) sequences with small amounts of short polynucleotides terminated with adenosine had to be considered.

A similar experiment (Table III) was carried out on both of the [^{14}C] adenosine-labeled poly(A)s present in nuclear RNA. As might have been predicted from the electrophoretic data of Fig. 3, end-group analysis of the long poly(A) sequence also shows it to be significantly longer than that from polysome-bound mRNA of the same cells. The short poly(A) sequence representing about 10% of

Table II.   Size of Purified Poly(A) Sequences in Messenger RNA

| | mRNA poly(A) | | | | |
| | HeLa (^{14}C cpm) (8) | | | Yeast ^{3}H cpm) (4) | |
	1	2	3	1	2^a
Adenosine	96	50	80	620	335
AMP	9700	8210	9536	29,000	17,200
Average length	102	165	120	48	52
Length estimated from electrophoretic mobility		150			50

^{a}Poly(A)-treated with *E. coli* alkaline phosphatase.

Table III.   Size of Purified Poly(A) Sequences in HnRNA of HeLa Cells

| | Nuclear poly(A) (8) | | |
| | Long (^{14}C cpm) | | Short (^{14}C cpm) |
	1	2	1
Adenosine	64	53	1
AMP	13,780	11,720	1,250
Average length	216	222	1,250
Length estimated from electrophoretic mobility	200		20

the total nuclear poly(A), however, showed no label in adenosine. It is therefore apparent that this poly(A) sequence is not at the 3′ end of HnRNA. Its length can only be estimated from its relative electrophoretic mobility in these experiments.

LOCATION OF POLY(A) SEQUENCES

The 3′ Termini of mRNA and HnRNA

Although the data cited above are consistent with a 3′-terminal locus for the poly(A) sequences of both mRNA and HnRNA, more decisive evidence on this point has been obtained by labeling the 3′ end of the parent RNA and by tracing the label into the 3' end of the poly(A) sequence released from it. Purified mRNA and HnRNA (>45S) from which ribosomal and preribosomal RNA had been removed were reduced with NaB ^{3}H$_4$ (9). Both the labeled mRNA, which showed almost no change in sedimentation after this treatment, and the HnRNA were purified and hydrolyzed in alkali. The radioactivities of the hydroxyl methyldiethylene glycol derivatives of each base purified from this alkaline hydrolysate are reported in Table IV.

It can be concluded from the data for mRNA that many mRNA molecules have poly(A) sequences at the 3' end, since more than 50% of the ^{3}H associated with the 3' termini of mRNA was recovered in the adenine derivative from the 3' terminus of the poly(A) sequence.

In a similar experiment with HnRNA (>45S), 15% of the ^{3}H in the 3' end of HnRNA was recovered in the adenine derivative at the 3' end of the poly(A) released from it. The high levels of ^{3}H found in the nucleoside derivatives of uracil, cytosine, and guanine in this RNA (Table IV) are explained by data to be reported later that show that no more than 40% of the >45S HnRNA molecules actually contain poly(A) sequences and most probably only about 20% contain the long poly(A) sequence.

The 3' Terminus of a Short Poly(A) Sequence in HnRNA

The evidence favoring an internal site for the short poly(A) sequence in HnRNA found in Table III has been confirmed by the NaB ^{3}H$_4$ end-group labeling technique. The distribution of ^{3}H in the adenosine derivative from the

Table IV. 3' Termini of HeLa mRNA and> 45S HnRNA and of Poly(A) Sequences Released from Them

Experiment	^{32}P (cpm)	[^{3}H] Nucleoside derivatives[a] (cpm)				Percent ^{3}H in poly(A)
		A'	U'	C'	G'	
22.5-hr label						
mRNA	136,900	770	125	27	82	
poly(A)	4,240	460	28	8	22	51.6
Percent poly(a)	3.1					
60 min. label						
45S HnRNA	1,405,000	1273	567	193	427	
poly(A)	6,800	343	5	2	4	14.4
Percent poly(A)	0.48					

[a]The hydroxyl methyldiethylene glycol derivative of each base of RNA (8).

long poly(A) sequence and the short poly(A) sequence, as well as in some heterogeneous AMP-rich material between these two peaks (see Fig. 6, A), is summarized in Table V.

Although the short poly(A) sequence accounts for but 10% of the total poly(A) sample, it is approximately one-tenth the length of the major poly(A) component and should therefore have an equivalent number of 3' ends. If a 3'-hydroxyl group of this poly(A) occupied the 3' terminus of the parent HnRNA, it would contain as much ^{3}H as the long poly(A) sequence. If it is assumed, for the sake of calculation, that each of these AMP-rich components is at the 3' ends of RNA, the projected distribution of ^{3}H among them, estimated from total tritium recovered and the quantity and average length of each poly(A), is shown in the last column of Table V. In contrast to these predictions, almost no ^{3}H was recovered in the adenine derivative (A') of the short poly(A) sequences. From this result, it can be concluded that, in contrast to the long poly(A) sequence, this short one did not have a free hydroxyl group at its 3' end. The existence of poly(A) sequences both with and without labeled 3' termini, which has been confirmed by the end-group labeling presented in Table V, demonstrates a significant degree of specificity for the labeling of the oxidized 3' termini of HnRNA with sodium borohydride.

POLY(A) SEQUENCES IN HETEROGENEOUS NUCLEAR RNA

Both the large (>45S) and the smaller (<45S) HnRNA fractions from the nucleus can be separated into two classes of RNA molecules, those with and those without poly(A) sequences. This separation can be achieved by hybridiza-

Table V. NaB ^{3}H$_4$-Labeled 3' Termini of the Major and Minor Poly(A) Sequences in> 45S HnRNA

Sample	AMP (%)	Average length (nucleotides)	Percent of total poly(A)	^{3}H in adenosine derivative (cpm)	
				Experiment	Predicted[a]
Total poly(A)	90	—	—	343	—
Long poly(A)	94	200	66	160	88
Medium poly(A)	70	60[b]	13	104	58
Short poly(A)	88	20[b]	10	14	133
Percent recovery			89	91[c]	

[a]From the assumption that all poly(A)s are at the 3' end of RNA with an unsubstituted 3'-hydroxyl group.

[b]Estimated from mobility on gel.

[c]Calculated for 89% recovery of poly(A)s. For details see ref. 8.

tion to oligo(dT)-cellulose without apparent degradation of either class of RNA molecule. The fraction of the total HnRNA found in each class is seen in Table VI. If the binding to oligo(dT)-cellulose is done without heat treatment, about 40% of the >45S HnRNA molecules bound contain essentially all of the poly(A) sequences. Both bound and unbound RNA can be recovered with apparently unaltered sedimentation properties. This is seen in the top panels of Fig. 7. If unfractionated >45S HnRNA (panel A) is compared with unbound (panel B) and bound (panel D), it is difficult to detect shifts in sedimentation velocities resulting from this treatment. This being the case, it can be concluded from the data of Table VI that about 60% of HnRNA molecules do not contain the long poly(A) sequence. Similar conclusions apply to the smaller HnRNA molecules (<45S). In this experiment, although many more poly(A) sequences were present in this fraction (Table VI), the presence of labeled preribosomal and ribosomal RNA in this fraction makes it impossible to estimate the number of HnRNA molecules that lack poly(A) sequences. Again, sedimentation analysis of these fractions (Fig. 7, bottom) shows almost no degradation (Fig. 7b,e). It should be noted that all of a 45S preribosomal RNA marker included in the unfractionated RNA prior to binding to oligo(dT)-cellulose was recovered from the <45S RNA in the unbound fraction. This verifies an earlier conclusion that ribosomal RNA does not contain poly(A) (1).

When the poly(A) sequences released from the >45S RNA were examined by electrophoresis in polyacrylamide gels (Fig. 6), the short poly(A) sequence discussed previously, and shown in Fig. 6A, was found in the RNA molecules binding to oligo(dT)-cellulose (Fig. 6C), although part of it was recovered in the unbound RNA (note difference in scales of B and C of Fig. 6). This latter observation suggested that the long and short poly(A) sequences might be in separate molecules and that conditions could be found for the oligo(dT) binding assay that would separate them.

Table VI. Isolation of HnRNA Molecules on Oligo(dT)-Cellulose: Effect of Preheating

	RNA (% bound)	Poly(A) in bound RNA	
		Cpm	Percent
> 45S HnRNA (4.67×10^6 cpm ^{32}P)			
Procedure 1 (not preheated)	39.1	18,817	1.0
Procedure 2 (preheated)	22.5	16,690	1.6
⩽ 45S RNA (16.6×10^6 cpm ^{32}P)			
Procedure 1	15.9	85,000	3.2
Procedure 2	11.9	83,500	4.2

Such conditions were found to be a brief heat treatment of the HnRNA in the presence of oligo(dT)-cellulose (3 min at 60°C) prior to the 60-min period at 23°C normally used for binding HnRNA RNA to oligo(dT)-cellulose. After such treatment, a poly(A) fraction devoid of the short poly(A) sequence can be recovered from the bound RNA fraction (Fig. 6D).

This mild heat step which separates the long and short poly(A) sequences is routinely accompanied by approximately a 50% decrease in the fraction of RNA bound to oligo(dT)-cellulose (Table VI). The relatively minor shift in sedimentation velocity observed in the >45S bound RNA resulting from this heat treatment (compare D with E in Fig. 7) makes it difficult to ascribe this drop to RNA degradation. Although activation of a specific RNase by heat must be considered here, such a ribonuclease attached to RNA would have to be resistant to hot phenol and detergents. RNases in oligo(dT)-cellulose appeared to be ruled out

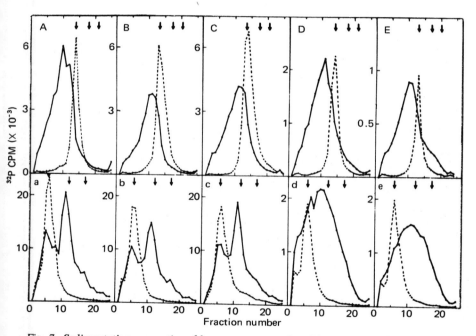

Fig. 7. *Sedimentation properties of heterogeneous nuclear RNA recovered from oligo(dT)-cellulose.* >45S [^{32}P] RNA and ⩽45S [^{32}P] RNA mixed with 45S preribosomal [^{3}H] RNA were fractionated on oligo(dT)-cellulose. The top row is >45S RNA. (A) Unfractionated RNA, (B) nonpreheated unbound RNA, (C) preheated unbound RNA, (D) nonpreheated bound RNA, (E) preheated bound RNA. The bottom row is ⩽45S RNA. (a) Unfractionated RNA, (b) nonpreheated unbound RNA, (c) preheated unbound RNA, (d) nonpreheated bound RNA, (e) preheated bound RNA. Solid lines, ^{32}P; . . . , ^{3}H.

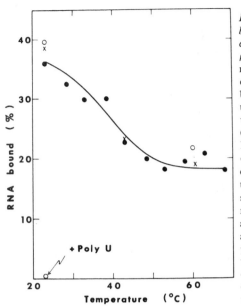

Fig. 8. Effect of heat treatment on the binding of >45S HnRNA to oligo(dT)-cellulose. >45S [³²P] RNA containing 15 μg unlabeled poly(A) was incubated for 3 min in binding mixture with oligo(dT)-cellulose, and the temperature during incubation was varied. Where indicated, 20 μg of unlabeled poly(U) was added to RNA solution before the mixture was added to oligo-(dT)-cellulose. ●, ○, ³²P recovery in bound RNA in different experiments; ×, ³²P recovery in bound RNA when diethyl pyrocarbonate treated oligo(dT)-cellulose was used for binding. [Oligo(dT)-cellulose was suspended in 10 ml of NETS containing 0.3 ml of diethyl pyrocarbonate. After shaking and boiling for 10 min, the mixture was autoclaved and washed.] In experiments expressed as ○ and ×, [³H]poly(A) was added to monitor recovery of poly(A). The recovery of ³H was more than 95% in all cases except when poly(U) was added (recovery was 1.5% in the latter case).

when the same decrease in RNA binding occurred after the cellulose had been treated with the protein denaturant diethyl pyrocarbonate (see Fig. 8).

A simple thermal rupture of phosphodiester bonds would seem to be ruled out by the data of Fig. 8 showing that temperatures as low as 40°C for the same time periods are sufficient to produce the same decrease in binding. Raising the temperature to as high as 70°C resulted in no further decrease in binding. HeLa messenger RNA also shows no decrease in binding when exposed to this identical heat treatment.

Although these data cannot eliminate phosphodiester bond cleavage as the explanation for this phenomenon, the reproducibility and well-defined nature of the transition indicate that some specific alteration of the HnRNA molecules is involved which is readily and reproducibly detected by the oligo(dT)-cellulose binding assay.

The effect of heat would not appear to be a simple melting of an intermolecular poly(A)·poly(U) duplex since, even without heating, all poly(A) sequences appear to be available for hybridization. This can be deduced from the fact that addition of poly(U) carrier to an unheated reaction can abolish all binding of HnRNA to oligo(dT) groups on cellulose (Fig. 8).

The separation of RNAs containing primarily long poly(A) sequences at the 3′ end from molecules containing the internal short poly(A) sequences achieved by this technique suggests that long and short poly(A)s either are in different HnRNA molecules or are widely separated if in the same molecule. This latter conclusion would follow from the fact that the RNA recovered after heat treatment is only slightly altered in sedimentation properties, essentially all of it remaining as very large molecules (Fig. 7E).

The poly(dT)-cellulose binding technique can thus be expected to serve as a useful probe of the structure of these large HnRNA molecules.

REFERENCES

1. M. Edmonds, M. H. Vaughan, and H. Nakazato. *Proc. Natl. Acad. Sci. (USA)* **68**:1336 (1971).
2. J. E. Darnell, R. Wall, and R. J. Tushinski. *Proc. Natl. Acad. Sci. (USA)* **68**:1321 (1971).
3. S. Y. Lee, J. Mendecki, and G. B. Brawerman. *Proc. Natl. Acad. Sci. (USA)* **68**:1331 (1971).
4. C. S. McLaughlin, J. R. Warner, M. Edmonds, H. Nakazato, and M. H. Vaughan. *J. Biol. Chem.,* **248**:1466 (1973).
5. R. A. Firtel, A. Jacobson, and H. F. Lodish. *Nature New Biol.* **239**:225 (1972).
6. J. A. Armstrong, M. Edmonds, H. Nakazato, B. A. Phillips, and M. H. Vaughan. *Science* **176**:526 (1972).
7. J. Mendecki, S. Y. Lee, and G. B. Brawerman. *Biochemistry* **11**:792 (1972).
8. H. Nakazato, D. W. Kopp, and M. Edmonds. *J. Biol. Chem.* **248**:1472 (1973).
9. R. DeWachter and W. Fiers. *J. Mol. Biol.* **30**:507 (1967).
10. H. Nakazato and M. Edmonds. *J. Biol. Chem.* **247**:3365 (1972).
11. G. Brawerman, J. Mendecki, and S. Y. Lee. *Biochemistry* **11**:637 (1972).

DISCUSSION

Question (Wickner): Have you looked for a poly(A) polymerase in the virion of reovirus?
Answer: We have not.

Question (Pradhan): Is poly(A) transcribed or added on later?
Answer: Evidence of several types suggests that it is added after transcription. Probably the most compelling is the apparent lack of oligo(dT) sequences of this length in some DNAs (e.g., adenovirus DNA) from which HnRNA molecules are transcribed and which contain poly(A) sequences. A variety of kinetic labeling experiments involving the drugs 3'-deoxyadenosine and actinomycin D are also suggestive.

Question (Pradhan): Could you comment on the method of isolating poly(A)-bearing HnRNA in which the RNA is held on membrane filters in the presence of high concentrations of potassium chloride?
Answer: We have not used this technique since the oligo(dT)-cellulose method offers so many advantages in terms of capacity and selectivity. The contamination of the messenger RNA fraction from animal cell polysomes with ribosomal RNA is significantly higher with the membrane filter method (11) than with the oligo(dT)-cellulose technique (10). It would be anticipated that the much larger HnRNA which contains double-stranded regions would present added obstacles to achieving a clean separation of RNAs containing poly(A) from those which do not.

Question (Mandal): Would you speculate about the function of poly(A) in polysomal mRNA?

Answer: At this time, it is difficult to assign any role to the poly(A) sequences. Their presence in animal RNA viruses (e.g., poliovirus) which replicate in the host cytoplasm encourages us to believe they have a role somewhere in the translation process, although apparently not the actual mechanism of translation itself, since histone mRNA which appears not to contain a poly(A) sequence can nonetheless be translated. A role in translation need not of course exclude a role for poly(A) in the processing and/or transport of mRNA from the nucleus to polyribosomes.

Comments (Sarkar): Using chicken embryonic polysomes, we have fractionated the polysomes into different sizes, each coding for distinct myofibrillar proteins of different polypeptide lengths such as myosin heavy chain (mol wt 200,000), actin (mol wt 46,000), and myosin light chains (average mol wt 20,000). We have determined the size of the poly(A) segments in messages isolated from these polysome fractions. Our conclusion is that the poly(A) segment of different messages is highly variable (varies from 75 to 200 nucleotides).

Answer: Our early results with the polysome-bound mRNA of HeLa cells labeled for brief periods indicated that the poly(A) sequence was strikingly homogeneous, and it was this property which encouraged us to investigate it further. Data from cells labeled for longer periods indicate that the poly(A) sequences in mRNA become more heterogeneous and shorter. This suggests that poly(A) sequences are being metabolized as messenger RNA ages. Although the poly(A) sequences in mRNAs of different species have been found to differ, i.e., that in yeast mRNA averages about 50 compared with 150 for HeLa mRNA, your data would be the first that I know of to suggest that the poly(A) sequences on specific mRNA molecules in the same cell have different lengths of poly(A).

26

Estradiol-Induced Expression of Genetic Information: Synthesis of Phosvitin in Birds

G. P. Talwar, B. L. Jailkhani, M. L. Sopori, S. Venkatesan, A. Grover, P. R. Narayanan, and C. Narasimhan

Department of Biochemistry
All-India Institute of Medical Sciences
New Delhi, India

Several growth-promoting and developmental hormones stimulate the synthesis of RNA in their target tissues (for review, see ref. 1). In some cases, such as those of growth hormone and thyroid hormones, the effect is noticed with a lag period of several hours, whereas steroid hormones influence transcriptional processes within minutes of their administration. We shall dwell here more particularly on estrogens, the female ovarian hormones that exercise a marked growth-promoting effect on the organs of the female reproductive tract.

FATE OF ESTRADIOL IN TARGET TISSUE

When estradiol 17B is injected into ovariectomized rats, it is rapidly concentrated and preferentially retained in its target organs, such as the uterus (2). Within the uterus, it is found noncovalently but tightly bound to protein "receptors" in the cytoplasm and the nucleus (3). In fact, the recognition of the hormone takes place initially in the cytoplasm. The hormone-receptor complex then migrates to the nucleus (4,5). Within the nucleus, the hormone, along with the "receptor" proteins, is associated with nonhistone acidic proteins of the chromatin. It is believed that the "acceptor" proteins of the chromatin are organ specific and are not present in organs that are not influenced by these hormones (6).

HORMONE EFFECT ON RNA SYNTHESIS

Estrogens induce, within 2 min of their administration in rats, an enhanced synthesis of RNA in the uterus (7). This is probably one of the earliest, if not the first, metabolic action provoked by the hormone. The activation of RNA synthesis is vital for the development of the biological effects of the hormone; actinomycin D if applied locally will block the biological response of the tissue to estradiol (8). Moreover, RNA from estrogen-primed tissues can simulate the hormone action (9).

How does the hormone activate the transcriptional processes? The precise answer to this question is not available. What is observed for estrogens is also found to be true for other steroid hormones. In each case, it is possible to identify a similar sequence of events, namely, (a) the presence of specific receptors in the cytoplasm, (b) their translocation to the nucleus along with the hormones, and (c) the synthesis of some early species of RNA. The steroid - receptor protein complex derepresses the transcription of a limited number of cistrons. In giant chromosomes of *Calliphora,* ecdysone induces discrete "puffs" of some segments (10). The puffs have been shown to be active sites of uridine incorporation into RNA.

A SYSTEM FOR ANALYSIS OF A SPECIFIC PROTEIN INDUCED BY ESTROGENS

In order to study the action of estrogens on expression of dormant gene information, we considered it appropriate to choose a system in which a specific product (protein) of hormone action could be looked for. Such a system was provided by an observation recorded earlier by Schjeide and Urist (11) showing that an egg-yolk protein phosvitin is produeed in male or immature chicks by the administration of estrogens. This protein is normally made by laying hens but requires female ovarian hormone action before the ability to synthesize it is induced in male birds. The protein is rich in serine (approximately 50% amino acid content), and much of it is phosphorylated. It has a sedimentation constant of 3-5S. The source of the protein is the liver.

Kinetics of Synthesis

The protein appears in the plasma about 24 hr after the administration of the hormone to an immature bird (Fig. 1). The plasma levels continue to rise until about the third day, after which decline sets in with low and insignificant levels being reached by about the sixth day.

What are the events that take place during the lag or latent period of several hours? Among others, RNA synthesis appears to be vital. If actinomycin D (11) or 8-azaguanine (Fig. 1) is given along with the hormone, the appearance of the protein in the plasma under hormonal influence is blocked.

RNA Synthesis in the Early Period

It is possible to detect a small but significant rise in the incorporation of radioactive precursors into RNA within 30 min after the administration of the hormone. This is followed by a more voluminous increase at about 4 hr. There are thus at least two phases detectable in the hormone-induced stimulation of RNA synthesis in the first 4 hr.

The initial 30-min rise is not dependent on the synthesis of any limiting protein(s), as cycloheximide sufficient to block over 90% of the incorporation of radioactive leucine into liver proteins does not prevent it.

Types of RNA Synthesized

Figure 2 gives the profile of RNA synthesized at 4 hr by the control and hormone-treated birds. There is a marked rise in the species of RNA having low sedimentation constants (around 4S). However, there is also an increase in other species—ribosomal as well as 4-18S fractions.

Two questions can be raised from these results. The first refers to the possible significance of the 4S peak, and the second to whether the species of RNA analyzed at the 4-hr period contains the messenger RNA for phosvitin.

The fact that phosvitin contains a large amount of serine, and also that

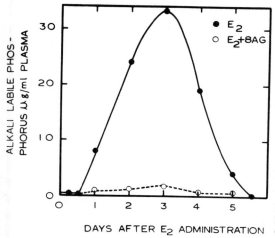

Fig. 1. Kinetics of induction of phosvitin in chickens following a single injection of estradiol 17B. Fourteen-day-old male chickens were given 1 mg estradiol alone (●) or together with 2 mg 8-azaguanine (○). At indicated times, the birds were killed by decapitation. Serum was collected and processed for determination of phosvitin phosphorus as described elsewhere (12).

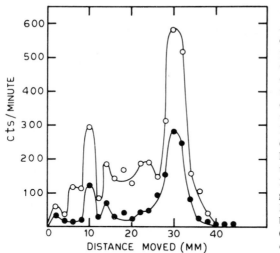

Fig. 2. *Electrophoresis of RNA on polyacrylamide gels.* RNA was prepared from the livers of roosters, by the hot-phenol and dodecylsulfate method, at 4 hr after they had received 2 mc of [^{32}P]-orthophosphate either alone or together with estradiol. Purified RNA (15 μg/gel) was subjected to electrophoresis on 2.4% gels for 1 hr 45 min. After electrophoresis, the gels were frozen and cut into 2-mm sections. Slices from three gels were pooled, dissolved in H_2O_2, and counted in a dioxan-based scintillation mixture. ●, Control RNA, input counts 1460; ○, E_2 RNA, input counts 3470.

serine, having six codons, would have as many isospecies of tRNA, raises the possibility that the lack of any one or more of these isoaccepting tRNAs could impose a restriction on the translation of phosvitin mRNA and that the hormonal induction may merely consist of supplying the missing species of tRNA for reading the message. That this is not the case seems evident from the following two experiments.

In the first experiment, tRNA prepared from control and estradiol-treated rooster liver was used to charge radioactive serine maximally and then subjected to fractionation by reverse-phase chromatography on freon-NH₄ columns. This procedure split the seryl-tRNA into five fractions. The data in Fig. 3 show that although there are quantitative differences and administration of estrogens has increased serine radioactivity in three of the five isoacceptors, there are no qualitative differences between the control and the hormone-treated rooster liver seryl-tRNA. No new species of seryl-tRNA are detectable, subject of course to the limitations, if any, of resolution by this method.

Another argument ruling out the vital requirement of hormone-treated bird liver tRNA for phosvitin synthesis is furnished by the second experiment, reported in Fig. 4. In this experiment, the incorporation of radioactive serine into proteins was studied *in vitro* utilizing a cell-free system composed of microsomes and cell sap of liver from chicks treated either with estrogens or with vehicle alone (controls). Serine incorporation was distinctly higher in the hormone-treated bird liver preparations. In a parallel experiment, the microsomes from hormone-treated birds were incubated with cell sap from the control birds, and *vice versa*. The enhanced ability to incorporate serine into proteins

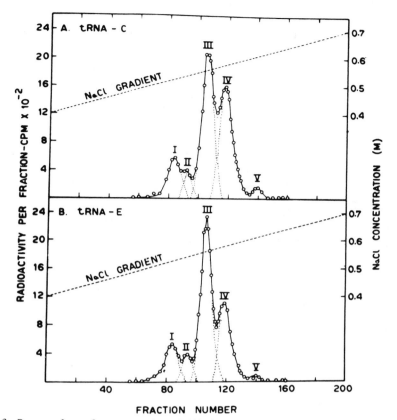

Fig. 3. Reverse-phase chromatography of [¹⁴ C] seryl-tRNA from control and estradiol-treated rooster liver. tRNA from control or hormone treated livers was incubated in a mixture containing ATP, [¹⁴ C] serine, and homologous aminoacyl-tRNA synthetases (DEAE-cellulose fraction) for 30 min at 30°C. The reaction mixture was extracted with water-saturated phenol, and the aqueous layer was dialyzed extensively. The dialyzed sample was applied to a freon column (3.4 by 45 cm) and eluted with a linear gradient of NaCl (0.4-0.7 M) in a buffer containing 0.01 M $MgCl_2$ and 0.05 M NaOAc (pH 4.5). Fractions (2.5 ml) were collected, and radioactivity was determined in 100-μl aliquots.

was found to be mainly dependent on the type of microsomal pellet utilized, the cell sap containing the tRNA and aminoacyl synthetase(s) from control bird liver being nearly as efficient as the hormone-treated preparations. The cell sap components are therefore not determinants of the ability to synthesize this protein, although they contribute somewhat to the quantity of the protein synthesized. Figure 5 gives the data on similar experiments performed with radioactive leucine as precursor, which measures the general protein synthesis in

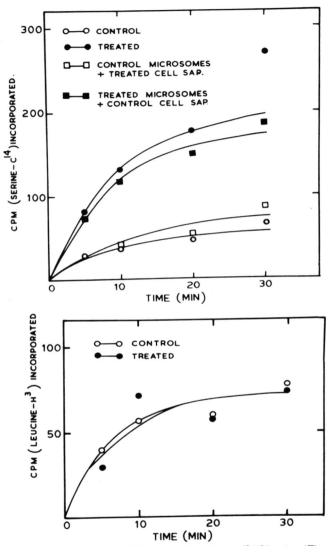

Figs. 4 and 5. *Incorporation of [^{14}C] serine (Fig. 4) and [^{3}H] leucine (Fig. 5) in protein-synthesizing systems derived from control and hormone-treated roosters.* Total incubation mixture (0.2 ml) contained 1 μmole ATP, 3 μmoles phosphoenolpyruvate, 10 μg pyruvate kinase, 0.1 μmole glutathione (reduced), 1 μmole GTP, 1 mg cell sap protein in 40 μl of medium A (tris, 35 mM, pH 7.8; MgCl$_2$, 10 mM; KCl, 25 mM, sucrose, 0.15 M), 0.2 μmole each of lysine, alanine, aspartic acid, glutamic acid, arginine, histidine, methionine, isoleucine, threonine, glycine, and phenylalanine, and 2.5 nmole (0.25 μc) of [^{14}C] serine or 0.33 μmole of [4,5-^{3}H] leucine. Estradiol (10 mg) was given intraperitoneally 24 hr before removal of liver.

the tissue, in contrast to that of serine, which serves as an index of the rate of synthesis of phosvitin, a protein especially rich in serine. It is apparent that the hormone treatment does not influence to any noticeable degree the synthesis of other proteins in this tissue.

POSSIBLE FUNCTION OF EARLY RNA SPECIES

It has been mentioned above that at 4 hr after the injection of the hormone, the incorporation of radioactive precursors into RNA is substantially stimulated. Is a new mRNA for phosvitin transcribed at this stage? To test this, two sets of experiments were performed. In the first set, the microsomes and cell sap preparations were obtained from birds at varying time intervals after the administration of the hormone and their ability to incorporate serine into proteins was measured. These experiments demonstrated that (a) the 4-hr RNA fractions were not competent for enhanced serine incorporation and (b) this ability was detectable only after 18-24 hr had elapsed since the injection of the hormone. In the second set of experiments, a short pulse of radioactive serine was given to birds treated with estrogens *in vivo,* and the cell sap was analyzed for polysomes with high radioactivity due to serine (Fig. 6). In both cases, it was evident that the early (up to 4 hr) species of RNA do not represent the message for phosvitin synthesis. It was also apparent from these studies that a number of other events preceded the induction of the ability to synthesize this protein. The RNA synthesized during the first 4 hr no doubt plays a crucial role in the subsequent ability to synthesize phosvitin, as actinomycin D and 8-azaguanine block almost completely the induction process. We would therefore like to believe that the RNA synthesized at this stage has an "organizer" role to determine the changes necessary in the tissue for the new task of the synthesis of egg-yolk proteins.

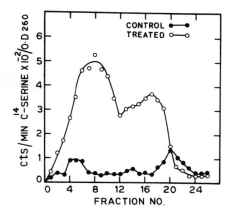

Fig. 6. Profile of liver polysomes engaged in synthesis of [^{14} C] serine-rich protein. [^{14} C] Serine (10 μc, 103 mc/mmole) was injected into birds at 48 hr after they had received either estradiol 17B or the vehicle. Four minutes later, the birds were killed and postmitochondrial supernatant fraction from liver was prepared. Aliquots were centrifuged in a linear gradient of sucrose (10-34%) for 4 hr at 25,000 rpm in an SW25 rotor in a Spinco model L. Fractions (1.0 ml) were collected and measured for absorbance at 260 mμ and for radioactivity.

DNA SYNTHESIS IMPLICIT IN THE INITIAL INDUCTION PROCESS

Following the first injection of estradiol to immature or male chicks, a period of enhanced incorporation of radioactive thymidine into DNA is observed in between 6 and 18 hr. The radioactivity is truly incorporated into a DNase-sensitive biopolymer located in the nuclei and not in the mitochondria. If the synthesis of the hormone-primed DNA is prevented by mitomycin C (Fig. 7), hydroxyurea, bromodeoxyuridine, or fluorodeoxyuridine, the appearance of phosvitin is also blocked (Table I). The action of these compounds in inhibiting phosvitin synthesis is exercised only if they are given during the critical period of the hormone-induced rise in DNA synthesis; their administration at later times has no effect on protein synthesis.

AMPLIFICATION OF THE CAPACITY TO SYNTHESIZE PHOSVITIN ON REPEATED ADMINISTRATION OF THE HORMONE

Figure 8 gives data on the plasma levels of phosvitin in a bird that received three sequential injections of the hormone. If the areas under these peaks are

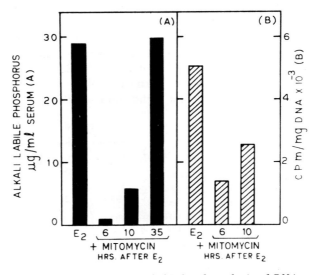

Fig. 7. Effect of mitomycin C on estradiol-induced synthesis of DNA and phosvitin in rooster liver. At indicated times after the administration of estradiol, birds were given mitomycin-C (1.5 mg/100 g) intraperitoneally. Then at 11.5 hr each bird received 50 μc of [³H]thymidine. Serum phosvitin (A) and radioactivity incorporated into DNA (B) were determined at 48 hr.

Table I. Effect of Bromodeoxyuridine, Fluorodeoxyuridine, and Hydroxyurea on Plasma
Phosvitin Levels[a]

Treatment	Hr after Estradiol	Phosvitin phosphorus (μg/ml plasma)
Estradiol (E$_2$)	–	45.9
E$_2$ + dBrUrd	6-10 48-52	8.5
E$_2$ + hydroxyurea	6-10 48-52	5.0 43.2
E$_2$ + F-dUrd	6-10	4.6

[a]Roosters (150 g) were given a single injection of 6.0 mg
estradiol 17B. Then 12.0 mg of other agents was injected
in three equal doses between the indicated times, and
plasma was measured for phosvitin at 70 hr.

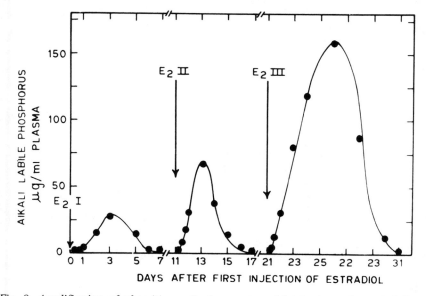

Fig. 8. Amplification of phosvitin synthesis on sequential injections of estradiol. Four-
month-old birds were given 2 mg/100 g of estradiol intraperitoneally. At indicated times,
blood was withdrawn into heparinized syringes and plasma obtained was measured for
phosvitin. Arrows indicate the times when second and third sequential injections of estradiol
were given to the same bird.

integrated, it will be observed that the capacity of the bird to synthesize phosvitin increases progressively until plateau levels are attained. Concomitant with the increase in phosvitin synthesis is an increase in the fresh, dry, and fat-free weight of the liver. It is also observed that mitotic inhibitors such as colcemid and vinblastine, if given at appropriate times, bring about an inhibition of phosvitin synthesis. It is therefore not unlikely that cell division is involved in the recruitment of the male or immature pullet liver for synthesis of this protein. However, the hormone is also required for the continuous functioning of "committed" cells to make phosvitin.

These observations suggest that the hormone has a dual role. Initially it acts as a differentiating agent, mobilizing the native but dormant potential of the tissue for synthesis of this protein. This takes place probably via a process of cell division. It is further required for continuous expression of the ability to synthesize the protein by these cells.

ACKNOWLEDGMENTS

This work has been supported by research grants from the Population Council, Inc., New York, The Council of Scientific and Industrial Research, New Delhi, and The World Health Organization, Geneva (Human Reproduction Division), and by PL-480 grant No. NR 108-892 of the Office of Naval Research.

REFERENCES

1. G. P. Talwar. *Internat. J. Biochem.* **3**:39 (1972).
2. E. V. Jensen and H. I. Jacobson. *Rec. Progr. Hormone Res.* **18**:387 (1962).
3. G. P. Talwar, S. J. Segal, A. Evans, and O. W. Davidson. *Proc. Natl. Acad. Sci. (USA)* **52**:1059 (1964).
4. G. Shyamala and J. Gorski. *J. Biol. Chem.* **244**:1097 (1969).
5. E. V. Jensen, T. Suzuki, T. Kwashima, W. E. Stumpf, P. W. Jungblut, and E. R. DeSombre. *Proc. Natl. Acad. Sci. (USA)* **59**:632 (1968).
6. T. C. Spelsberg, A. W. Steggles, and B. W. O'Malley. *J. Biol. Chem.* **246**:4188 (1971).
7. A. R. Means and T. H. Hamilton. *Proc. Natl. Acad. Sci. (USA)* **56**:686,1594 (1966).
8. G. P. Talwar and S. J. Segal. *Proc. Natl. Acad. Sci. (USA)* **50**:226 (1963).
9. S. J. Segal, O. W. Davidson, and K. Wada. *Proc. Natl. Acad. Sci. (USA)* **54**:782 (1965).
10. U. Clever. *Exptl. Cell Res.* **20**:623 (1960).
11. O. A. Schjeide and M. R. Urist. *Science* **124**:1242 (1956).
12. O. Greengard, A. Sentenac, and G. Acs. *J. Biol. Chem.* **239**:2079 (1964).

DISCUSSION

Question (Sarkar): In your system, do you see sequential DNA, RNA, and protein synthesis or does the synthesis of these macromolecules show independent kinetics?

Answer: The tissue is synthesizing more than one type of RNA and protein. These are also the biopolymers synthesized continuously in the liver of control birds. Study of the kinetics of their synthesis is thus not meaningful.

Question (Sarkar): With respect to your early (0-4 hr) macromolecule synthesis, are the RNA and protein syntheses independent?

Answer: The first rise in RNA synthesis noticed within 30 min of estradiol administration appears to be independent of protein synthesis and is not prevented by cycloheximide.

Question (Das): I would like to know whether radioautography of liver cells during DNA synthesis is indicated to quantitate the number of nuclei that are incorporating radioactive precursor. If this is compared with number of cells dividing, then it might give an idea whether DNA synthesis is an expression of gene amplification or whether it indicates division before differentiation.

Answer: The preliminary data that we have at the moment suggest that the synthesis of DNA does not represent the amplification of genes but is related to the division of cells.

27

Comparison of Biochemical Characteristics of Reverse Transcriptase from Human Acute Leukemic Cells and Several RNA Tumor Viruses

P. S. Sarin, [*]
National Institutes of Health
Bethesda, Maryland, U.S.A.

J. W. Abrell,
Litton Bionetics
Bethesda, Maryland, U.S.A.

and

R. C. Gallo [*]
National Institutes of Health
Bethesda, Maryland, U.S.A.

The presence of reverse transcriptase in RNA tumor viruses (oncornaviruses) is well documented (1,2). We recently described the purification and characterization of reverse transcriptase activity from the blood leukocytes of some patients with acute lymphocytic and acute myelocytic leukemia (3). The enzyme isolated from human acute leukemic cells has both biochemical and immunological characteristics of the reverse transcriptase from oncornaviruses. For example, (a) the enzyme is located in a particulate fraction, requiring high salt and/or non-ionic detergent for solubilization; (b) it catalyzes a ribonuclease-sensitive endogenous DNA synthesis; (c) the DNA product of the endogenous reaction is a DNA·RNA hybrid and is covalently attached to RNA; and (d) the purified

[*] Laboratory of Tumor Cell Biology, National Cancer Institute.

enzyme transcribes heteropolymeric portions of 70S RNA isolated from avian myeloblastosis virus (AMV)[1] and Rauscher leukemia virus (RLV) and prefers $(rA)_n \cdot (dT)_{12\text{-}18}$ over $(dT)_{12\text{-}18} \cdot (dA)_n$ as a template-primer. The purified enzyme from the human acute leukemic cells does not possess any terminal transferase activity. Recently, in collaboration with G. Todaro, we showed that the enzyme we isolated from human acute leukemic cells with the biochemical properties of viral reverse transcriptase is also immunologically related to the enzyme from mammalian type-C leukemia virus, especially to reverse transcriptase from a primate type-C virus, gibbon ape virus (4).

In this chapter, we present a summary comparison of the biochemical properties of this human leukemic enzyme with DNA polymerases isolated from human normal blood lymphocytes (5,6), AMV, RLV, woolly monkey virus, and Mason Pfizer monkey virus (MPMV).

Human leukemic lymphoblasts were obtained by leukophoresis from patients with acute leukemia. The human normal blood lymphocytes were stimulated for 72 hr with phytohemagglutinin (PHA) and used for the extraction of DNA polymerases I and II (5) and a particulate (cytoplasmic high-speed pellet) DNA polymerase (6). The viral enzymes from AMV (7), RLV, woolly monkey, and MPMV were prepared by extraction of the virus with KCl and Triton followed by chromatography on DEAE and phosphocellulose columns (8).

CHARACTERISTICS OF VARIOUS DNA POLYMERASES

A summary comparison of the biochemical properties (Table I) of the human leukemic enzyme and the human normal lymphocyte DNA polymerases with viral DNA polymerases shows that the leukemic enzyme (like the viral enzymes) catalyzes a RNase-sensitive endogenous DNA synthesis from a particulate fraction that bands at 1.16 g/cm^3 in a sucrose-density gradient (Fig. 1). For comparison, the banding of Rauscher leukemia virus is also presented. The leukemic enzyme purified from the banded cytoplasmic pellet prefers $(dT)_{12\text{-}18} \cdot (rA)_n$ over $(dT)_{12\text{-}18} \cdot (dA)_n$ (3), utilizes $(dG)_{12\text{-}18} \cdot (rC)_n$ as a template-primer (3), and transcribes heteropolymeric regions of AMV 70S RNA and RLV 70S RNA (3), also all characteristics of the viral enzyme (1,7). The enzymes isolated from normal lymphocytes, on the other hand, show marked preference for $(dT)_{12\text{-}18} \cdot (dA)_n$ over $(dT)_{12\text{-}18} \cdot (rA)_n$ (5,6), are unable to utilize $(dG)_{12\text{-}18} \cdot (rC)_n$ as a template-primer (5,6), and do not transcribe heteropolymeric regions of AMV 70S RNA or RLV 70S RNA (5,6). [The normal DNA polymerases, however, transcribe poly(A) regions of AMV 70S

---

[1] AMV, avian myeloblastosis virus; FeLV, feline leukemia virus; RLV, Rauscher leukemia virus; gibbon, gibbon ape lymphosarcoma virus; woolly, simian sarcoma virus, type 1; MPMV, Mason Pfizer monkey virus; RNase, ribonuclease; PHA, phytohemagglutinin.

Table I. Some Characteristics of DNA Polymerases in Human Cells and RNA Tumor Viruses

Property	Leukemic cells (3)	Normal cells (5, 6)			AMV (7)	RLV (8)	WOOLLY (8)	MPMV (8)
		Pellet	DNAP-I[a]	DNAP-II[a]				
RNase-sensitive endogenous reaction	+	±	-	-	+	+	+	+
Density of pellet or virus in sucrose gradient	1.16	1.1			1.16	1.16	1.16	Not tested
Elution from phosphocellulose column at pH 7.9[b]	Low salt	Low salt	Low salt	High salt	Low salt	Low salt	Low salt	Low salt
pH optimum	Neutral	Neutral	Neutral	Alkaline	Neutral	Neutral	Neutral	Neutral
Molecular weight	70,000	170,000	160,000	30,000	160,000	70,000	70,000	110,000
Response to $(dG)_{12-18} \cdot (rC)_n$	+	-	-	-	+	+	+	+
$(dT)_{12-18} \cdot (rA)_n > (dT)_{12-18} \cdot (dA)_n$	+	-	-	-	+	+	+	+
Response to AMV 70S RNA + $(dT)_{10}$ ($[^3H]$dCTP incorporation)	+	-	-	-	+	+	+	+

[a] DNAP-I is DNA polymerase I, and DNAP-II is polymerase II. These DNA polymerases were not isolated from particulate components of the cell; therefore, densities in sucrose gradients are not given.

[b] Low salt is less than 0.4 M concentration, and high salt is more than 0.4 M concentration.

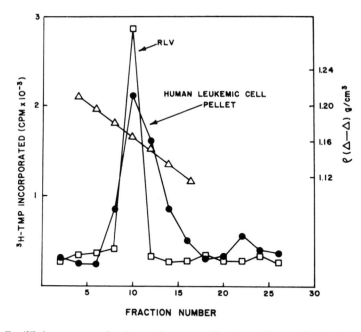

Fig. 1. *Equilibrium sucrose density gradient centrifugation of human leukemic pellet and RLV.* One milliliter of the sample was layered on 10 ml of 20-50% (w/w) linear sucrose gradient prepared in 0.01 M tris-Cl (pH 7.5), 0.1 M NaCl, and 1 mM EDTA. The samples were centrifuged for 22 hr at 60,000 × g in a Spinco SW41 rotor. After centrifugation, 0.4-ml fractions were collected, and the density of every other fraction was determined from refractive index measurements. An aliquot of 10 μl from every other fraction was assayed for endogenous DNA polymerase activity in a 0.05-ml standard reaction mixture. The reaction mixture contained 50 mM tris-Cl (pH 7.5), 60 mM NaCl, 5 mM dithiothreitol, 0.05% Triton X100, 80 μM each of dATP, dCTP, and dGTP, and 5.6 μM[^{3}H]dTTP (8100 cpm/pmole). Five-millimolar magnesium chloride was used for assay of the leukemic pellet fractions, and 1 mM manganese chloride was used for RLV. The samples were incubated at 37°C for 1 hr.

RNA in the presence of oligo(dT).] All these DNA polymerases are bound at low salt on a phosphocellulose column.

TEMPLATE-PRIMER RESPONSE

Template-primer response of the various human and viral DNA polymerases is given in Table II. All the values reported in this table are based on experiments carried out in the presence of magnesium as the divalent cation. Some of the viral enzymes (RLV, FeLV, woolly, and gibbon) have optimum values for the various template-primers with managanese as the divalent cation. The leukemic

Table II. Template-Primer Characteristics of DNA Polymerases from Human Blood Lymphocytes and RNA Tumor Viruses

DNA polymerase[d]	$(dT)_{12-18} \cdot (rA)_n / (dT)_{12-18} \cdot (dA)_n$ [a]	$(dT)_{12-18} \cdot (rA)_n$ / act. DNA [a]	$(dG)_{12-18} \cdot (rC)_n$ [b]
Human cell			
Normal:			
60K pellet enzyme	1:5	1:20	< 0.01
DNA polymerase I	1:12	< 1:100	< 0.01
DNA polymerase II	< 1:100	< 1:100	< 0.01
Leukemic:			
60K pellet enzyme	3:1–60:1	1:3	4.26
RNA tumor viruses			
AMV	37:1	4:1	133
RLV[c]	20:1	1:1	24
FeLV	12:1	1:1	47
Woolly	10:1	1:1	46.8
Gibbon	1:2	1:5	38.0
MPMV	110:1	55:1	142

[a] DNA polymerase assays were carried out at 37°C for 1 hr in a standard reaction mixture (0.05 ml) that contained 50 mM tris (pH 7.5), 60 mM NaCl, 5 mM dithiothreitol, 5 mM MgCl$_2$, 80 μM dATP, and 5.6 μM dTTP (8100 cpm/pmole) for $(dT)_{12-18} \cdot (rA)_n$ and $(dT)_{12-18} \cdot (dA)_n$ reactions. For reactions containing activated DNA as a template (primer), the reaction mixture also contained 80 μM each of dCTP and dGTP.

[b] DNA polymerase assays were carried out as in footnote a, except 80 μM dCTP and 6.5 μM [^{3}H]dGTP (6930 cpm/pmole) were used in place of dATP and [^{3}H]dTTP. Values are expressed in pmoles/10 μg protein/hr.

[c] The viral enzymes (RLV, FeLV, woolly, and gibbon) prefer manganese as the divalent cation; e.g., $(dT)_{12-18} \cdot (rA)_n / (dT)_{12-18} \cdot (dA)_n$ ratios are RLV, 1400:1; FeLV, 150:1; woolly, 320:1; and gibbon virus, 7:1.

[d] There is no activity with primers alone [$(dT)_{12-18}$ or $(dG)_{12-18}$ with [^{3}H]TTP or [^{3}H]dGTP as substrates] with any of these polymerases.

enzyme and the viral enzymes have preference for $(dT)_{12\text{-}18} \cdot (rA)_n$ over $(dT)_{12\text{-}18} \cdot (dA)_n$. Response to $(dG)_{12\text{-}18} \cdot (rC)_n$ is a very sensitive probe for detection of the viral DNA polymerase. However, a low response to this template-primer should be treated with caution, since variable results are usually obtained with an enzyme preparation under different reaction conditions. The enzyme purified from human acute leukemic cells, like the viral enzymes, utilizes $(dG)_{12\text{-}18} \cdot (rC)_n$ as a template-primer. The normal human blood lymphocyte DNA polymerases, on the other hand, show no activity with $(dG)_{12\text{-}18} \cdot (rC)_n$.

RESPONSE TO AMV 70S RNA

The purified leukemic enzyme transcribes heteropolymeric regions of AMV 70S RNA, and this reaction is completely sensitive to pretreatment of the 70S RNA with ribonuclease (3). Table III shows that the leukemic enzyme and the viral enzymes from AMV, RLV, FeLV, woolly, and MPMV will incorporate $[^3H]\,dCTP$ with AMV 70S RNA primed with oligo(dT). The normal cell poly-

Table III. AMV 70S RNA Directed DNA Synthesis by the Human and Viral DNA Polymerases

DNA polymerase	AMV 70S RNA + dT_{10}[a]
Human cell	
Normal:	
60K pellet enzyme	< 0.01
DNA polymerase I	< 0.01
DNA polymerase II	< 0.01
Leukemic:	
60K pellet enzyme	4.9
RNA tumor viruses	
AMV	81.5
RLV	9.1
FeLV	19.8
Woolly	17.3
MPMV	24.0

[a]DNA polymerase assays were carried out at $37°C$ for 1 hr in a standard reaction mixture (0.05 ml) that contained 50 mM tris-Cl (pH 7.5), 30 mM NaCl, 5 mM MgCl$_2$, 5 mM dithiothreitol, 80 μM each of dATP, dGTP, and dTTP, and 8 μM $[^3H]\,dCTP$ (12,700 cpm/pmole).

merases did not incorporate $[^3H]$ dCTP with AMV 70S RNA in the presence of oligo(dT) (only dTTP was incorporated).

REVERSE TRANSCRIPTASE PROPERTIES OF LEUKEMIC ENZYME

The various properties common to the leukemic enzyme and the viral reverse transcriptases are summarized in Table IV. These comparisons show that the leukemic enzyme is related both biochemically and immunologically to viral reverse transcriptases and is distinct from the major DNA polymerases isolated from human normal blood lymphocytes. Antibody prepared against reverse

Table IV. Summary of Reverse Transcriptase Properties of the Human Leukemic Particulate DNA Polymerase

1.[a,b] Isolated from a cytoplasmic particulate (60,000 × g) fraction that bands at a density of 1.16 g/ml in an equilibrium sucrose gradient density centrifugation.

2.[a] Catalyzes RNase-sensitive endogenous DNA synthesis, i.e., dependent on a natural and endogenous RNA. Requires all four dNTPs and Mg^{2+}.

3.[a,b] Analysis of the endogenous reaction product on Cs_2SO_4 shows the presence of RNA·DNA hybrid structures.

4.[b] The RNA template appears to be a 70S molecule.

5.[a] The purified polymerase, like the viral reverse transcriptase, has a greater preference for $(dT)_{12-18} \cdot (rA)_n$ over $(dT)_{12-18} \cdot (dA)_n$, whereas the major normal leukocyte DNA polymerases prefer $(dT)_{12-18} \cdot (dA)_n$ over $(dT)_{12-18} \cdot (rA)_n$.

6.[a] The purified polymerase is able to utilize $(dG)_{12-18} \cdot (rC)_n$ as a template primer, whereas the major normal leukocyte DNA polymerases are unable to utilize $(dG)_{12-18} \cdot (rC)_n$ as a template-primer.

7.[a] The purified polymerase transcribes heteropolymeric portions of the 70S RNA from animal tumor viruses (AMV and RLV). Under these conditions (and with polymerase activities standardized with a DNA template which each enzyme is able to utilize), the major normal leukocyte DNA polymerases do not transcribe heteropolymeric regions of 70S RNA.

8.[a,c] The leukemic enzyme is inhibited specifically by antibody (IgG) to the reverse transcriptase of mammalian type-C RNA tumor virus and most significantly by antibody to reverse transcriptase from primate type-C virus.

[a] Data from our laboratory (3,5,6,15).
[b] Data from Spiegelman's laboratory (11,12).
[c] Data from our laboratory, in collaboration with Todaro (4).

transcriptase from the gibbon ape leukemia virus inhibits the human leukemic enzyme to the same degree that it inhibits the gibbon virus polymerase (the enzyme to which the antibody was prepared). In contrast, this antibody does not inhibit the activity of the DNA polymerases from *avian* type-C virus or from mammalian type-B virus, nor does it inhibit any of the three DNA polymerases isolated from normal human cells (ref. 4 and unpublished results of G. Todaro and R. Gallo). This antibody cross-reaction clearly demonstrates that the leukemic enzyme is related to primate type-C viruses.

CONCLUSIONS

Recently, a terminal transferase activity has been reported (9) to be present in one patient with acute lymphocytic leukemia. The separation of this transferase activity from cellular polymerases has not been achieved. The enzyme we have isolated and purified from the white blood cells of patients with acute lymphocytic and acute myelocytic leukemia does not contain any terminal transferase activity (see Table II, footnote d).

A DNA polymerase activity (10) in HeLa cells has been described that shows considerable activity with $(dT)_{12-18}$ $\cdot$ $(rA)_n$, and preference for this template-primer over $(dT)_{12-18}$ $\cdot$ $(dA)_n$ is found with manganese. However, preference for $(dT)_{12-18}$ $\cdot$ $(dA)_n$ is found with magnesium (R. G. Smith, P. S. Sarin, and R. C. Gallo, unpublished observation), a finding so far not compatible with the properties of viral reverse transcriptase. Moreover, this enzyme does not utilize $(dG)_{12-18}$ $\cdot$ $(rC)_n$ as a template-primer and fails to transcribe heteropolymeric regions of AMV 70S RNA (P. S. Sarin and R. C. Gallo, unpublished observation). Thus the reverse transcriptase purified from human acute leukemic cells is distinct from this polymerase.

The presence of an RNA-dependent DNA polymerase activity in human leukemic cells has also recently been demonstrated by the simultaneous detection method by Spiegelman and associates (11). Also, Baxt and Spiegelman (12) recently reported that nuclear DNA of human leukemic cells contains viral RNA related sequences absent in the DNA of normal leukocytes.

These results combined with the findings of immunological cross-reactivity of the leukemic enzyme with the antibody prepared against mammalian and particularly primate virus reverse transcriptase (4) strongly suggest that the leukemic enzyme we have purified is at least in part viral in origin. Although we have detected a particulate and RNase-sensitive endogenous DNA polymerase activity in normal phytohemagglutinin-stimulated human lymphocytes, we have not been able to demonstrate that this reaction is, in fact, RNA directed (6). The data are so far compatible with an RNA-primed DNA-directed DNA synthesis. Moreover, the biochemical properties of this enzyme after purification do not resemble those of reverse transcriptase (6), and no immunological relatedness to viral reverse transcriptase has been found (G. Todaro and R. C. Gallo, unpublished results). On the other hand, it is possible that a cellular reverse transcriptase exists in normal human lymphocytes with the biochemical and immunological properties of primate type-C virus that we have failed to detect. Recently, a reverse transcriptase activity has been described in normal, presumably virus-free chicken cells (13,14). However, this enzyme is both biochemically and immunologically *distinct* from the known avian type-C viruses.

The detection of reverse transcriptase in human leukemia obviously does not establish the mechanism of the cause of cancer but provides evidence that human leukemic cells contain at least one expression of type-C virus related information.

REFERENCES

1. R. C. Gallo. *Nature* **234**:194 (1971).
2. H. M. Temin and D. Baltimore. *Advan. Virus Res.* **17**:129 (1972).
3. M. G. Sarnagadharan, P. S. Sarin, M. R. Reitz, and R. C. Gallo. *Nature New Biol.* **240**:67 (1972).
4. G. Todaro and R. C. Gallo. *Nature.* **244**:206 (1973).
5. R. G. Smith and R. C. Gallo. *Proc. Natl. Acad. Sci. (USA)* **69**:2879 (1972).
6. S. N. Bobrow, R. G. Smith, M. S. Reitz, and R. C. Gallo. *Proc. Natl. Acad. Sci. (USA)* **69**:3228 (1972).
7. M. Robert, R. G. Smith, R. C. Gallo, P. S. Sarin, and J. W. Abrell. *Science* **176**:798 (1972).
8. J. W. Abrell and R. C. Gallo. *J. Virol.* **12**:431 (1973).
9. R. McCaffrey, D. F. Smoler, and D. Baltimore. *Proc. Natl. Acad. Sci. (USA),* **70**:521 (1973).
10. B. Fridlender, M. Fry, A. Bolden, and A. Weissbach. *Proc. Natl. Acad. Sci. (USA)* **69**:452 (1972).
11. W. Baxt, R. Hehlmann, and S. Spiegelman. *Nature New Biol.* **240**:72 (1972).
12. W. G. Baxt and S. Spiegelman. *Proc. Natl. Acad. Sci. (USA)* **69**:3737 (1972).
13. C. Y. Kang and H. M. Temin. *Proc. Natl. Acad. Sci. (USA)* **69**:1550 (1972).
14. C. Y. Kang and H. M. Temin. *Nature,* **242**:206 (1973).
15. R. C. Gallo, P. S. Sarin, A. M. Wu, M. G. Sarngadharan, M. Reitz, M. S. Robert, N. Miller, W. C. Saxinger, and D. Gillespie. In L. Silvestri (ed.), *Possible Episomes in Eukaryotes,* Fourth Lepetit Colloquium on Biology and Medicine, North-Holland, Amsterdam, in press.

DISCUSSION

Question (Sambrook): Do the people who show reverse transcriptase activity in leukemic cells also show any antibody activity against the woolly monkey C-type RNA tumor virus?

Answer: That's a good question. We do not as yet have this information. However, it would be surprising if they did have antibody, since in animals carrying tumor cells induced by virus derived from the same species, antibodies to reverse transcriptase have not been found. Antibodies to reverse transcriptase have been isolated from a small percentage of animals treated with tumor cells derived from a different species.

Question (Mitra): How much of the virion RNA is transcribed? Do you think the DNA product is big enough to be integrated into the host chromosome as a provirus?

Answer: A variable amount of the virion RNA is transcribed by virion reverse transcriptase. In some studies, it appears that, to a small extent, all the RNA is transcribed, but the vast majority of the DNA is transcribed from a limited segment of the viral genome (about 10%). No, I do not think the DNA product is big enough to be integrated—the size that we get from *in vitro* results may not be an accurate reflection of the *in vivo* size. Another possibility is that the small products are joined by DNA ligase, resulting in a product big enough to be integrated.

Question (Burma): You mentioned that RNase H of the virus differs from host RNase H. What is the difference in specificity of the two enzymes?

Answer: The major difference appears to be the ability of the cellular but not the viral RNase H to attack RNA·DNA hybrid circles. Leis and Hurwitz have indicated that viral RNase H is a processive exonuclease whereas RNase H from other sources appears to be an endonuclease on the basis of its capacity to hydrolyze hybrid circles, which the viral enzymes do not do. Perhaps it should be emphasized at this point that these observations are limited to a few systems; for example, the only viral RNase H significantly studied to date is from avian RNA tumor viruses.

28

Synthesis by Reverse Transcriptase of DNA Complementary to Globin Messenger RNA

Inder M. Verma, Gary F. Temple, Hung Fan, and David Baltimore

Department of Biology
Massachusetts Institute of Technology
Cambridge, Massachusetts, U.S.A.

RNA tumor viruses contain a DNA polymerase that can synthesize a faithful DNA copy of viral RNA (1,5,23,25,26,31,32). This enzyme is easily released and purified from virions and can utilize a wide variety of polymers as templates (6,7,13,14,18,35,38). In order for a template to be copied, a primer or initiator that binds to the template by hydrogen bonds is required (3). The 3'-OH end of the primer is then covalently attached to the newly synthesized DNA (29). When the 60–70S tumor viral RNA is transcribed, the primer is apparently a short polyribonucleotide that is found attached to the DNA product (10,18,35,37).

One use of the RNA tumor virus DNA polymerase could be the synthesis of DNA complementary to messenger RNA (28). Most eukaryotic messenger RNAs (mRNA) contain adenine-rich sequences [poly(A)] as an integral part of their structure (9,16,19,22). For an up-to-date reference list of poly(A)-containing metazoan genetic messages, see Slater *et al.* (34). Because these sequences are apparently present at or near the 3'-end of the mRNA, an oligomer of dT that can hydrogen-bond to the poly(A) segment can be used as a primer for transcription of mRNA into DNA. The mRNA for rabbit globin can be partially purified from rabbit recticulocytes (12,17,20) by sucrose-gradient rate-zonal centrifugation. The identity of the RNA recovered from the 10S region has been established by its ability to direct synthesis of globin in a cell-free protein-synthesizing system (12,20). It contains poly(A) sequences, at least some of which are at the 3'-end of the molecule (4,19). Reticulocyte 10S RNA therefore appears to be a good model RNA for transcription into DNA by the tumor virus DNA polymerase. The successful synthesis of DNA complementary to 10S RNA can be achieved (15,24,36) as described diagrammatically in Fig. 1. Table I describes the requirements for DNA synthesis from 10S RNA. Following are some of the salient features of this system:

a. The synthesis of complementary DNA is primer-dependent.
b. The DNA synthesized is approximately 450 nucleotides long.
c. The DNA transcript is a faithful copy of 10S RNA, because it will hybridize to the 10S RNA.
d. If actinomycin D is omitted from the reaction mixture, double-stranded DNA is obtained, as characterized by its resistance to single-strand-specific nuclease (8).
e. Both the single-stranded and double-stranded DNA products can be transcribed back into RNA by *Escherichia coli* RNA polymerase.
f. Isolated single-stranded DNA can be used as a template for further DNA synthesis. The newly synthesized DNA is covalently linked to the template. The product is mostly double-stranded.

In this chapter, we shall describe some of these properties in details.

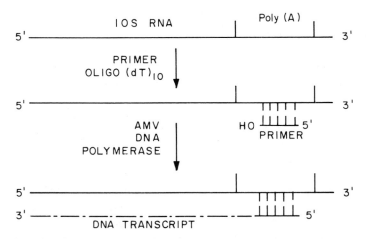

Fig. 1. *Diagrammatic model for the synthesis of complementary DNA from 10S globin messenger RNA.*

Table I.   Requirements for DNA Synthesis Using 10S Reticulocyte RNA as Template[a]

Experiment	Pmoles dGMP incorporated in 90 min
1. Complete	225
Without $(dT)_{10}$	10
With ribonuclease	2
With actinomycin D	150
2. Complete	90
Without dTTP	3
Without dCTP	3
Without dATP	4
3. Complete	112
Without $(dT)_{10}$, with $(dT)_{12-16}$	119
Without $(dT)_{10}$, with $(dG)_{12-16}$	39
Without $(dT)_{10}$, with $(dC)_{12-16}$	8
Without $(dT)_{10}$, with $(dA)_{12-16}$	9

[a]The complete reaction mixture consisted of the following in 0.1 ml: 50 mM Tris-HCl (pH 8.3), 10 mM dithiothreitol, 6 mM magnesium acetate, 60 mM NaCl, 20 μg/ml actinomycin D, 1 mM dATP, 1 mM dCTP, 1 mM dTTP, 160 μM [^{3}H]dGTP (40 cpm/pmole), 14.2 pmoles $(dT)_{10}$ (concentrations given in terms of monomer concentration), 1000 pmoles rabbit reticulocyte 10S RNA, 0.20-0.50 μg of AMV DNA polymerase (38). For experiment 1, actinomycin was omitted from the reaction mixture except where indicated. Ribonuclease-treated samples were prepared by diluting 2 μl of sample containing 1000 pmoles of rabbit reticulocyte 10S RNA to 10 μl with 0.01 M Tris-HCl (pH 7.6) and 0.01 M NaCl and adding 2 μl of ribonuclease reagent. The ribonuclease reagent contained 400 μg of pancreatic ribonuclease A/ml (Worthington Biochemical), 80 μg of ribonuclease T$_1$/ml (Calbiochem, 5000 U/mg), and 1 mg of bovine serum albumin/ml in 0.01 M Tris-HCl (pH 7.6) and 0.01 M NaCl. The samples were incubated at 37°C for 30 min, and the RNA was then used in a standard reaction mixture. In experiment 3, we compared $(dT)_{10}$ and $(dT)_{12-16}$, because they came from different sources. The amounts of $(dT)_{12-16}$, $(dG)_{12-16}$, $(dC)_{12-16}$, and $(dA)_{12-16}$ used in experiment 3 were 1420 pmoles of nucleotides/reaction mixture. Reactions were carried out in sealed tubes under an N$_2$ atmosphere and incubated at 37°C for 90 min. Acid-precipitable radioactivity was determined as previously described (2).

REQUIREMENT OF PRIMER

It is clear from Table I that there is little detectable synthesis of complementary DNA in the absence of primer. Although oligo(dT) is the most efficient primer, it can be replaced by a less efficient primer, oligo(dG). Figure 2a compares the rate of synthesis of DNA using oligo(dT) or oligo(dG) primer. The oligo(dT)-stimulated reaction reaches saturation in 90-120 min, whereas the

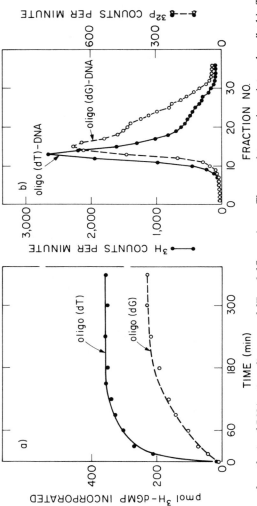
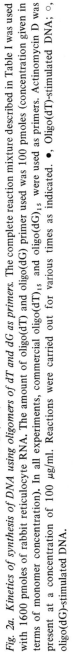

Fig. 2a. Kinetics of synthesis of DNA using oligomers of dT and dG as primers. The complete reaction mixture described in Table I was used with 1600 pmoles of rabbit reticulocyte RNA. The amount of oligo(dT) and oligo(dG) primer used was 100 pmoles (concentration given in terms of monomer concentration). In all experiments, commercial oligo(dT)$_{15}$ and oligo(dG)$_{15}$ were used as primers. Actinomycin D was present at a concentration of 100 μg/ml. Reactions were carried out for various times as indicated. ●, Oligo(dT)-stimulated DNA; ○, oligo(dG)-stimulated DNA.

Fig. 2b. Size comparison of oligo(dT)- and oligo(dG)-stimulated DNA on alkaline sucrose gradients. Linear sucrose gradients (5-20%) containing 0.7 M NaCl, 0.3 M NaOH, and 0.005 M EDTA (pH 12.6) were prepared. ³H-Labeled oligo(dT)-DNA and ³²P-labeled oligo(dG)-DNA were made 0.3 M with NaOH and boiled for 5 min at 100°C. The product was neutralized with 3 N HCl and purified from unincorporated radioactivity by gel filtration on G50 Sephadex columns as described earlier (35). ³H-Labeled oligo(dT)-DNA and ³²P-labeled oligo(dG)-DNA were made up to 0.1 ml in gradient buffer and layered on the gradient. The gradients were centrifuged at 45,000 rpm in a SW50.1 rotor for 16 hr at 4°C. Two-drop fractions were collected by puncturing the bottom of the gradient tube and were neutralized by adding 1 N acetic acid followed by 3.0 ml of distilled water and 10.0 ml of Aquasol (from N.E.N.) and shaken thoroughly to make a gel. ●, [³H]Oligo(dT)-DNA; ○, [³²P]oligo(dG)-DNA.

oligo(dG)-stimulated reaction proceeds at a slower rate. At saturation, about 40% of input nucleotides of the template are transcribed into complementary DNA with oligo(dG) primer. Under similar conditions, using oligo(dT), about 60% of the input nucleotides are transcribed into DNA. The respective sizes of oligo(dT)- and oligo(dG)-stimulated complementary DNA are compared in Fig. 2b. Oligo(dG)-primed DNA is slightly smaller and more heterogeneous. Oligo (dG)-DNA, upon hybridization to 10S globin RNA, is rendered completely resistant to the S_1 nuclease from *Aspergillus* that degrades single-stranded DNA selectively. In order to eliminate the possibility that oligo(dG) serves as primer for the transcription of either a- or β-10S RNA exclusively, we compared the stimulation of DNA synthesis with oligo(dG) and oligo(dT) using isolated a- and β-10S RNA from rabbit reticulocytes (33). Table II shows that both a- and β-10S RNA are transcribed with the same efficiency using oligo(dG) and oligo (dT) primers; β-10S RNA appears to be transcribed more extensively than a-10S RNA. Table II also shows that oligo(dG) does not stimulate any DNA synthesis when 28S RNA and 18S RNA from rabbit reticulocytes are presented as

Table II[a]

Template	Primer	Pmoles dGMP incorporated	Percent of input nucleotides transcribed
Rabbit reticulocyte 10S RNA	Oligo(dT)	350	58
	Oligo(dG)	235	39
Rabbit reticulocyte a-10S RNA	Oligo(dT)	80	13
	Oligo(dG)	68	11
Rabbit reticulocyte β-10S RNA	Oligo(dT)	216	36
	Oligo(dG)	192	32
Rabbit reticulocyte 28S RNA		6	< 2
	Oligo(dG)	8	< 2
	Oligo(dT)	9	< 2
Rabbit reticulocyte 18S RNA		4	< 2
	Oligo(dG)	2	< 1
	Oligo(dT)	7	< 2

[a]The complete reaction mixture as described in Table I and the caption of Fig. 2a was used. The concentration of rabbit reticulocyte 10S RNA was 2400 pmoles, a-10S RNA 2400 pmoles, β-10S RNA 2400 pmoles, 28S RNA 1700 pmoles and 18S RNA 1500 pmoles. The percent of input nucleotides transcribed has been determined by multiplying pmoles of dGMP incorporated by 4 (assuming that all four deoxyribonucleoside triphosphates have been incorporated in equimolar ratios).

templates. Thus, like oligo(dT) (Table I), oligo(dG) specifically utilized the 10S RNA from rabbit reticulocytes as template to synthesize complementary DNA.

The role of oligo(dG) as primer for the synthesis of complementary DNA is puzzling because there are no known poly(C)-rich regions in the 10S RNA. However, regions of RNA containing five or six residues of cytidylic acid could well exist and act as sites for primer attachment. Because the oligo(dG)-DNA is quite long, some of the primer binding sites must be near the 3'-end of the template. Thus, it might be expected that oligo(dT)-primed DNA synthesis, which starts at the 3'-end, would cover the oligo(dG) binding sites and prevent any oligo(dG)-stimulated synthesis. This conjecture has been confirmed by showing that addition of oligo(dG) at the end of an oligo(dT)-primed synthesis leads to little further DNA synthesis. If, however, oligo(dT) is added after maximal oligo(dG)-stimulated synthesis has occurred, further stimulation of DNA synthesis is detected.

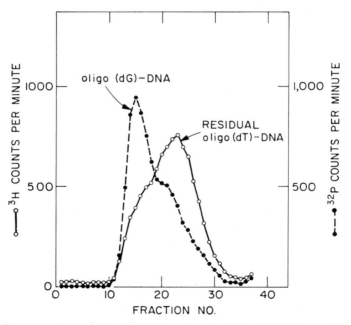

Fig. 3. Size comparison of oligo(dG)-DNA and residual oligo(dT)-DNA on alkaline sucrose gradients. Oligo(dG)-primed reaction mixture (as in Fig. 2a) was incubated for 7 hr, and then oligo(dT) (as in Fig. 2a) was added along with [3H]-labeled deoxyguanosine triphosphate (600 cpm/pmole). The reaction was further incubated for 180 min and the product purified by gel filtration as described before. The product was analyzed by centrifugation on an alkaline sucrose gradient as described in Fig. 2b along with [32P]-labeled oligo(dG)-DNA as marker. ○, Residual [3H] oligo(dT)-DNA; ●, [32P] oligo(dG)-DNA.

If oligo(dT)-DNA is a nearly complete transcript of 10S RNA, then the sum total of the sizes of oligo(dG)-DNA and residual oligo(dT)-DNA [i.e., where oligo(dG) is used as primer and, at the end of the incubation, oligo(dT) is added] should not exceed the size of oligo(dT)-DNA. Figure 3 portrays sedimentation patterns of oligo(dG)-DNA and residual oligo(dT)-DNA on alkaline sucrose gradients. By using the method of Studier (30), the size of the largest species of residual oligo(dT)-DNA was determined to be approximately 150-160 nucleotides long and that of oligo(dG)-DNA to be approximately 350-370 nucleotides long. Together they represent a size approximately 500-550 nucleotides long, as compared to oligo(dT)-DNA which is approximately 450 nucleotides long. Thus the size of oligo(dG)-DNA plus residual oligo(dT)-DNA is approximately 10-20% larger than that of oligo(dT)-DNA alone. This suggests that some nucleotide sequences in oligo(dG)-DNA are unique. In order to investigate this further, competition-hybridization studies were carried out, and the results show that approximately 30% of the sequences in oligo(dG)-DNA do not compete with oligo(dT)-DNA and appear to be unique. So it appears that oligo(dT)-primed DNA synthesis is initiated near the 3'-end of the RNA, while oligo(dG)-stimulated DNA synthesis is initiated from regions [presumably oligo(C)-rich] situated internally in the RNA, and the DNA transcript includes some sequences analogous to oligo(dT)-DNA and some unique sequences. A tentative model to explain oligo(dT)- and oligo(dG)-primed synthesis of complementary DNA is proposed in Fig. 4. This model can explain satisfactorily a number of the properties of the oligo(dG)-stimulated reaction: (a) the slower kinetics of oligo (dG)-primed DNA is a result of the binding of oligo(dG) to short cytidylic acid-rich regions, which are not very stable; (b) at saturation, oligo(dG)-DNA is only slightly shorter than oligo(dT)-DNA; (c) if oligo(dG) is added to oligo(dT)-primed reaction mixture, no detectable enhancement of incorporation is observed, and conversely, if oligo(dT) is added to a reaction mixture that has previously been incubated with oligo(dG), significant enhancement in incorporation is observed; (d) the sum total of the sizes of oligo(dG)-DNA and residual oligo(dT)-DNA

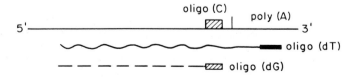

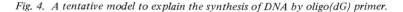

Fig. 4. A tentative model to explain the synthesis of DNA by oligo(dG) primer.

barely exceeds the size of oligo(dT)-DNA. However, the model is unable to explain competition-hybridization results, which suggest that either the oligo(dG)-DNA is transcribed more extensively near the 5′-end of the 10S RNA or oligo(dG) is priming the transcription of some unknown species of RNA present in the 10S RNA preparation.

TRANSCRIPTION OF RNA FROM COMPLEMENTARY GLOBIN DNA

The DNA transcript of 10S RNA can be used for RNA synthesis *in vitro* by *E. coli* RNA polymerase. Figure 5 shows the rate of incorporation of GMP into acid-insoluble material. Table III summarizes the requirements for RNA synthesis. The reaction requires all four ribonucleoside triphosphates for synthesis of RNA. Rifampicin (20 μg/ml) inhibits about 85% of RNA synthesis. Both oligo(dT)-DNA and oligo(dG)-DNA can act as templates for the synthesis of RNA. Figures 6a,b depict the sedimentation patterns on neutral sucrose gradients of the RNA synthesized using oligo(dT)-DNA and oligo(dG)-DNA tem-

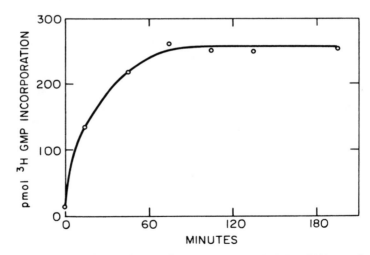

Fig. 5. Kinetics of synthesis of RNA from single-stranded globin DNA template. The complete reaction mixture consisted of the following in 0.1 ml: 50 m*M* Tris-HCl (pH 7.9), 50 m*M* magnesium acetate, 0.4 m*M* dithiothreitol, 150 m*M* KCl, 0.4 m*M* ATP, 0.4 m*M* CTP, 0.4 m*M* UTP, 160 μM [³H] GTP (40 cpm/pmole), 1500 pmoles of single-stranded globin DNA, and 10 μg of *E. coli* RNA polymerase (gift of Dr. R. A. Firtel). The reaction mixture was incubated at 37°C, and aliquots of 10 μl were withdrawn at the times indicated and acid-precipitable radioactivity was determined as described before (Table I).

Table III. Requirements for RNA Synthesis Using
8S Single-Stranded Globin DNA[a]

Experiment	Pmoles of GMP incorporated
1. Complete	32
Without ATP	6
Without CTP	4
Without UTP	3
2. Complete	310
Rifampicin (20 μg/ml)	50

[a]The complete reaction mixture as described in Fig. 5 was used except that 200 pmoles of 8S single-stranded globin DNA in experiment 1 and 1600 pmoles in experiment 2 were added. Reactions were carried out in sealed tubes under an N_2 atmosphere and incubated at 37°C for 120 min. Acid-precipitable radioactivity was determined as previously described.

plates, respectively. Although some of the RNA synthesized sediments faster, the majority of the RNA synthesized sediments between 5 and 6S.

Using the complementary DNA made from 10S RNA isolated from patients with sickle-cell anemia and separate reaction mixtures containing one of the four α-P^{32}-labeled nucleoside triphosphates, ^{32}P-labeled RNA sedimenting at 6S in DMSO gradients has been obtained (11,21). The T_1 ribonuclease fingerprint pattern of the purified ^{32}P-labeled synthetic 6S RNA is compatible with the fingerprint of original 10S RNA treated with T_1 RNase and then with polynucleotide kinase. Many T_1 RNase sequences were identical with oligopeptides found in the α and β chains of globin. Similar comparisons are in progress with RNA synthesized from DNA complementary to rabbit reticulocyte 10S RNA.

The majority of the RNA synthesized from oligo(dT)-stimulated single-stranded rabbit globin DNA hybridizes back to the template DNA and is efficiently competed out with excess unlabeled 10S RNA. Double-stranded DNA made in the absence of actinomycin D is also a good template for RNA synthesis, except that the size of the RNA synthesized is much smaller. Detailed studies of the hybridization properties of these synthetic RNAs are in progress.

SYNTHESIS OF DOUBLE-STRANDED DNA FROM THE SINGLE-STRANDED GLOBIN DNA TRANSCRIPT

If actinomycin D is omitted from the reaction mixture containing globin mRNA (Table I), double-stranded DNA is synthesized as measured by enhanced incorporation of deoxyribonucleoside triphosphates and resistance to single-

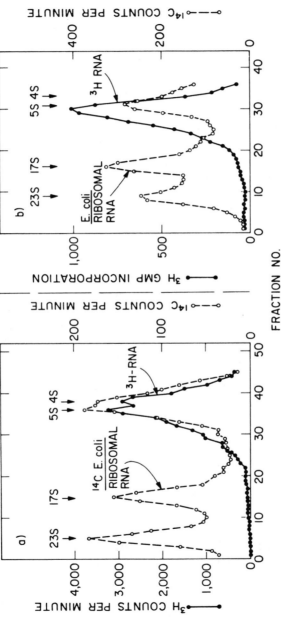

Fig. 6. Sedimentation patterns of RNA synthesized from (a) oligo(dT)- and (b) oligo(dG)-stimulated single-stranded rabbit globin DNA. The complete reaction mixture described in Fig. 5 was used except that the specific activity of [³H]GTP was 600 cpm/pmole and the amount of DNA used in each case was approximately 800 pmoles. The reactions were terminated at 180 min by addition of Sarkosyl at a final concentration of 1%. The products were separated from the unincorporated radioactivity on Sephadex G75 columns. The column-purified products were then treated with deoxyribonuclease (Worthington) at a concentration of 10 μg/ml in a buffer containing 1 mM Mg²⁺ and incubated at 37°C for 10 min. The DNase was inactivated by adding 10 mM EDTA and diluted in the gradient buffer. Two 4.8-ml 5-20% sucrose gradients made in 0.1 M NaCl, 0.01 M tris-Cl (pH 7.5), and 0.001 M EDTA were prepared. The products in volumes of 100 μl were layered separately on two gradients along with ¹⁴C-labeled E. coli ribosomal RNA as marker (provided by Dr. A. Jacobson). The gradients were centrifuged for 4½ hr at 45,000 rpm at 4°C in a SW50.1 rotor. Gradients were collected and radioactivity was counted as described in Fig. 2b. •, [³H] RNA; ○, E. coli ribosomal [¹⁴C] RNA.

stranded DNA-specific nucleases. Figure 7 shows the analysis of double-stranded DNA on alkaline sucrose gradients. The double-stranded DNA sediments slightly slower than the single-stranded DNA made in the presence of actinomycin D. This suggests the following three mechanisms of synthesis of double-stranded DNA: (a) there is some primer attached at or near the 3'-OH end of the single-stranded DNA that serves as initiator for the synthesis of the second strand of DNA; (b) the 3'-OH end of nascent single-stranded DNA chains supports the synthesis of the second strand; (c) the synthesis of the second strand of DNA does not require a primer.

In order to rule out the possibility that some primer is fortuitously attached at the 3'-OH end of the single-stranded DNA, we purified the single-stranded DNA made in the presence of actinomycin D on alkaline sucrose gradients. Peak fractions were pooled and excess sucrose and alkali removed by gel filtration on G50 Sephadex columns. This is referred to as "purified single-stranded DNA." When purified single-stranded DNA is incubated with the four deoxyribonucleoside triphosphates, and purified avian myeloblastosis virus (AMV) DNA polymerase, double-stranded DNA is synthesized. The product has been analyzed on alkaline

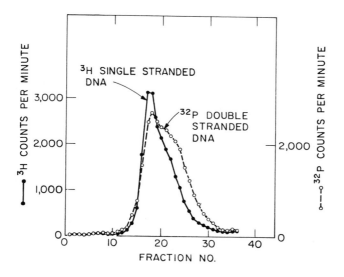

Fig. 7. Alkaline sucrose gradient profile of double-stranded DNA made from 10S rabbit reticulocyte RNA in the absence of actinomycin D. The complete reaction mixture as described in Table I was used except that actinomycin D was omitted and [³H] dGTP was replaced with [³²P] dGTP. The reaction was carried out for 6 hr, and the product was purified by gel filtration and analyzed on a 5-20% alkaline sucrose gradient as described in Fig. 2b. ●, ³H-Labeled single-stranded globin DNA marker; ○, ³²P-labeled double-stranded DNA.

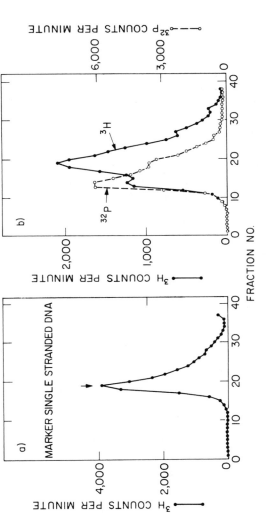

Fig. 8. Sedimentation profiles of purified single-stranded globin DNA before and after incubation with ^{32}P-labeled deoxyribonucleoside triphosphates. Single-stranded DNA was made as described before in Table I and then purified further by sedimentation on an alkaline sucrose gradient. Peak fractions were collected and excess alkali and sucrose removed by gel filtration. Panel (a) shows the sedimentation profile. The arrow shows the position of a marker ^{32}P-labeled 8S single-stranded DNA. Panel (b) depicts the sedimentation pattern after incubating 2100 pmoles of ^{3}H-labeled purified single-stranded DNA (1236 cpm/pmole of dGMP) with 50 mM Tris-HCl (pH 8.3), 5 mM dithiothreitol, 6 mM magnesium acetate, 60 mM NaCl, 0.6 mM each of dATP, dCTP, and dTTP, ^{32}P-labeled dGTP (specific activity 12,000 cpm/pmole), and AMV DNA polymerase for 6 hr at 37°C. The product was purified by gel filtration and part of it analyzed on the alkaline sucrose gradients described in Fig. 2b. ●, ^{3}H-Labeled single-strand globin DNA; ○, ^{32}P-labeled second strand of DNA.

sucrose gradients. Figure 8a,b shows the profile of ^{3}H-labeled single-stranded DNA before incubation and after incubation with ^{32}P-labeled deoxyribonucleoside triphosphates. The ^{32}P-labeled second strand of DNA sedimented faster than the majority of ^{3}H-labeled single-stranded DNA template. About 20-30% of the input nucleotides of the template strand were transcribed, and about that amount of ^{3}H-labeled DNA sedimented coincidentally with ^{32}P-labeled DNA. Since the new strand of DNA sedimented faster than the template strand and carried with it some template strand, it appears that the second strand was covalently linked to the 3'-OH end of the template strand.

When the product was chromatographed on hydroxylapatite columns, the majority of the unreacted template strand was eluted by 0.12 M phosphate buffer, whereas the ^{3}H and ^{32}P covalently linked double-stranded DNA eluted at 0.48 M phosphate buffer concentration. S1 nuclease digestion of the 0.48 M phosphate buffer eluate of hydroxylapatite columns showed that 100% of the ^{32}P label remained acid insoluble, whereas only 70% of the ^{3}H label remained acid precipitable. This suggests that the ^{3}H-labeled template strand was not completely copied.

Analysis of the product by formamide gel electrophoresis showed that the 3H- and ^{32}P-labeled double-stranded DNA migrated more slowly than the marker ^{32}P-labeled single-stranded DNA (figure not shown), suggesting that the double-stranded DNA was larger in size than the single-stranded DNA.

Thus, from the above results, it appears that (a) the purified single-stranded DNA acts as a template for the synthesis of a second strand of DNA, (b) the second strand is covalently linked to the template strand, and (c) the second strand is not a complete transcript of the template strand.

As mentioned before, double-stranded DNA synthesized in the absence of actinomycin D is smaller in size than the single-stranded DNA. We are now investigating this reaction in detail to determine if the nascent growing chain of DNA forms a "hairpin" and provides the 3'-OH end for the synthesis of the second strand, or whether there is another mechanism of synthesis of this double-stranded DNA.

TRANSCRIPTION OF VARIOUS OTHER RNA TEMPLATES BY AMV DNA POLYMERASE

In addition to reticulocyte 10S RNA, several other natural RNAs have been successfully transcribed into complementary DNA in our laboratory and in others. Table IV summarizes the efficiency of various RNAs as templates with and without primers. The properties of some of these systems will be described in detail elsewhere (40,41).

Table IV[a]

	Template	Primer[b]	Efficiency[c]
1.	70S AMV RNA		++
2.	70S hamster leukemia virus RNA		++
3.	70S murine leukemia virus RNA		++
4.	35S heat-denatured AMV RNA		+
	35S heat-denatured AMV RNA	oligo(dT)	++
5.	Polio 35S RNA		+
	Polio 35S RNA	oligo(dT)	++
		oligo(dG)	++
6.	Phage f2 RNA		+
	Phage f2 RNA	oligo(dT)	++
		oligo(dG)	++
7.	28S rabbit reticulocyte ribosomal RNA	oligo(dT)	+
8.	18S rabbit reticulocyte ribosomal RNA	oligo(dT)	+
9.	10S rabbit, duck, or human reticulocyte RNA		+
	10S rabbit, duck, or human reticulocyte RNA	oligo(dT)	+++
	10S rabbit, duck, or human reticulocyte RNA	oligo(dG)	+++
10.	26S myosin RNA		+

Table IV (Continued)[a]

Template	Primer[b]	Efficiency[c]
26S myosin RNA	oligo(dT)	++
11. 10S histone RNA		+
10S histone RNA	oligo(dT)	++
12. Silk worm mRNA		+
Silk worm mRNA	oligo(dT)	++
	oligo(dC)	++
13. 14S crystalline lens mRNA		+
14S crystalline lens mRNA	oligo(dT)	+++
14. *E. coli* 5S RNA		+
E. coli 5S RNA	oligo(dT)	+
	oligo(dG)	+
15. Yeast fMet-tRNA	oligo(dT)	+
16. Crude *E. coli* 4S RNA	oligo(dT)	+
17. Slime mold mRNA	oligo(dT)	+++
18[d] Vaccinia mRNA	oligo(dT)	+++
19. Single-stranded 8S globin DNA		+++
20. Commercial calf thymus and salmon sperm DNA		+++

[a]The conditions employed were the same as described for the assay of the fractions, except for substituting appropriate template and primer. The incubation time was 90-120 min. This represents the yield but not the rate of reaction. The change of ionic medium can alter the efficiency of certain templates.

[b]The oligomer primers have a chain length of 12-18 nucleotides.

[c]+++, Excellent template, approximately 20-80% of nucleotides of the input template are transcribed; ++, fair template, approximately 1-20% of nucleotides of the input template are transcribed; +, poor template, less than 1% of nucleotides of the input template are transcribed.

[d]Zassenhaus and Kates (39).

ACKNOWLEDGMENTS

This work was supported by a contract from the Special Virus Cancer Program of the National Cancer Institute awarded to D. Baltimore and by NIH grant No. GM-17151 awarded to Dr. U. L. RajBhandary. I. M. V. and G. F. T. were fellows of the Jane Coffin Childs Memorial Fund for Medical Research. H. F. was a Helen Hay Whitney fellow, and D. B. was an American Cancer Society Professor of Microbiology. The avian myeloblastosis virus was generously supplied by Dr. J. Beard.

REFERENCES

1. D. Baltimore. RNA-dependent DNA polymerase in virions of RNA tumor viruses. *Nature* **226:**1209-1211 (1970).
2. D. Baltimore, A. S. Huang, and M. Stampfer. Ribonucleic acid synthesis of vesicular stomatitis virus. II. An RNA polymerase in the virion. *Proc. Natl. Acad. Sci. (USA)* **66:**572 (1970).
3. D. Baltimore and D. Smoler. Primer requirement and template specificity of the RNA tumor virus DNA polymerase. *Proc. Natl. Acad. Sci. (USA)* **68:**1507-1511 (1971).
4. H. Burr and J. B. Lingrel. Poly A sequences at the 3'-termini of rabbit globin mRNAs. *Nature New Biol.* **233:**41 (1971).
5. P. H. Duesberg and E. Canaani. Complementarity between Rous sarcoma virus (RSV) RNA and the *in vitro*-synthesized DNA of the virus-associated DNA polymerase. *Virology* **42:**783-788 (1970).
6. P. Duesberg, K. V. D. Helm, and E. Canaani. Properties of a soluble DNA polymerase isolated from Rous sarcoma virus. *Proc. Natl. Acad. Sci. (USA)* **68:**747-751 (1971).
7. P. Duesberg, K. V. D. Helm, and E. Canaani. Comparative properties of RNA and DNA templates for the DNA polymerase of Rous sarcoma virus. *Proc. Natl. Acad. Sci. (USA)* **68:**2505-2509 (1971).
8. H. Fan and D. Baltimore. *J. Mol. Biol.,* in press (1973).
9. R. A. Firtel, A. Jacobson, and H. F. Lodish. Isolation and hybridization kinetics of messenger RNA from *Dictyostelium discoideum. Nature New Biol.* **239:**225 (1972).
10. R. M. Flugel and R. D. Wells. Nucleotides at the RNA-DNA covalent bonds formed in the endogenous reaction by the avian myeloblastosis virus DNA polymerase. *Virology* **48:**394-401 (1972).
11. B. G. Forget, C. Marotta, I. M. Verma, R. P. McCaffrey, D. Baltimore, and S. M. Weissman. Nucleotide sequence analysis of human globin messenger RNA. *Blood* **40:**961 (1972).
12. D. Housman, R. Pemberton, and R. Taber. Synthesis of a and β chains of rabbit hemoglobin in a cell-free extract from Krebs II ascites cells. *Proc. Natl. Acad. Sci. (USA)* **68:**2716 (1971).
13. J. Hurwitz and J. P. Leis. RNA-dependent DNA polymerase activity of RNA tumor viruses. 1. Directing influence of DNA in the reaction. *J. Virol.* **9:**116-129 (1972).
14. D. L. Kacian, K. F. Watson, A. Burny, and S. Spiegelman. Purification of the DNA polymerase of avian myeloblastosis virus. *Biochim. Biophys. Acta* **246:**365-383 (1971).
15. D. L. Kacian, S. Spiegelman, A. Bank, M. Terada, S. Metafora, L. Dow, and P. A. Marks. *In vitro* synthesis of DNA components of human genes for globins. *Nature New Biol.* **235:**167-169 (1972).

16. J. Kates. Transcription of vaccinia virus genome and the occurrence of polyriboadenylic acid sequences in messenger RNA. *Cold Spring Harbor Symp. Quant. Biol.* **35**:743 (1970).

17. F. Labrie. Isolation of an RNA with the properties of haemoglobin messenger. *Nature* **221**:1217 (1969).

18. J. P. Leis and J. Hurwitz. RNA-dependent DNA polymerase activity of RNA tumor viruses. II. Directing influence of RNA in the reaction. *J. Virol.* **9**:130-142 (1972).

19. L. Lim and E. S. Canellakis. Adenine rich polymer associated with rabbit reticulocyte messenger RNA. *Nature* **227**:710 (1970).

20. R. E. Lockard and J. B. Lingrel. The synthesis of mouse haemoglobin β-chains in a rabbit reticulocyte cell-free system programmed with mouse reticulocyte 9S RNA. *Biochem. Biophys. Res. Commun.* **37**:204 (1969).

21. C. Marotta, B. G. Forget, I. M. Verma, and R. P. McCaffrey. Nucleotide sequence analysis of human globin messenger RNA. *Fed. Proc.,* **32**:455 (1973).

22. L. Philipson, R. Wall, G. Glickman, and J. E. Darnell. Addition of polyadenylate sequence to virus specific RNA during adenovirus replication. *Proc. Natl. Acad. Sci. (USA)* **68**:2806 (1971).

23. M. Rokutanda, H. Rokutanda, M. Green, K. Fujinaga, R. K. Ray, and C. Gurgo. Formation of viral RNA-DNA hybrid molecules by the DNA polymerase of sarcoma-leukaemia viruses. *Nature* **227**:1026 (1970).

24. J. Ross, H. Aviv, E. Scolnick, and P. Leder. *In vitro* synthesis of DNA complementary to purified rabbit globin mRNA. *Proc. Natl. Acad. Sci. (USA)* **69**:264-268 (1972).

25. S. Spiegelman, A. Burny, M. R. Das, J. Keydar, J. Schlom, M. Travnicek, and K. Watson. Characterization of the products of RNA-directed DNA polymerases in oncogenic RNA viruses. *Nature* **227**:563-567 (1970).

26. S. Spiegelman, A. Burny, M. R. Das, J. Keydar, J. Schlom, M. Travnicek, and K. Watson. DNA-directed DNA polymerase activity in oncogenic RNA viruses. *Nature* **227**:1029-1031 (1970).

27. S. Spiegelman, A. Burny, M. R. Das, J. Keydar, J. Schlom, M. Travnicek, and K. Watson. Synthetic DNA-RNA hybrids and RNA-RNA duplexes as templates for the polymerases of the oncogenic RNA viruses. *Nature* **228**:430-432 (1970).

28. S. Spiegelman, K. F. Watson, and D. L. Kacian. Synthesis of DNA complements of natural RNA's: A general approach. *Proc. Natl. Acad. Sci. (USA)* **68**:2843-2845 (1971).

29. D. Smoler, I. Molineux, and D. Baltimore. Direction of polymerization of the avian myeloblastosis virus DNA polymerase. *J. Biol. Chem.* **246**:7697-7700 (1971).

30. W. F. Studier. Sedimentation studies of the size and shape of DNA. *J. Mol. Biol.* **11**:373 (1965).

31. H. Temin and D. Baltimore. RNA-directed DNA synthesis and RNA tumor viruses. *Advan. Virus Res.* **17**:129 (1972).

32. H. Temin and S. Mizutani. RNA-dependent DNA polymerase in virions of Rous sarcoma virus. *Nature* **226**:1211-1213 (1970).

33. G. F. Temple and D. E. Housman. Separation and translation of the mRNAs coding for α and β chains of rabbit globin. *Proc. Natl. Acad. Sci. (USA)* **69**:1576 (1972).

34. D. W. Slater, I. Slater, and D. Gillespie. Post fertilization synthesis of adenylic acid in sea urchin embryos. *Nature* **240**:333 (1972).

35. I. M. Verma, N. L. Meuth, E. Bromfeld, K. F. Manly, and D. Baltimore. A covalently-linked RNA-DNA molecule as the initial product of the RNA tumor virus DNA polymerase. *Nature New Biol.* **233**:131 (1971).

36. I. M. Verma, G. F. Temple, H. Fan, and D. Baltimore. *In vitro* synthesis of DNA complementary to rabbit reticulocyte 10S RNA. *Nature New Biol.* **235**:163-167 (1972).

37. I. M. Verma, N. L. Meuth, and D. Baltimore. The covalent linkage between RNA primer and DNA product of the avian myeloblastosis virus DNA polymerase. *J. Virol.* **10:**622-627 (1972).
38. I. M. Verma and D. Baltimore. Purification of the RNA-directed DNA polymerase from avian myeloblastosis virus and its assay with polynucleotide templates. *Meth. Enzymol.,* in press (1973).
39. Zassenhaus and Kates. *Nature New Biol.,* **238:**139 (1972).
40. A. J. M. Berns, H. Blomendal, S. Kaufman, and I. M. Verma. *Biochem. Biophys. Res. Commun.* **52:**1013 (1973).
41. I. M. Verma, R. A. Firtel, H. F. Lodish, and D. Baltimore, in preparation (1973).

DISCUSSION

Question (Edmonds): Have you transcribed heterogeneous nuclear RNA with reverse transcriptase? What sizes of heterogeneous nuclear RNA have you transcribed?
Answer: No, we have not used heterogenous nuclear RNA as template.

Question (Dutta): What kind of slime mold did you use?
Answer: We used cellular slime mold.

Question (Dutta): Is it *in vivo* or *in vitro* labeling?
Answer: The labeling of mRNA was *in vivo*.

Question (Mehrotra): How do you account for the long time taken for transcribing your message in the presence of oligo(dG) as the primer?
Answer: I don't know, but I think most likely the answer lies in the fact that there is a very small stretch of oligo(C) and the binding of oligo(dG) to such a stretch of oligo(C) is not very stable.

Question (Mitra): What is the stoichiometry of the DNA product and 10S messenger RNA template at saturation?
Answer: At best, about 80% of the input nucleotides of the template are transcribed into the DNA product.

29

Investigations on Reverse-Transcribed DNA from RNA Templates

M. R. Das

Tata Institute of Fundamental Research
Bombay, India

Following the discovery of reverse transcriptase by Temin and Mizutani (1) and Baltimore (2), it was shown by Spiegelman *et al.* (3), using molecular hybridization experiments, that the DNA strand synthesized by a tumor virus reverse transcriptase is complementary to the viral RNA.

It was also realized that labeled DNA of this type can be used as an analytical probe for the corresponding gene in the host chromosome, or for its message in a mixture of RNA molecules. An elegant series of experiments based on this principle by Spiegelman and coworkers (4-7) revealed several interesting facts. They looked for evidence of a possible viral etiology of several types of human cancers making use of radioactive DNA products from murine RNA tumor viruses. These experiments were designed to exploit the possible presence of transcripts in human tumors that possess at least some sequences in common with those of the homologous murine viruses. It was observed that human leukemias (4), sarcomas (5), and lymphomas (6) contain RNA that exhibits homology to the DNA product synthesized by the Rauscher leukemia virus (RLV).

Axel *et al.* (7) used this technique for studying human breast carcinomas. These tumors were found to contain RNA homologous to the DNA product of the mouse mammary tumor virus (MMTV). However, no such RNA was found in normal breast tissue, or in benign pathologies such as fibrocystic disease and fibroadenoma. It was also noted that the breast cancer RNA did not hybridize to DNA complementary to the RNA of RLV.

Meanwhile, Schlom *et al.* (8) had already demonstrated the presence of reverse transcriptase in B-type particles isolated from human milk. The presence of a high molecular weight RNA, either 70S or 35S, which might be a subcomponent of a 70S RNA, and the synthesis of nascent DNA on the RNA template were also shown (9,10) in *in vitro* reactions using these particle isolates. It is of obvious interest to characterize these particles and to examine the DNA product synthesized from these virus-like particles of human origin for homology with RNA from breast tumors. But this type of experiment has some limitations, owing to the limited availability of milk samples having the particles. Nevertheless, such experiments are of great importance in examining possible links between these human milk particles containing reverse transcriptase and human mammary neoplasia. We report here our results showing the presence, in malignant human breast tumors, of polysomal RNA that has sequences homologous with DNA products synthesized using the reverse transcriptase reaction of human milk particle isolates.

MATERIALS AND METHODS

Several samples of milk obtained from Parsi and Hindu women were screened for the presence of reverse transcriptase. Attempts were made to work with fresh samples as far as possible. The samples were received in containers cooled in ice and were kept cold in ice. The purification procedures were started as soon as the samples were received in the laboratory. ^{3}H-Labeled thymidine-5' -triphosphate was obtained from the Radiochemical Centre, Amersham, and all the unlabeled deoxynucleoside triphosphates were purchased from P-L Biochemicals. Enzymes such as RNase, trypsin, and trypsin inhibitor used in our experiments were obtained from Sigma. For equilibrium gradients, Optical Grade cesium sulfate from Schwartz/Mann was employed.

The detailed method of isolation of the virus-like particles has been described elsewhere (10).

Reverse Transcriptase Assay

The assay of reverse transcriptase was carried out using purified particle isolates by methods that have already been described (3,8-10). Two types of assay procedures were employed. In a large number of samples, the temporal synthesis of radioactive DNA by the enzyme obtained by breaking open the milk particles with Nonidet P40 was followed (10). The reactions were carried out using methods described before (8-10). Control experiments in which the NP40-broken virus preparations were treated with RNase to check whether an observed DNA synthesis was truly RNA dependent were also carried out. An alternative method (9-11) was employed for all samples in the later part of our investigation. After enzyme reaction had been carried out for an hour, the total nucleic acid present in the mixture was extracted using the phenol method. A portion of this was examined using velocity sedimentation in a 10-30% glycerol gradient or a 5-20% sucrose gradient. The gradients were analyzed to determine the position of banding of the radioactive DNA. Banding of nascent radioactive DNA attached to a high molecular weight RNA (either 70S or 35S) was taken as evidence for reverse transcriptase and the presence of high molecular weight RNA in the milk particle isolates. Prior treatment of the nucleic acid extracts with RNase and the consequent disappearance of counts in the RNA density region with the simultaneous appearance of more counts in the DNA region (8-9S region) was taken as confirmatory evidence of the above conclusion.

Hybridization

The DNA·RNA hybridization experiments were carried out using purified DNA products. The aqueous extract of nucleic acids obtained by phenol extraction of the reaction mixture was dialyzed for 24 hr against 0.002 M EDTA (pH 7.2) to remove labeled nucleoside triphosphates. *Escherichia coli* ribosomal RNA was added as carrier, and the nucleic acids were precipitated after making the solution 0.4 M with respect to NaCl and adding 2 vol of ethanol. After keeping the solution at $-20°$C overnight, the precipitated nucleic acids were collected by centrifugation at 10,000 rpm in an SS34 rotor. The pellet was taken up in 0.1 ml of 0.002 M EDTA (pH 7.2) and was treated with 0.3 M KOH at 37°C for 18 hr to destroy all the RNA. Polysomal RNA was isolated (7) from human breast tumors after dispersing the tissues with a Silverson homogenizer at 4°C in 2 vol of 5% sucrose in 0.01 M tris (pH 7.2), 0.15 M naCl, 0.002 M MgCl$_2$. The suspension was centrifuged at 15,000 × g for 30 min at 0°C. The pellet was discarded, and 5 ml each of the supernatant was layered on 5 ml of 25% sucrose in the same buffer and spun for 3 hr at 48,000 rpm in a Spinco 50Ti rotor. The pellets were dissolved in the same buffer, and the RNA was extracted using phenol-cresol (7:1, v/v) after making the solution 1% with respect to sodium dodecylsulfate. From the aqueous extract, RNA was precipitated by the addition of 2 vol of ethanol and 1/10 vol of 4 M LiCl. The purified DNA (4000 cpm) was incubated at 80°C for 10 min in 50% formamide to denature the DNA and was quickly cooled in ice and mixed with 500 μg polysomal RNA. The mixture was brought to 0.4 M NaCl and 50% formamide in a final volume of 0.15 ml and incubated for 24 hr at 37°C. The contents were diluted to 2.5 ml using 0.002 M EDTA and mixed with 2.56 ml of saturated Cs$_2$SO$_4$ solution. It was centrifuged at 36,000 rpm in an SW39 rotor for 60 hr at 20°C. Ten-drop fractions were collected (0.4 ml) and assayed for trichloroacetic acid precipitable radioactivity.

Analysis of Results

In the kinetic method, the reaction was carried out as described earlier (10) in a total reaction volume of 250 μl, and 50-μl aliquots of the reaction mixture were assayed for acid-precipitable radioactivity at definite time intervals. Using this method, if the incorporation of the labeled nucleotide is greater than 0.2 pmole in 60 min, the reaction is designated as strong. If the incorporation increases with time up to at least 40 min and the amount of incorporation is at least up to 0.1 pmole, the reaction is designated positive but weak. In the velocity-gradient method, the reaction was carried out for 1 hr and the nucleic acid products were subjected to velocity-gradient centrifugation. For analyzing the data, we have used a method similar to the one used by Spiegelman and coworkers (4,5,7) for equilibrium density gradients. The sums of the 10-min counts for three samples in the 67-70S region and 33-36S region were taken after subtracting the background counts in each fraction. Using background counts (from between the 45S and 55S region in our gradients, which did not show much radioactivity above average background) in three samples from each of 15 gradients, the standard deviation, S, in the background was calculated. The sums of the counts above background obtained for the 70S and 35S region were divided by the standard deviation. If this ratio is greater than 3, the reaction is termed positive but weak. When the ratio is above 50, the reaction is designated strong.

Results of DNA·RNA hybridization experiments between radioactive DNA products synthesized by the reverse transcriptase reaction and polysomal RNA extracted from different sources were analyzed using the method employed by Axel *et al.* (7). The 10-min counts from fractions of the Cs_2SO_4-density gradients were corrected for background, and the counts in fractions between the densities of 1.63 g/cm^3 and 1.68 g/cm^3 (for three samples) were summed and expressed as the counts in the RNA density region. A standard deviation, S, in the 10-min background counts was determined using the first three fractions of ten difficult gradients. If the ratio of the counts in the RNA density region to the standard deviation is greater than 3, the reaction is considered positive.

RESULTS AND CONCLUSIONS

Several milk samples obtained from women belonging to both the Parsi and Hindu communities were analyzed according to methods described above. The results have been described elsewhere (12). Figure 1a shows the velocity-gradient profile of the nucleic acids isolated from the reverse transcriptase reaction of a Hindu milk sample, H1. This is a typical example of a strong reaction. It shows, in addition to a major peak at the 70S region, a minor peak near the 35S region. A part of the same product after RNase treatment, when analyzed in an identical

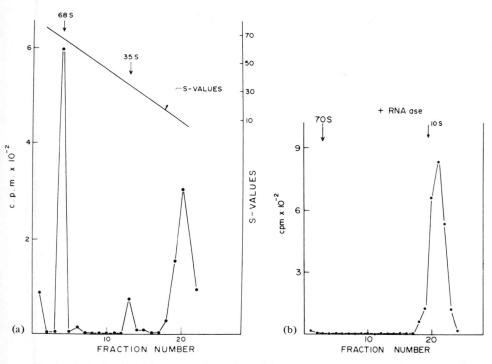

Fig. 1. Analysis of nucleic acid products formed from the reverse transcriptase reaction of human milk particle isolate H1 (see Table I) on a 10-30% glycerol gradient. (a) Without RNase treatment; (b) after RNase treatment (see text).

manner, gave the profile shown in Fig. 1b, thereby demonstrating the fact that the DNA is originally attached to an RNA template.

After the presence of a strong reverse transcriptase reaction had been ascertained using small portions of the nucleic acid products, the remaining part of the nucleic acid extracts from two enzyme-positive samples, H1 and H9, was carefully purified for hybridization experiments. It should be emphasized that extreme care must be taken in the purification and characterization of the DNA products (3,4,7) used for hybridization experiments with polysomal RNA from different sources. Contamination of the product with any RNA·DNA hybrid structures from the reaction mixture will give false positives. Consequently, we have taken all the necessary precautions, such as treatment of the product with 0.3 M KOH for 18 hr at 37°C followed by extensive dialysis (13) and testing the banding of the product in a Cs_2SO_4 gradient before the DNA products were used for hybridization experiments. Polysomal RNAs from different sources were prepared and purified according to methods already described (4,7). The

Table I. Results of DNA · RNA Hybridization Experiments[a]

| Tissues | | DNA product | Counts/ 10 min | Counts/ 10 min/S | Reaction |
Source	No.				
Undifferentiated carcinoma with fibroblastic metaplasia	AC12928	H1	960	16.8	+
Infiltrating duct carcinoma III	AC13883	H1	102	1.8	-
Human placenta	–	H1	64	1.1	-
Mouse embryos	–	H1	51	0.9	-
Undifferentiated carcinoma	AC12928	H9	7832	137.7	+
Infiltrating duct carcinoma III	AC13883	H9	39	0.7	-
Infiltrating duct carcinoma III	AD305	H9	96	1.7	-
Infiltrating duct carcinoma III	AD3558	H9	225	3.9	+
Infiltrating duct carcinoma III	AD2268	H9	170	3.0	+
Infiltrating duct carcinoma II	AD569	H9	20	0.4	-
Colloid carcinoma of breast	C296	H9	119	2.1	-
Normal breast	N1	H9	0	0.0	-
Normal breast	N2	H9	11	0.2	-
Undifferentiated carcinoma	AC12928	MMTV	749	13.1	+
Undifferentiated carcinoma	AC12928	AMV	80	1.4	-

[a]H, Hindu milk samples; MMTV, mouse mammary tumor virus; AMV, avian myeloblastosis virus; S, standard deviation (see text).

annealing reactions were carried out at 37°C in 50% formamide to minimize the degradation of the RNAs.

Polysomal RNAs from several breast carcinomas were used for hybridization experiments. RNAs extracted from human placenta and from mouse embryos were also used with the DNA products for hybridization. Of all the hybridization experiments listed in Table I, positive results were observed in five individual experiments. Both the human DNA products from H1 and H9 and the DNA obtained from the MMTV reverse transcriptase reaction, which was purified in a manner identical to that used for the human products, hybridized in a clear-cut fashion with the polysomal RNA isolated from an undifferentiated carcinoma of the human breast (AC12928). The tumor has been diagnosed as an undifferentiated carcinoma with fibroblastic metaplasia. This has been a rather unusual case, and the ultrastructural pathology is under careful investigation. In addition, two other infiltrating duct carcinomas showed weak but positive hybridizations (see Table I).

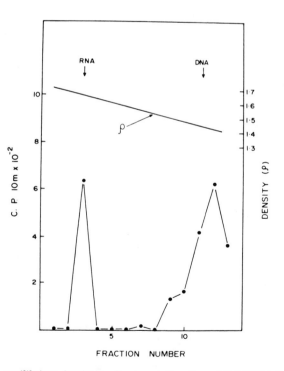

Fig. 2. *Cs$_2$SO$_4$ equilibrium density gradient centrifugation of [^{3}H]DNA from the reaction of human milk H1 (see Table I) after annealing to polysomal RNA from human breast tumor AC12928 (see text).*

Figure 2 shows the Cs_2SO_4 equilibrium density gradient profile of the hybridization between the polysomal RNA AC12928 and the DNA product obtained from milk sample H1. Figure 3 shows hybridization results using the DNA product made from mouse milk (MMTV DNA), and Fig. 4 shows the result when H9 DNA product was hybridized with polysomal RNA isolated from mouse embryos. In addition to demonstrating the negative result, Fig. 4 gives an indication of the purity of the DNA product used.

In Table I, the presentation of the data is according to the method adopted by Axel *et al.* (7). It may be noted that our positive results with AC12928 RNA are beyond any experimental error. Further, the negative results from the hybridization of the same polysomal RNA and the DNA product obtained from the reverse transcriptase reaction using avian myeloblastosis virus (AMV) (see Table I) rules out any artifact resulting from the polysomal RNA preparation.

At the moment, it is difficult to interpret why homology has been observed in the case of only some malignant tumors and not all RNAs from tumors, in the light of hybridization experiments (7) with MMTV in which the mouse DNA product hybridized with RNAs from as many as 67% of the total number of

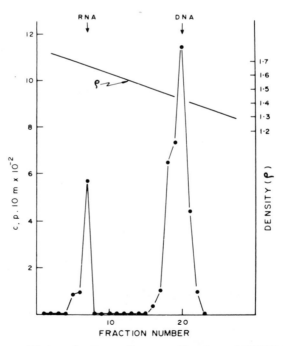

Fig. 3. Cs_2SO_4 equilibrium density gradient centrifugation of MMTV [³H] DNA after annealing to polysomal RNA from human breast tumor AC12928 (see text).

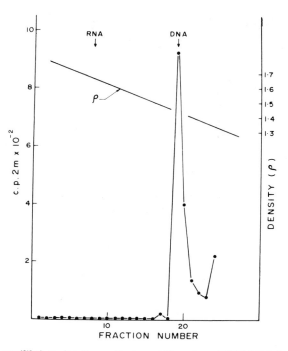

Fig. 4. Cs$_2$SO$_4$ equilibrium density gradient centrifugation of [^{3}H] DNA from the reaction of human milk H9 (see Table I) after annealing to polysomal RNA isolated from mouse embryos.

malignant human tumors examined. However, this point need not be emphasized too much, as the total number of polysomal RNAs from malignant tumors that we have examined is small. The observation that the hybrid structures are found mainly in the RNA density region implies that the RNA is much larger than the DNA product and only a small fraction of the base sequences in the RNA has hybridized with complementary DNA. In order to do saturation experiments and provide even an approximate figure for the extent of homology between the polysomal RNA and the human milk DNA product, one would have to make large amounts of the product. However, on a qualitative level it can be noted that the fraction of counts moved into the RNA density region when H9 was used is much larger than the fraction moved when the MMTV product was used with the same polysomal RNA (see Table I). The results of the present experiments provide suggestive evidence regarding the possible expression of viral-specific information from particles containing reverse transcriptase that are found in human milk in at least some types of breast tumors.

ACKNOWLEDGMENTS

The author wishes to thank Professors S. Spiegelman and G. Beaudreau for gifts of AMV.

REFERENCES

1. H. M. Temin and S. Mizutani. *Nature* **226**:1211 (1970).
2. D. Baltimore. *Nature* **226**:1209 (1970).
3. S. Spiegelman, A. Burny, M. R. Das, J. Keydar, J. Schlom, M. Travnick, and K. Watson. *Nature* **227**:563 (1970).
4. R. Hehlman, D. Kufe, and S. Spiegelman. *Proc. Natl. Acad. Sci. (USA)* **69**:435 (1972).
5. D. Kufe, R. Hehlman, and S. Spiegelman. *Science* **175**:182 (1972).
6. R. Hehlman, D. Kufe, and S. Spiegelman. *Proc. Natl. Acad. Sci. (USA)* **69**:1727 (1972).
7. R. Axel, J. Schlom, and S. Spiegelman. *Nature* **235**:32 (1972).
8. J. Schlom, S. Spiegelman, and D. H. Moore. *Nature* **231**:97 (1971).
9. J. Schlom, S. Spiegelman, and D. H. Moore. *Science* **175**:542 (1972).
10. M. R. Das, A. B. Vaidya, S. M. Sirsat, and D. H. Moore. *J. Natl. Cancer Inst.* **48**:1191 (1972).
11. J. Schlom and S. Spiegelman. *Science* **174**:840 (1971).
12. M. R. Das, E. Sadasivan, R. Koshy, A. B. Vaidya, and S. M. Sirsat. *Nature New Biol.* **239**:92 (1972).
13. M. Green, H. Rokutanda, and M. Rokutanda. *Nature New Biol.* **230**:229 (1971).

DISCUSSION

Question (Gallo): What criteria do you use for positive reverse transcriptase assays in the human milk particles?

Answer: The criteria that are used for judging positive reaction are several. The major one is, of course, RNase sensitivity of the reaction. That is to say, after purifying the "milk particle isolates" when the reverse transcriptase reaction is carried out, a control is always done in which part of the sample is subjected to RNase treatment for 30 min prior to the assay. If this treatment fails to produce a peak in the 70S or 35S region and at the same time there is a positive reaction when no RNase treatment is done, then only the original sample is judged positive. Toward the later stages of our investigations, the reactions were carried out in the presence of actinomycin D to prevent DNA-dependent DNA synthesis. In some of the positive reactions, we did try leaving out one of the four deoxynucleoside triphosphates in turn and made sure that the presence of all four triphosphates was required for the reaction to proceed. However, this latter test could not be done for all the samples because we did not always have enough of the sample material.

30

Transcriptional Control
of M13 Phage DNA Replication

Sankar Mitra

Biology Division
Oak Ridge National Laboratory
Oak Ridge, Tennessee, U.S.A.

M13 belongs to the group of small filamentous coliphages containing single-stranded circular DNA of 2×10^6 molecular weight (1). The phage does not kill the host but leaks out of intact and multiplying cells (2,3). Thus it behaves like an autonomously multiplying lytic phage except for lysis of the host. Jaenisch *et al.* (4) showed that M13 messenger RNA has an unusually long half-life of at least 18 min. On the other hand, Roy (5) showed that rifampicin and actinomycin D inhibit phage synthesis almost immediately after addition to the infected culture. It appeared reasonable to us to look into the effects of rifampicin on M13 DNA replication in wild-type and rifampicin-resistant strains of *Escherichia coli.*

The spontaneous rifampicin-resistant strain *E. coli* H491 was isolated by S. Adhya from wild-type *E. coli* HfrH and is able to grow in the presence of 200 µg/ml rifampicin.

RESISTANCE OF BACTERIAL GROWTH AND OF RNA POLYMERASE TO RIFAMPICIN

We compared the growth properties of both uninfected and infected wild-type and rifampicin-resistant strains in the presence of rifampicin (Fig. 1). *E. coli* is not highly permeable to rifampicin, but permeability increases after infection with M13 as in the case of actinomycin D (6). Both turbidity and cell count

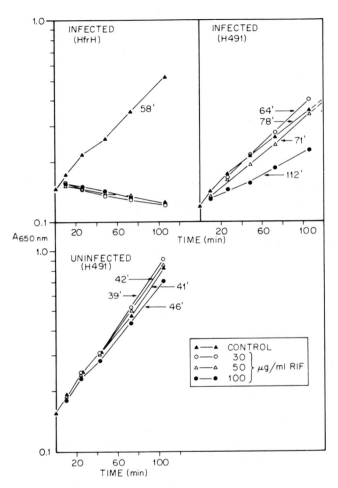

Fig. 1. Growth rate of Escherichia coli HfrH and H491 in the presence of rifampicin.
Rifampicin was added to log-phase cultures of bacteria in supplemented M9 medium at zero
time, and growth was measured by turbidity at 650 nm. For infected cultures, M13 phage
(m.o.i. = 100-200) was added 5 min before the drug. The numbers on the curves indicate
generation time.

measurements showed that H491, whether infected or not, is resistant to ten
times the minimum inhibitory concentration of the drug for HfrH. The rate of
uridine incorporation in these strains also showed that while in *E. coli* HfrH 200
μg/ml rifampicin inhibited [^{3}H] uridine incorporation by 95% in the first 3 min,
in agreement with the published report (7), there was a transient inhibition in

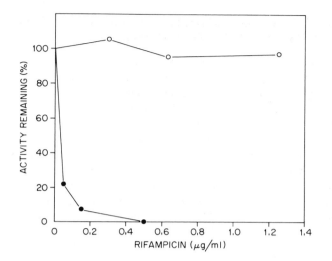

Fig. 2. Rifampicin inhibition of RNA polymerases. RNA polymerases from *E. coli* HfrH and H491 were partially purified and assayed in the presence of various concentrations of rifampicin (11). The inhibition by the drug is expressed as the percentage of activity in the control. •, HfrH polymerase; ○, H491 polymerase.

H491 by about 30% after the addition of the drug, from which the cells recovered in about 20 min.

Although it is unlikely that rifampicin resistance of *E. coli* H491 is due to altered permeability, since no such case is known (8), the partially purified RNA polymerases from HfrH and H491 were tested for sensitivity to rifampicin (Fig. 2). It is evident that H491 polymerase is far more resistant than HfrH polymerase to the drug.

INHIBITION OF PHAGE SYNTHESIS BY RIFAMPICIN

When rifampicin was added to the M13-infected H491 cultures at different times after infection, phage synthesis was inhibited, particularly at late times after infection (Fig. 3). It was also found that 30-40 μg/ml rifampicin, which hardly affected the bacterial growth, caused maximum inhibition (11). The more complete inhibition at later times after infection is presumably due to increased permeability of the infected cells. Rifampicin prevents release of RNA phages from *E. coli* (9). *E. coli* normally does not have an intracellular phage pool after infection with M13 (10). We have found that M13-infected H491 does not accumulate any intracellular phage pool after addition of rifampicin. The inhibition of phage synthesis by the drug is also reversed after its removal (11).

RESISTANCE OF PARENTAL RF SYNTHESIS TO RIFAMPICIN IN RIFAMPICIN-RESISTANT MUTANT

The general mechanism of M13 DNA replication is the same as that established for ϕX174 phage DNA (12). Parental single-stranded circular DNA (SS) is replicated by the host enzymes to parental double-stranded circular DNA, i.e., replicative form (RF). The parental RF replicates semiconservatively to progeny RF, which then gives rise to the pool of progeny SS DNA. The synthesis of parental RF does not involve any phage-coded protein, while M13 gene-2 and gene-5 proteins are required for progeny RF and SS synthesis (12). Brutlag *et al.* (13) showed that synthesis of M13 RF involves the synthesis of an RNA primer for the product strand. In a rifampicin-sensitive strain, parental RF synthesis is rifampicin sensitive, whereas it is not in the rifampicin-resistant mutant. In *E. coli* H491, therefore, parental M13 RF synthesis should be rifampicin resistant as opposed to the situation in HfrH. This is actually shown to be true (Fig. 4).

INHIBITION OF PROGENY RF AND SS DNAS BY RIFAMPICIN AND CHLORAMPHENICOL

It is thus evident that rifampicin inhibits M13 DNA replication beyond the stage of parental RF synthesis. Hence we investigated the replication of M13 progeny RF and SS DNAs in the presence of rifampicin (Fig. 5). The host DNA,

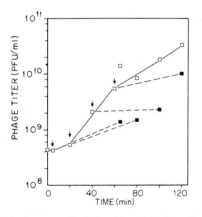

Fig. 3. Inhibition of M13 phage synthesis by rifampicin. Log-phase culture of *E. coli* H491 was infected at zero time, and aliquots were taken out at various times (indicated by arrows) to be treated with 50 µg/ml rifampicin. The phage yield was determined after 60 min incubation in the treated and in the control cultures. The solid line connecting the open squares indicates growth curve of M13 in the control. The dashed lines indicate the increase in phage titer after drug addition.

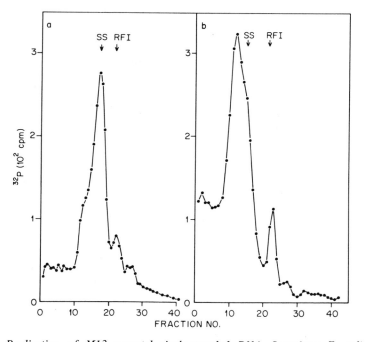

Fig. 4. Replication of M13 parental single-stranded DNA. Log-phase *E. coli* H491 (thymine-requiring auxotroph) in supplemented M9 medium was treated with 200 μg/ml rifampicin, and 10 min later was infected with ^{32}P-labeled M13 phage (6 × 10⁴ pfu/cpm) (at m.o.i. = 100-200). Ten minutes later, growth was stopped by adding KCN (10^{-2} *M*) and chilling in ice. Cells were harvested, washed by vigorous shaking with 0.1 *M* NaCl, 0.01 *M* tris-Cl (*p*H 8.0), 0.001 *M* EDTA. Finally, the cells were lysed in the same buffer with 100 μg/ml lysozyme and 0.5% sodium dodecylsulfate. The host DNA was removed by precipitation in 1 *M* NaCl (14). The supernatant was analyzed in a 5-20% sucrose gradient in 1 *M* NaCl, 0.01 *M* tris-Cl, 0.001 *M* EDTA (*p*H 8.0) in a Spinco SW41 swinging-bucket rotor for 5 hr at 39,000 rpm at 5°C. Fractions were assayed for acid-insoluble radioactivity. (a) H491 control; (b) H491 pretreated with rifampicin. The positions of SS and RF DNAs are indicated on the graphs. The large peaks of SS DNAs are due to incomplete removal of unadsorbed phage.

which was also labeled with radioactive thymidine used to label the phage DNA, was removed quantitatively by Hirt's procedure (14). It is evident that rifampicin inhibits synthesis of both progeny RF and SS DNAs. The inhibition of the latter is more significant.

Chloramphenicol also inhibits the synthesis of progeny RF and SS DNAs, presumably by inhibiting the synthesis of phage-coded proteins, which are required for phage DNA synthesis. However, rifampicin, unlike chloramphenicol,

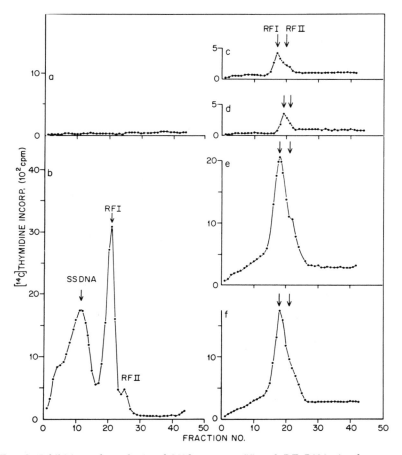

Fig. 5. Inhibition of synthesis of M13 progeny SS and RF DNAs in the presence of rifampicin and chloramphenicol. E. coli H491 in log phase in supplemented M9 was infected with M13. Forty minutes later, rifampicin and chloramphenicol were added to 20-ml aliquots, and 5 min afterward the cultures were treated with [^{14}C] thymidine (0.5 μc/ml) and deoxyadenosine (50 μg/ml) for 5 min. The cells were then lysed and the lysates analyzed for incorporation of label in RF and SS DNAs as in Fig. 4. (a) Uninfected culture; (b) infected control culture; (c) infected culture in the presence of 50 μg/ml rifampicin; (d) infected cells in the presence of 100 μg/ml rifampicin; (e) infected cells + 10 μg/ml chloramphenicol; (f) infected cells + 30 μg/ml chloramphenicol.

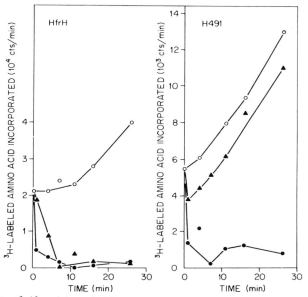

Fig. 6. Effects of rifampicin and chloramphenicol on rate of amino acid incorporation by Escherichia coli HfrH and H491. Aliquots of HfrH and H491 cultures in log phase in M9 medium containing 0.1% Casamino acid were treated with chloramphenicol (100 μg/ml) and rifampicin (200 μg/ml). At different times, 1-ml aliquots were treated with 10 μc ³H-labeled protein hydrolysate for 2 min at 37°C. The cells were precipitated with 5% trichloroacetic acid, collected and washed on Whatman GF/C paper, and counted for radioactivity. ○, Control; ▲, rifampicin treated; ●, chloramphenicol treated.

does not inhibit protein synthesis in H491, although in the case of HfrH both inhibit amino acid incorporation almost completely within 5 min after addition (Fig. 6). Thus rifampicin inhibition of progeny M13 DNA synthesis is not due to inhibition of protein synthesis in general but due to either inhibition of M13 messenger RNA synthesis or inhibition of primer RNA synthesis, which may be required for progeny RF (13) or SS DNA synthesis or both. It may be pointed out here that rifampicin inhibits M13 RF replication earlier than chloramphenicol (data not shown). This suggests that the synthesis of primer RNA is necessary for RF replication, as proposed earlier (13).

Chloramphenicol inhibits total DNA synthesis in both uninfected and infected cells after about a 30-min lag, due to prevention of a new round of replication (15). However, rifampicin does not significantly inhibit DNA synthesis in the uninfected cells and prevents the increased rate of DNA synthesis in the infected cells, presumably by preventing M13 RF DNA replication (1).

INHIBITION OF M13 mRNA SYNTHESIS BY RIFAMPICIN

That rifampicin specifically inhibits M13 messenger RNA synthesis as compared to the total host messenger RNA synthesis was shown by isolating pulse-labeled RNA from the infected H491 cells pretreated with rifampicin and by hybridizing with M13 RF (Table I). It is clear that rifampicin inhibits synthesis of M13 mRNA by about 80%. Whether the residual M13 mRNA synthesized in the presence of rifampicin is due to a unique species of RNA is not known.

ALKALI-LABILE NUCLEOTIDES IN M13 RF

While rifampicin specifically inhibits the synthesis of M13 mRNA, it is also possible that rifampicin may inhibit the replication of M13 RF by inhibiting the synthesis of primer RNA attached to the replicating DNA molecules, as suggested above. In order to test this possibility, we pulse-labeled M13-infected cells with $^{32}PO_4$ in the presence of rifampicin, purified M13 RF by equilibrium centrifugation in Cs_2SO_4, removed nascent mRNA chains by heating at $100°C$ for 5 min, and finally rebanded the DNA in Cs_2SO_4 equilibrium centrifugation. The amount of alkali-labile ^{32}P in the two peaks of DNA corresponding to SS and renatured RF with buoyant densities of 1.457 and 1.435 g/cm^3, respectively, is presumably a measure of RNA primer covalently attached to the DNA (Fig. 7). The ^{32}P counts are normalized with respect to $[^3H]$ thymidine counts, which served as the internal control and with which the DNA was labeled. It is quite suggestive from these preliminary data that the replicating M13 had

Table I. Inhibition of M13 mRNA Synthesis by Rifampicin in *Escherichia coli* H491

$[^3H]$ Uridine pulse-labeled RNA	Total input (cpm $\times 10^{-5}$)	Specific activity (cpm/A_{260} unit)	RNA bound to M13 RF fixed to membrane
Uninfected cells	1.3 2.6	8.0×10^4	0 0
Infected cells	1.2 2.4	8.8×10^4	527 880
Infected cells pretreated with rifampicin	1.2 2.4	5.2×10^4	135 180

[a]The detailed procedures for extraction and purification of pulse-labeled RNA, for purification of M13 RF, and for DNA · RNA hybridization have been described elsewhere (11).

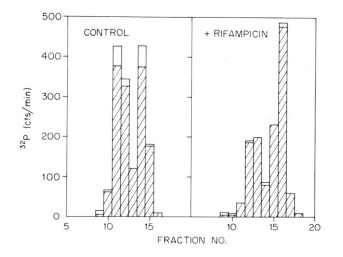

Fig. 7. Effect of rifampicin on incorporation of $^{32}PO_4$ into alkali-labile material in M13 RF. E. coli H491 grown to log phase in low-phosphate tris - Casamino acid - glucose medium was infected with M13. Five minutes later, [^{3}H] thymidine (2 μc/ml) was added. Three minutes afterward, rifampicin (200 μg/ml) was added to the experimental sample, and after 2 min both the control and the experimental cultures were treated with $^{32}PO_4$ (50 μc/ml) for 2 min. The cultures were treated with KCN, chilled, centrifuged, washed, and lysed as already described. After removal of host DNA by sodium dodecylsulfate + NaCl (14), the lysate was extracted with phenol and M13 RF was purified from the total nucleic acid by equilibrium ultracentrifugation in Cs_2SO_4. The purified RF after removal of CS_2SO_4 was heated at 100°C for 5 min and quickly chilled and rebanded in Cs_2SO_4 by equilibrium ultracentrifugation. Aliquots of fractions of the RF peak in duplicate were assayed for total and alkali-stable (0.3 N NaOH, 18 hr at 37°C) radioactivity of both ^{3}H and ^{32}P. After precipitation with trichloroacetic acid, ^{32}P counts were normalized with respect to ^{3}H counts. The total ^{32}P counts are represented by the bars, and the hatched part indicates the radioactivity remaining after alkali treatment.

alkali-labile nucleotides that were absent in rifampicin-treated cells. Further characterization of this material is in progress.

Thus we may tentatively conclude that (a) M13 directs most of its messenger RNA synthesis and (b) M13 RF DNA replication is directly dependent on transcription over and above the synthesis of phage-coded proteins.

ACKNOWLEDGMENT

This research was sponsored by the U.S. Atomic Energy Commission under contract with the Union Carbide Corporation.

REFERENCES

1. D. A. Marvin and B. Hohn. *Bacteriol. Rev.* **33:**172 (1969).
2. L. R. Brown and C. E. Dowell. *J. Virol.* **2:**1290 (1968).
3. A. Roy and S. Mitra. *J. Virol.* **6:**333 (1970).
4. R. Jaenisch, E. Jacob, and P. H. Hofschneider. *Nature* **227:**59 (1970).
5. A. Roy. Biochemical studies of *Escherichia coli* infected with bacteriophage M13. I. Altered surface structure of the infected host. Doctor of Science Thesis, Calcutta University, India (1972).
6. A. Roy and S. Mitra. *Nature* **228:**365 (1970).
7. P. Reid and J. Speyer. *J. Bacteriol.* **104:**376 (1970).
8. R. J. White and G. Lancini. *Biochim. Biophys. Acta* **240:**429 (1971).
9. H. Engelberg and E. Soudry. *J. Virol.* **7:**847 (1971).
10. E. Trenkner. *Virology* **40:**18 (1970).
11. S. Mitra. *Virology* **50:**422 (1972).
12. D. Pratt and W. S. Erdahl. *J. Mol. Biol.* **37:**181 (1968).
13. D. Brutlag, R. Schekman, and A. Kornberg. *Proc. Natl. Acad. Sci. (USA)* **68:**2826 (1971).
14. B. Hirt. *J. Mol. Biol.* **26:**365 (1967).
15. P. C. Hanawalt, O. Maaløe, D. J. Cummings, and M. Schaechter. *J. Mol. Biol.* **3:**56 (1961).

DISCUSSION

Question (Sarkar): Could you tell us what is the size of the ribopolynucleotide involved in the replication of M13 DNA?

Answer: No. I mentioned at the beginning that these data are very preliminary, and we are further investigating the nature and size of this putative RNA primer.

Question (Bautz): One problem in interpreting your results is that it is difficult to show that RNA polymerase activity on denatured DNA template is as sensitive to rifampicin as on native DNA, as you are looking at small differences in sensitivity.

Answer: I used double-stranded DNA (calf thymus) as template for assaying RNA polymerase activity, and although the difference in sensitivity of wild-type and mutant RNA polymerase to rifampicin is not very large, this was reproducible.

Question (Chakravorty): In your thymidine-pulsing experiment, you used rifampicin at a concentration of 200 μg/ml. Do you really need such a high concentration?

Answer: As I pointed out, even infected *E. coli* cells are poorly permeable to rifampicin. Although 200 μg/ml of the drug is higher than the minimum inhibitory concentration for M13-infected cells, RNA and DNA synthesis of the host cell is only slightly inhibited by this concentration.

Question (Pradhan): Could it be possible that for phage DNA replication binding of RNA polymerase to DNA is necessary but not RNA synthesis *per se?*

Answer: It is possible, but it has been shown that initiation of DNA synthesis by RNA primer is necessary for replication of M13 single-stranded DNA, and my preliminary data also suggest the presence of *de novo* synthesized RNA in replicating RF DNA.

Question (Sambrook): Although you have made a strong case for the involvement of RNA in M13 DNA synthesis, I think that the data shown in the last two figures should be interpreted with care. It seems to me that you could explain the density shift of SS M13 DNA in Cs_2SO_4 gradients by hybridization of the DNA with phage-specific RNA that is contaminating the DNA preparation. In order to eliminate this possibility, you could run the Cs_2SO_4 gradients in the presence of DMSO or treat the pulse-labeled DNA with RNase H.

Answer: This is a very good point, and we are in the process of doing the experiments you have suggested.

Question (Mandal): Are all the progeny RF molecules synthesized on the single parental RF molecules, one after another?

Answer: No. The progeny RF replication occurs semiconservatively.

31

Conversion of φX174 and fd DNA to Their Replicative Forms by Two Enzyme Systems in *Escherichia coli*

S. Wickner, R. B. Wickner, M. Wright, I. Berkower, and J. Hurwitz

Department of Developmental Biology and Cancer
Albert Einstein College of Medicine
Bronx, New York, U.S.A.

Extracts of *Escherichia coli pol* A1 strains catalyze the conversion of φX174 or fd (M13) single-stranded circular DNA to the replicative form (1,2,). The fd DNA dependent reaction is sensitive to rifampicin and requires all four ribonucleoside triphosphates, but does not involve the products of the *dna*A or *dna*B gene. The reaction with φX174 DNA, in contrast, is rifampicin resistant and is temperature sensitive in extracts of *dna*B[ts] cells (1,2).

This chapter concerns our studies on the macromolecular and nucleoside triphosphate requirements of these reactions (3) and the purification of various components that may be involved in these reactions (4,5).

Extracts capable of carrying out the conversion of φX174 or fd single-stranded circular DNA to RF II are prepared by treating thawed concentrated cell suspensions with lysozyme and either gentle warming or addition of Brij-58 (1,3). These extracts incorporate base label or α-^{32}P label from dTTP into an alkali-resistant, RNase-resistant, DNase-sensitive product that, with either template, sediments in neutral gradients as RF II and in alkaline gradients at the size of full-length linear molecules (1-3). On alkaline CsCl equilibrium centrifugation, the product bands at the density of complementary strand (1,2).

The requirements of the fd and φX174 DNA dependent activities in the dialyzed ammonium sulfate fraction have been studied. The fd DNA dependent

Table I. Conversion of ϕX174 or fd (M13) Single-
Stranded Circular DNA to the Replicative Form[a]

	Requirements	
Omissions	ϕX174 DNA dependent activity (%)	fd DNA dependent activity (%)
Complete	100	100
-DNA	5	2
-Mg^{2+}	4	4
-dATP, dCTP, dCTP	0	0
-dATP	1	–
-dCTP	4	–
-dGTP	1	–
-ATP	0	10
-UTP, CTP, GTP	100	12

[a]*Preparation of extracts (1, 3):* Cells *(E. coli* H560F$^+$ *pol* A$_1$, *thy$^-$, endoI$^-$)* were grown to an OD$_{595}$ of 0.45 at 30°C in Hershey broth supplemented with 10 μg/ml of thiamine and 20 μg/ml of thymine, centrifuged at room temperature, and resuspended by vortexing in 0.002 vol of 10% sucrose containing 50 mM Tris-C1 (pH 7.5) at room temperature. The cell suspension was quick-frozen in a dry ice isopropanol bath and stored at -20°C until use. Frozen cells were thawed in an ice-water bath and treated in one of the following ways: (A) One-tenth volume of a lysozyme solution (2 mg/ml in 0.25 M Tris-C1, pH 7.6) and 0.025 vol of 4 M KC1 were added to 1 vol of cell suspension. The mixture was incubated at o°C for 30 min and then warmed for 90 sec in a 30-37°C water bath. (B) One-tenth volume of the lysozyme solution and 0.05 vol of 10% Brij-58 were added to 1 vol of cell suspension, and the mixture was incubated for 30 min at 0°C. With either procedure A or B, the lysate was then centrifuged at 2°C for 20 min at 50,000 $\times$ *g*, and the supernatant fluid was saved.

Ammonium sulfate precipitation: To a crude extract prepared by method A was added 0.656 vol of an ammonium sulfate solution, saturated at 4°C and adjusted to pH 7.5 with tris base. After 10 min at 0°C the suspension was centrifuged for 15 min at 10,000 $\times$ *g*, and the pellet was dissolved in the original volume of 0.05 M tris-Cl (pH 7.6) containing 1 mM EDTA and 1 mM dithiothreitol. This procedure was repeated, and the pellet was dissolved in 0.2 vol of the same buffer. The sample was then dialyzed for 1-2 hr at 4°C against 200 vol of the same buffer.

Assay conditions: In reactions containing fd DNA, additions were as follows: each reaction mixture (0.05 ml) contained 20 mM tris-C1 (pH 7.6), 10 mM MgCl$_1$, 4 mM dithiothreitol, 500 pmoles (as nucleotides) of fd single-stranded circular DNA, 2 mM ATP, 0.08 mM each of UTP, GTP, and CTP, 0.04 mM dATP, dCTP, dGTP, and [a-^{32}P]dTTP (300 cpm/pmole), 0.5 unit of RNA polymerase, 0.08 μg of *E. coli* unwinding protein (17), and 50 μg of protein of ammonium sulfate fraction. The mixture was incubated for 20 min at 25°C and acid-precipitable radioactivity was measured. In these experiments, *E. coli* unwinding protein was added before addition of the ammonium sulfate fraction, while RNA polymerase was added last. In experiments with ϕX174 DNA, all additions were the same except that RNA polymerase and *E. coli* unwinding protein were omitted and rifampicin (10 μg/ml) was added to the extract before addition of the extract to other components. One-hundred percent activity for the ϕX174 DNA dependent reaction was equivalent to the incorporation of 24 pmoles of dTMP; for fd DNA, this value was 45 pmoles of dTMP.

activity required all four deoxynucleoside triphosphates and all four ribonucleoside triphosphates (Table I) (1). With the same enzyme fraction, ϕX174 DNA
dependent activity, in contrast, required all four deoxynucleoside triphosphates
and only ATP of the ribonucleoside triphosphates (Table I). The ATP requirement in the ϕX174 DNA dependent reaction could not be replaced by comparable amounts of dATP, AMP, ADP, and a,β- or β,γ-methylene analogs of ATP, or
any of the other common ribonucleoside triphosphates. The ATP requirement of
the ϕX174 system was relatively high, with maximal activity observed at 5 mM.
In the presence of an ATP-generating system, the optimal concentration of ATP
was reduced to 0.2 mM. There was no requirement for CTP, UTP, or GTP, even
in fractions that were treated with DEAE-cellulose in the presence of 0.2 M
KCl to remove nucleic acids, precipitated with ammonium sulfate, and dialyzed.
Thus the ATP requirement of the ϕX174 system resembles the ATP requirement
for DNA synthesis in toluenized cells (6).

While the fd DNA dependent activity was sensitive to rifampicin (1) or to
antibody to RNA polymerase (Table II), the ϕX174 reaction was insensitive to
both of these agents (Table II) (1). This result suggests that at least the β subunit
of RNA polymerase is involved in the fd reaction, but RNA polymerase is
probably not involved in the ϕX174 reaction.

Table II. Effect of Inhibition of RNA Polymerase on
ϕX174 and fd *in Vitro* DNA Synthesis[a]

Inhibitor	Activity (%)	
	ϕX174	fd
None	100	100
Rifampicin (10 μg/ml)	138	8
Control γ-globulin (30 μg)	100	91
Antibody to RNA polymerase (40 μg)	90	13

[a]Crude extract of *E. coli* H560F$^+$ (400 μg of protein) prepared by method A (Table I) was incubated 15 min at 25°C
with rifampicin, control γ-globulin, or antibody to RNA
polymerase. The reaction mixture was added, and the incubation was continued for 15 min at 25°C. One-hundred
percent activity with ϕX174 DNA was equivalent to the
incorporation of 68 pmoles of dTMP, and with fd DNA it
was 44 pmoles. Control γ-globulin was prepared from serum
removed from a rabbit before immunization with *E. coli*
RNA polymerase.

GENE PRODUCTS

Involvement of the *dna* Gene Products in Conversion of fd and φX174 DNA to RF II

The *dna*B product of *E. coli* are required for the φX174 reaction, but not for the fd reaction (1). We have extended these studies to other *dna* ts mutants.

Extracts of *E. coli* strain NY73 (*dna*G ts, *pol* A1) (7,8), when compared with extracts from a temperature-insensitive revertant, showed thermolability in the φX174 reaction when incubated at 30°C (Fig. 1). In contrast, the activity with fd DNA was stable in extracts of both temperature-sensitive and revertant strains. An equal mixture of heat-treated extracts of the mutant and revertant shows more than additive activity (Fig. 1), suggesting that the extract of the revertant contained an excess of *dna*G product.

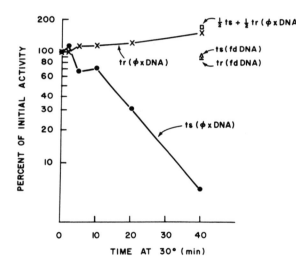

Fig. 1. Heat inactivation of extracts of *Escherichia coli* strain NY73 (pol A1, dnaG ts) and a temperature-insensitive revertant of strain NY73. Extracts of each strain were prepared by method B (Table I). Mutant and revertant extracts were incubated at 30°C, and, at the times indicated, 0.03-ml aliquots were withdrawn and placed in assay tubes at 0°C. The mixing experiment was done with 15 μl of each extract. Each assay (0.05 ml) contained 0.5 μmole of MgCl₂, 2.5 μmoles of tris·Cl (pH 7.6), 0.75 nmole of φX174 DNA or fd DNA, 2.5 nmoles each of dATP, dCTP, dGTP, and [α-³²P]dTTP, 30 nmoles of ATP, 5 nmoles each of GTP, CTP, and UTP, and cell extract. Reactions were incubated for 20 min at 20°C, and acid-insoluble radioactivity was measured. One-hundred percent activity for the extract of *E. coli* strain NY73 was 22 pmoles of dTMP per 20 min with φX174 DNA and 48 pmoles with fd DNA; for the temperature-resistant revertant of NY73, 100% activity was 48 pmoles with φX174 DNA and 43 pmoles with fd DNA. All values represent rates of synthesis since incorporation under the conditions used was essentially linear for 60 min. •, φX174 DNA dependent activity in extract of *dna*G ts cells; ×, φX174 DNA dependent activity in extract of temperature-insensitive revertant; □, φX174 DNA dependent activity in mixture of extracts (one-half ts plus one-half revertant); △ fd DNA dependent activity in extract of *dna*G ts cells; ▲, fd DNA dependent activity in extract of revertant.

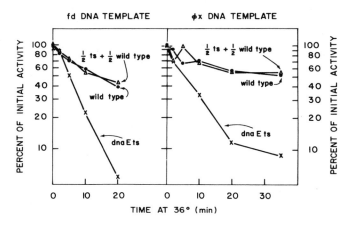

Fig. 2. Heat inactivation at 36°C of extracts of Escherichia coli strain BT1040 (pol A1, dnaE ts, end) and strain H560 (pol A1, end). Experimental details were as in Fig. 1. One-hundred percent activity for the extract of strain BT1040 was 11 pmoles of dTMP incorporated per 20 min with φX174 DNA, and 12 pmoles with fd DNA; for strain H560, 100% activity was 7 pmoles of dTMP incorporated per 20 min at 20°C with φX174 DNA, and 9 pmoles with fd DNA. Left, fd DNA template; right, φX174 DNA template. ×, *dna*E ts strain; •, wild-type strain; △, one-half *dna*E ts strain plus one-half wild-type strain.

The *dna*F gene product is not involved in either the φX174 or the fd DNA dependent systems (3) and has been shown to be ribonucleotide reductase (9).

Extracts of *E. coli* strain BT1026 (*dna*E ts, *pol* A1), when compared with either the wild-type or a temperature-insensitive revertant of strain BT1026, showed increased thermolability of both the φX174 and fd DNA dependent activities. This analysis was also performed with another *dna*E allele, *E. coli* strain BT1040 (Fig. 2), with similar results. An equal mixture of heated mutant and wild-type extracts had greater activity than expected, indicating the presence in the wild-type extract of an excess of DNA polymerase III with respect to its requirement in these reactions.

While DNA polymerase III seems to be involved in both the fd and φX174 DNA dependent systems, DNA polymerase II is not necessary for either. Extracts of *E. coli* strain HMS-83, a strain that has no detectable DNA polymerase I or DNA polymerase II measured *in vitro* (10), have the same amount of both the fd and φX174 DNA dependent activities as strains with normal amounts of DNA polymerase II.

Extracts of *E. coli* strain PC79 (7,8) (*dna*D ts, *pol* A1) or strain PC22 (7,8) (*dna*C ts, *pol* A1) cells showed no detectable activity with φX174 DNA, while temperature-insensitive revertants showed normal amounts of activity (Fig. 3). In contrast, activity with fd DNA was identical in both mutant and revertant extracts.

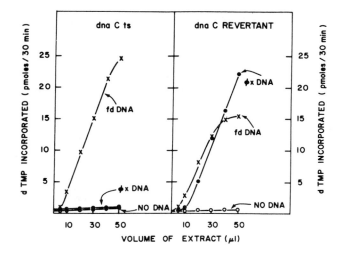

Fig. 3. φX174 and fd DNA-dependent activity of extracts of Escherichia coli strain PC22 (pol A1, dnaC ts) and a temperature-resistant revertant. Extracts of each strain were prepared by method B in the presence of 0.1 *M* NaCl and tested for activity at 20°C under the standard assay conditions, with φX174 DNA (●) or fd DNA (×) or without added DNA (○).

In summary, the two systems are distinct in at least seven components and in their rNTP requirements.

Purification of *dna* Gene Products Using the φX174 DNA Dependent System

Mixtures of extracts of different *dna* ts mutants that have been heat-inactivated show greater φX174 DNA dependent activity than the sum of the individual extracts. This *in vitro* "complementation" presumably is the result of each mutant extract supplying the component missing from the other. Thus this is an assay for each of the *dna* gene products. Barry and Alberts (11) have used this type of *in vitro* complementation assay to purify a complex of two proteins involved in T4 DNA replication. Nüsslein *et al.* (12,13), using a complementation assay in the cellophane disc system (14), have purified both the *dna*E gene product and the *dna*G gene product.

We have purified the *dna*G product about 10,000-fold using the complementation assay in the φX174 DNA dependent system (Table III) (4).

The ability of two fractions in the purification of the *dna*G gene product to stimulate receptor crude extracts from *dna*A, B, C, D, E, and G ts cells is shown in Table IV (4). While the ammonium sulfate fraction complements each of the

Table III. Purification of *dna*G Gene Product[a]

Fraction	Total protein (mg)	Total U	Specific activity (U/mg)	Percent recovery
High-speed supernatant	59,500			
20-30% ammonium sulfate fraction	3,240	1375	0.37	100
DNA agarose eluate	100	727	6.7	53
DEAE-cellulose eluate	28.8	650	22.6	47
DEAE-Sephadex eluate	3.8	270	74	20
Glycerol gradient[b]	1.3	270	222	20

[a]*Complementation assay:* Each assay (0.075 ml) contained 20 mM tris-C1 (pH 7.6), 10 mM MgCl$_2$, 4 mM dithiothreitol, 0.04 mM each of dATP, dGTP, dCTP, and [α-^{32}P]dTTP, (300-500 cpm/pmole), 1.5 mM ATP, 0.05 mM each of UTP, CTP, and GTP, 10 μg/ml rifampicin, 2 mM spermidine-HC1, 500 pmoles ϕX174 DNA, 0.05 ml of ts receptor crude extracts (15 mg/ml of protein) prepared by method B (Table I) and inactivated by freezing and thawing or by heating 30 min at 30°C, and protein fraction. After incubation at 30°C for 20 min, the acid-insoluble radioactivity was measured. One unit (U) stimulates a receptor crude extract to incorporate 1 nmole of dTMP in 20 min at 30°C.

Purification of dnaG gene product: E. coli HMS-83 (400 g) suspended in 400 ml of 0.02 M potassium phosphate (pH 7.5), 0.5 M KC1, 5 × 10^{-4} M EDTA, 10^{-3} M dithio-threitol, and 10% glycerol was broken in the Gaulin French press and centrifuged at 100,000 × g for 60 min. The supernatant was adjusted to 4% with streptomycin sulfate and centrifuged at 10,000 × g for 15 min. The supernatant was adjusted to 40% saturation with solid ammonium sulfate. This pellet was washed successively with 200 ml each of 40%, 30%, and 20% saturated ammonium sulfate solution in 0.02 M potassium phosphate (pH 7.5), 10^{-3} M dithiothreitol, and 5 × 10^{-4} M EDTA. The supernatant obtained after extraction with 20% ammonium sulfate was adjusted to 40% saturation with solid ammonium sulfate (11.3 g/100 ml). The precipitate was dissolved in 100 ml of 0.02 M Tris-C1 (pH 7.5), 10^{-3} M dithiothreitol, 5 × 10^{-4} M EDTA, and 20% glycerol (buffer A) and dialyzed against buffer A. The dialyzed sample was diluted to 250 ml with buffer A minus glycerol and applied to a 6 by 40-cm column of denatured calf thymus DNA-agarose (15). The column was washed with 500 ml of buffer A containing 10% glycerol, and the *dna*G activity was eluted with buffer A containing 1 M NaCl. The 1 M NaCl eluate was adjusted to 50% saturation with solid ammonium sulfate (29.1 g/100 ml); the precipi-tate was dissolved in 14 ml of 0.05 M tris-C1 (pH 7.8), 10^{-3} M dithiothreitol, 5 × 10^{-4} M EDTA, and 20% glycerol (buffer B). The enzyme was dialyzed against buffer B and applied to a DEAE-cellulose column (2.2 by 19 cm) equilibrated with the same buffer. The column was washed with 35 ml of buffer B and then with a 600-ml linear gradient from 0 to 0.35 M KCl in buffer B. The active fractions (36 ml) were pooled, dialyzed against 2 liters of buffer B, and applied to a DEAE-Sephadex column (2 by 24 cm) equilibrated with the same buffer. The column was washed with 20 ml of buffer B and then with a 400-ml linear gradient from 0 to 0.2 M KCl in buffer B. Active fractions were pooled and adjusted to 50% saturation with solid ammonium sulfate. The pellet was dissolved in 3 ml of buffer B. A portion of the DEAE-Sephadex fraction was dialyzed against 0.05 M tris-C1 (pH 7.8), 0.2 M KCl, 10^{-3} M dithiothreitol, 5 × 10^{-4} M EDTA, and 5% glycerol. The dialyzed sample was layered on a 6-ml 10-30% glycerol gradient in the same buffer and centrifuged in the Spinco SW50.1 rotor at 50,000 rpm for 35 hr. The *dna*G activity sedimented through two-thirds of the gradient.

[b] This step was carried out with only part of the DEAE-Sephadex eluate. The values reported are calculated assuming that the yield would be the same if all of this fraction were subjected to the glycerol gradient procedure.

mutant extracts, the purified *dna*G-complementing activity was usually specific in complementing only extracts of *dna*G ts cells.

When the *dna*G-complementing activity was purified from *dna*G ts cells, it was found to be thermolabile in comparison with that purified from wild-type cells (Fig. 4) (4). This shows that the *dna*G-complementing activity was the product of the *dna*G gene. This experiment is especially important because some purified fractions stimulated receptor crude extracts of both *dna*G and *dna*A cells.

If the stimulation of the *dna*A receptor crude extract were due to the *dna*A gene product, it should be thermolabile in comparison with wild-type activity when prepared from *dna*A ts cells. Using the procedure described in Table III, the *dna*G activity was purified from *dna*A ts cells through the DEAE-cellulose step. Stimulation of neither *dna*A nor *dna*G receptor crude extracts by this fraction was thermolabile when compared with a wild-type preparation.

To determine if the stimulation of the *dna*A receptor crude extract were due to the *dna*G gene product, the thermolabilities of *dna*A- and *dna*G-complementing activities were compared in material purified from wild-type cells with that purified from *dna*G ts cells. Both activities were more thermolabile in the preparation from *dna*G ts cells than in that from wild-type cells. Thus the *dna*G

Table IV. Stimulation of Various Receptor Crude Extracts by *dna*G Gene Product[a]

Receptor crude used	pmoles dTMP incorporated	
	Ammonium sulfate fraction	DEAE-sephadex fraction
*dna*G	18.2	10.3
*dna*A	17.8	0.8
*dna*B	33.7	0.2
*dna*C	16.8	0.2
*dna*D	19.6	0.5
*dna*E	17.0	0.2

[a]The ammonium sulfate fraction was prepared by lysing wild-type cells frozen in sucrose (as described in Table I) with 0.2% Brij and 0.2 mg/ml lysozyme on ice 30 min, centrifuging at 100,000 $\times$ g for 30 min, and making the supernatant (20 ml) 40% saturated with saturated neutralized ammonium sulfate. The pellet was dissolved in 0.05 M tris-Cl (pH 7.5), 10^{-3} M dithiothreitol, 5 $\times$ 10^{-4} M EDTA, and 10% glycerol (2 ml) and dialyzed 2 hr against this buffer; 0.12 of this fraction and 0.14 µg of the DEAE-Sephadex fraction were assayed under the conditions described in Table III. The ammonium sulfate fraction incorporated no dTMP in the absence of ϕX DNA and incorporated 0.9 pmole in the presence of DNA minus any receptor crude extract; the DEAE-Sephadex fraction incorporated no dTMP in the presence or absence of ϕX DNA in the absence of receptor crude. The receptor crude extract of *dna*A, B, C, D, or G ts cells incorporated 0.2-1 pmole of dTMP dependent on ϕX DNA in the absence of added ammonium sulfate or DEAE-Sephadex fraction, while that of *dna*E ts cells incorporated 4.9 pmoles. The values given have been corrected for this endogenous activity of the receptor crudes.

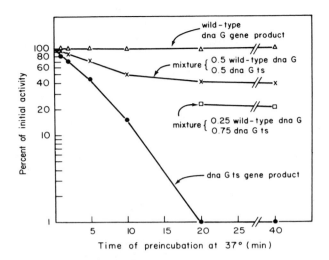

Fig. 4. Temperature sensitivity of dnaG activity isolated from Escherichia coli dnaG ts and wild-type cells. Preparations containing 0.02 U of *dna*G-stimulating activity purified from either *dna*G ts cells (9 U/mg protein) or wild-type cells (23 U/mg protein) were preincubated at 37°C for the times indicated. Mixtures containing 0.01 U of ts *dna*G activity and 0.01 U of wild-type *dna*G activity and others containing 0.015 U of ts *dna*G activity and 0.005 U of wild-type *dna*G activity were also preincubated at 37°C. After preincubation, the samples were assayed for *dna*G activity at 30°C using the conditions described in Table III.

product is capable of complementing extracts from *dna*A ts cells, and it is clear that complementing activity alone is not sufficient to determine what gene product(s) has been purified.

The *dna*G product has a molecular weight of about 60,000, as determined by glycerol-gradient centrifugation (4). It is *N*-ethylmaleimide insensitive and binds only weakly to DNA (4). No enzymatic activity attributable to the *dna*G product has yet been detected.

Using a similar assay, we have partially purified the *dna*B gene product and the *dna*D gene product, and the former has been shown to be thermolabile when purified from *dna*B ts cells.

*dna*E-Complementing activity has been purified extensively using the complementation assay as above (4) from wild-type and *dna*E ts cells. The *dna*E-complementing activity and DNA polymerase III activity were similarly thermolabile in the mutant (compared with the wild-type) in an experiment analogous to that shown in Fig. 4 for *dna*G activity. Moreover, in the final chromatographic stage of purification, the *dna*E-complementing activity and DNA polymerase III activity coincided. Thus, in agreement with the earlier results of

Gefter *et al.* (8), Nüsslein *et al.* (12), and Richardson *et al.* (16), the *dna*E gene product is DNA polymerase III.

This system has the advantage that, since a defined DNA is used as template, once all the protein components of the system have been isolated one can hope that analysis of the mechanism of the reaction may be possible.

DNA POLYMERASE STIMULATORY FACTOR

Isolation of a Protein that Stimulates dNMP Incorporation by DNA Polymerases of *E. coli* (5)

As mentioned above, the fd DNA dependent system requires four rNTPs and four dNTPs, involves RNA polymerase and DNA polymerase III, and is specific for fd DNA.

In an attempt to purify enzymes involved in this pathway, we have constructed a system containing fd DNA, RNA polymerase, *E. coli* unwinding protein (17), and DNA polymerase III. These enzymes, under the conditions used, carry out only a limited deoxynucleotide incorporation (Table V, line 2) but the addition of a factor isolated as described in the footnote to Table V stimulates the activity twentyfold (Table V, lines 1 and 2). The reaction with "stimulatory protein" requires DNA, DNA polymerase III, RNA polymerase, and all four rNTPs and dNTPs. The reaction was blocked by the addition of rifampicin prior to the addition of RNA polymerase. As has been shown for the fd DNA dependent system in crude extracts (1), the RNA polymerase is probably providing primer RNA for DNA polymerase III in this reconstructed system. The reason for the inclusion of unwinding protein in this system is made clear below. The reaction shown in Table V is linear with time and amount of stimulatory protein added.

Properties of Stimulatory Factor

Stimulatory factor is *N*-ethylmaleimide insensitive, has no RNA polymerase, DNA polymerase, or RNase H activity, and does not complement extracts of *dna* A, B, C, D, E, or G cells in the ϕX174 DNA dependent system (5). The factor partially purified from *dna*A, B, C, D, E, or G^{ts} cells was not thermolabile in comparison to that purified from wild-type cells. The factor has not yet been completely freed of DNase and RNase activity.

The stimulatory protein, unlike *E. coli* unwinding protein (17), does not bind to DNA-agarose columns and does not render ϕX174 DNA or fd DNA resistant to the action of the *Neurospora* nuclease (20). The factor had no effect on ribonucleotide incorporation by RNA polymerase primed with fd or ϕX174 DNA and if, in the "reconstituted system" of Table V, fd DNA, RNA polymer-

Table V. Requirements for Effect of Stimulatory Protein[a]

	Additions or omissions	dTMP incorporated (pmoles/20 min)
1.	Complete	10.2
2.	Omit stimulatory protein	0.74
3.	Omit DNA, or omit all rNTPs, or omit three unlabeled dNTPs	< 0.1
4.	Omit DNA polymerase III	0.74
5.	Omit RNA polymerase	1.12
6.	Omit UTP, GTP, CTP	1.02
7.	Omit ATP	1.75
8.	Omit spermidine and *E. coli* unwinding protein	3.6
9.	Omit *E. coli* unwinding protein	7.8
10.	Omit spermidine	3.9
11.	Complete + rifampicin (25 μg/ml)	0.85

[a]*Assay of stimulatory protein:* Reaction mixtures (0.05 ml) contained 5 nmoles each of dATP, dCTP, dGTP, and [^{3}H]dTTP (200-300 cpm/pmole), 5 nmoles each of UTP, GTP, and CTP, 250 nmoles of ATP, 0.5 μmole of MgCl$_2$, 1.5 μmoles of tris-Cl (pH 7.5), 10 nmoles of dithiothreitol, 500 pmoles of fd DNA, 60 nmoles of spermidine, stimulatory protein as indicated, 0.05 unit (5) of *E. coli* unwinding protein (17), 0.35 unit of DNA polymerase III [prepared by a modification of the method of Kornberg and Gefter (18)], and 0.1 unit of RNA polymerase [purified as described (19)]. Reactions were initiated by the addition of RNA polymerase and incubated for 20 min at 30°C, and acid-insoluble radioactivity was measured. Two control mixtures were incubated simultaneously, one without stimulatory protein and one without stimulatory protein and DNA polymerase III. A unit of stimulatory protein is defined as the incorporation of 1 nmole of dTMP under the above conditions.

Purification of stimulatory protein (5): A column of DE52 (3 by 21 cm) was equilibrated with 0.02 M potassium phosphate buffer (pH 7.5), 10^{-3} M dithiothreitol, 10^{-3} M EDTA, and 10% glycerol (buffer B). Half of the material not adhering to DNA-agarose (Table III) (150 ml) was applied to the column, which was then successively washed with 75-ml volumes of buffer B, buffer B containing 0.2 M potassium phosphate (pH 7.5), buffer B containing 0.3 M potassium phosphate (pH 7.5), and buffer B containing 0.5 M potassium phosphate (pH 7.5). Approximately 70% of the activity applied to the column was eluted with 0.3 M potassium phosphate (700 units, 7.3 units/mg protein).

Phosphocellulose chromatography: The DEAE-cellulose fraction was precipitated with solid ammonium sulfate, dialyzed for 2 hr against 500 ml of 10% glycerol, 0.02 M potassium phosphate buffer (pH 6.4), 10^{-3} M 2-mercaptoethanol (buffer C). The dialyzed fraction was then diluted two-fold with buffer C and loaded slowly onto a phosphocellulose column (P11, 3 by 18 cm) equilibrated with buffer C, and the column was successively washed with 30 ml of buffer C, 50 ml of buffer C containing 0.05 M potassium phosphate (pH 6.4), and 50 ml of buffer C containing 0.3 M potassium phosphate (pH 6.4). The 0.05 M phosphate eluate was collected in three fractions; all fractions were precipitated with ammonium sulfate (50% saturation, 29.1 g/100 ml) and dissolved with 1 ml of buffer C. The activity eluting with the 0.05 M phosphate buffer was heated at 50°C for 4 min and centrifuged for 15 min at 100,000 × g in the Spinco ultracentrifuge and the supernatant retained (293 units, 22 units/mg protein).

G100 Sephadex chromatography: A column of G100 Sephadex (1 by 32 cm) was equilibrated with buffer C containing 20% glycerol; 1 ml of the phosphocellulose fraction was applied to the column. The column was washed with buffer C (containing 20% glycerol, and 1-ml fractions were collected. Those fractions purified between three- and six-fold were combined, adjusted to 50% saturation with solid ammonium sulfate (29.1 g/100 ml), and dissolved in 1 ml of buffer C with 20% glycerol (120 units, 83 units/mg protein). The concentrated preparation was heated at 50°C for 5 min; while this treatment did not lead to further purification, it resulted in the complete inactivation of traces of DNA polymerase III activity.

ase, and rNTPs were replaced by preformed fd DNA·RNA hybrids (made by RNA polymerase and isolated by isopycnic banding), the reaction still depended on both DNA polymerase III and stimulatory protein, but was no longer inhibited by rifampicin. Thus the stimulatory protein seems to act after the formation of the RNA primer (5).

Each of the three *E. coli* DNA polymerases is stimulated by the factor in either the "reconstituted system" (Table VI) or using poly(dA)·oligo(rU) as primer-template (Table VI). The mechanism of this stimulation is unclear at this time.

As previously mentioned, the fd DNA dependent system in crude extracts is incapable of utilizing ϕX174 DNA. In extracts of *dnaC* ts cells, for example, rifampicin-sensitive activity with fd DNA is normal, but no activity (either sensitive or resistant to rifampicin) is detected with ϕX174 DNA as template (Fig. 3). The "reconstituted system," however, can utilize either ϕX174 or fd DNA with equal efficiency (Table VII, lines 1 and 3, column B). A second factor has been found in an eluate of a DNA-agarose column that appears to allow the "reconstituted system" to differentiate between fd and ϕX174 DNA, largely by inhibiting the activity with ϕX174 DNA (Table VII, lines 2 and 4, column B). If

Table VI. Influence of Stimulatory Protein on dNMP Incorporation by DNA Polymerases of *Escherichia coli*

DNA polymerase added	dTMP incorporated (pmoles/20 min)	
	+ stimulatory Protein	− stimulatory Protein
"Reconstituted system" as described in Table V[a]		
I (0.12 unit)	21.6	8.3
II (0.10 unit)	5.7	0.36
III (0.14 unit)	7.6	<.2
Poly(dA) · oligo(rU) primer-template[b]		
I (0.12 unit)	144	8.8
II (0.11 unit)	18.4	< 0.2
III (0.28 unit)	31.5	< 0.2

[a] Reactions were carried out as described in Table V, except that the DNA polymerase used was as indicated.

[b] Reaction mixtures (0.1 ml) contained 5 nmoles of [^{3}H]dTTP (190 cpm/pmole), 5 nmoles of dATP, 0.5 μmole of MgCl$_2$, 2 μmoles of tris-Cl (pH 7.5), 10 nmoles of DTT, 400 pmoles of poly(dA) (chain length 1700), 340 pmoles of poly(U) (chain length 100), 0.044 unit of stimulatory protein where indicated, and DNA polymerase. Reaction mixtures were incubated for 30 min at 30°C, and nucleotide incorporation was measured.

Table VII. Specific Inhibition of ϕX DNA Dependent dNMP Incorporation[a]

	Incorporation of dTMP after preincubation of DNA	
Additions	A. With RNA polymerase (pmoles)	B. Without RNA polymerase (pmoles)
1. Complete with fd DNA	12.0	9.0
2. As in (1) + DNA-agarose eluate	9.8	9.1
3. Complete with ϕX DNA	14.9	13.4
4. As in (3) + DNA-agarose eluate	11.4	0.4

[a]Reaction mixtures containing buffer, MgCl$_2$, dithiothreitol, ribonucleoside triphosphates, 200 pmoles of DNA, and either 0.1 unit or no RNA polymerase were incubated 10 min at 30°C. After incubation, dNTPs, spermidine, 0.05 unit of unwinding protein, 0.044 unit of stimulatory protein, 0.70 unit of DNA polymerase III, 6 μg of DNA-agarose eluate, and 0.1 unit of RNA polymerase (where not previously added) were added. Nucleotide incorporation was measured. The DNA-agarose fraction was prepared by passing a crude extract (3) of *E. coli* strain PC79 cells through a DEAE-cellulose column in 0.1 *M* KCl, adsorbing the eluate to a denatured calf thymus DNA-agarose column, eluting the material with 2 *M* NaCl, precipitating the eluate with ammonium sulfate (60% saturation), and dialyzing the dissolved pellet.

Table VIII. Summary of the Requirements for fd and ϕX174 DNA Dependent *in vitro* DNA Synthesis[a]

Component(s)	ϕX174 DNA dependent system	fd DNA dependent system
ϕX174 DNA	Utilized	Not Utilized
fd DNA	Not utilized	Utilized
4 dNTP	+	+
ATP	+	+
UTP, CTP and GTP	−	+
RNA polymerase	−	+
dna A	−	−
dna B	+	−
dna C	+	−
dna D	+	−
dna E (DNA polymerase III)	+	+
dna G	+	−
DNA polymerase II	−	−
DNA polymerase I	−	−

[a]+, Required for activity; −, not required for activity.

a preliminary incubation of the DNA with RNA polymerase and rNTPs is carried out, allowing production of a DNA·RNA hybrid, this differentiating effect is abolished (Table VII, column A). Moreover, this effect is seen only at a critical ratio of unwinding protein to DNA.

CONCLUSION

The nucleoside triphosphate and macromolecular requirements of the ϕX174 and fd DNA dependent systems are summarized in Table VIII. The ϕX174 DNA dependent system may be a good model for study of the mechanism of DNA replication in *E. coli*. The fd DNA dependent system, on the other hand, may be composed of elements from another of the cell's DNA synthetic systems. Both systems are proving very useful in the study of the enzymology of DNA metabolism.

NOTE ADDED IN PROOF

Recent experiments in our laboratory have shown that:

1. The *dna*A gene product is not involved in either the ϕX174 or fd DNA dependent reactions (21,22). *In vivo* results of Taketo are consistent with this conclusion (23).
2. The *dna*C product has been purified extensively by complementation (21).
3. The *dna*B product has been purified extensively and contains a DNA dependent ribonucleoside triphosphatase activity (22,24).
4. The stimulatory factor described here has been resolved into two factors, both of which must be present for the stimulatory effect to be observed (25).
5. The stimulatory effect requires either ATP or dATP, even on templates (such as poly dA·oligo dT) where dAMP incorporation is not necessary (and does not, in fact, occur) (25).

REFERENCES

1. W. T. Wickner, D. Brutlag, R. Schekman, and A. Kornberg. *Proc. Natl. Acad. Sci. (USA)* **69**:965-969 (1972).
2. R. Schekman, W. T. Wickner, O. Westergaard, D. Brutlag, K. Geider, L. L. Bertsch, and A. Kornberg. *Proc. Natl. Acad. Sci. (USA)* **69**:2691-2695 (1972).
3. R. B. Wickner, M. Wright, S. Wickner, and J. Hurwitz. *Proc. Natl. Acad. Sci. (USA)* **69**:3233-3237 (1972).
4. S. Wickner, M. Wright, and J. Hurwitz. *Proc. Natl. Acad. Sci. (USA)* **70**:1613-1618 (1973).
5. J. Hurwitz, S. Wickner, and M. Wright. *Biochem. Biophys. Res. Commun.* **51**:257-267 (1973).

6. D. Pisetsky, I. Berkower, R. B. Wickner, and J. Hurwitz. *J. Mol. Biol.* **71**:557-571 (1972).

7. P. L. Carl. *Mol. Gen. Genet.* **109**:107-122 (1970).

8. M. L. Gefter, Y. Hirota, T. Kornberg, J. Wechsler, and C. Barnoux. *Proc. Natl. Acad. Sci. (USA)* **68**:3150-3153 (1971).

9. J. A. Fuchs, H. O. Karlstrom, H. R. Warner, and P. Reichard. *Nature New Biol.* **238**:69-71 (1972).

10. J. L. Campbell, L. Soll, and C. C. Richardson. *Proc. Natl. Acad. Sci. (USA)* **69**:2090-2094 (1972).

11. J. Barry and B. Alberts. *Proc. Natl. Acad. Sci. (USA)* **69**:2717-2721 (1972).

12. V. Nüsslein, B. Otto, F. Bonhoeffer, and H. Schaller. *Nature New Biol.* **234**:285-286 (1971).

13. V. Nüsslein, F. Bonhoeffer, A. Klein, and B. Otto. In R. Wells and R. Inman (eds.), *The Second Annual Harry Steenbock Symposium,* University Park Press, Maryland, in press (1972).

14. H. Schaller, B. Otto, V. Nüsslein, J. Huf, R. Herrmann, and F. Bonhoeffer. *J. Mol. Biol.* **63**:183-200 (1972).

15. H. Schaller, C. Nüsslein, F. J. Bonhoeffer, C. Kurz, and I. Neitzschmann. *Europ. J. Biochem.* **26**:474-481 (1972).

16. C. C. Richardson, J. L. Campbell, J. W. Chase, D. C. Hinkle, D. M. Livingston, H. L. Mulcahy, and H. Shizuya. In R. Wells and R. Inman (eds.), *The Second Annual Harry Steenbock Symposium,* University Park Press, Maryland, in press (1972).

17. N. Sigal, H. Delius, T. Kornberg, M. L. Gefter, and B. Alberts. *Proc. Natl. Acad. Sci. (USA)* **69**:3537-3541 (1972).

18. T. Kornberg and M. L. Gefter. *J. Biol. Chem.* **247**:5369-5375 (1972).

19. J. Hurwitz, L. Yarbrough, and S. Wickner. *Biochem. Biophys. Res. Commun.* **48**:628-635 (1972).

20. E. Z. Rabin, M. Mustard, and M. J. Frazer. *Can. J. Biochem.* **46**:1285 (1968).

21. S. Wickner, I. Berkower, M. Wright, and J. Hurwitz. *Proc. Natl. Acad. Sci. (USA)* **70**:1613-1618 (1973).

22. M. Wright, S. Wickner, and J. Hurwitz. *Proc. Natl. Acad. Sci. (USA)* in press (1973).

23. A. Taketo. *Mol. Gen. Genet.* **122**:15 (1973).

24. S. Wickner, M. Wright, and J. Hurwitz. *Proc. Natl. Acad. Sci. (USA)* in press (1973).

25. J. Hurwitz, and S. Wickner. *Proc. Natl. Acad. Sci. (USA)* in press (1973).

DISCUSSION

Question (Burma): Do you know whether *dna*G product (which is highly purified) acts in a catalytic fashion? Is it sensitive to -SH agents or any other inhibitor which acts with the active centers of the enzyme?

Answer: The *dna*G product is insensitive to the action of N-ethylmaleimide, a -SH reagent. We have no evidence on the question of whether G acts catalytically or stoichiometrically.

Question (Sambrook): Do the factors have any effect on RNA-dependent DNA polymerase?

Answer: We have not yet detected any such effect.

32

A Quantitative Estimate of DNA·RNA Hybridization in *Neurospora crassa*

S. K. Dutta and D. R. Jagannath

Department of Botany
Howard University
Washington, D.C., U.S.A.

Britten and Kohne (1) have shown that the presence of repeated DNA sequences in eukaryotic organisms interferes with the true estimates of DNA·DNA and DNA·RNA reactions in annealing experiments. *Neurospora crassa* DNA has been reported to contain repeated DNA sequences (2). This might account for why no more than 20% DNA·DNA (3) and 9% DNA·RNA (Mahadevan and Bhagwat, this volume, Chapter 18) reactions were obtained using unfractionated DNA and RNA of the same *N. crassa* mycelial cells. A true estimate of the transcription of genetic information from DNA into complementary RNA in eukaryotic cells is needed for a better understanding of the control of cell and tissue differentiation. Using the conditions described in this chapter, it has been possible to arrive at an almost complete (98%) DNA·DNA and about 30% (where the theoretically maximum possible estimate is 50%) DNA·RNA hybridization in *N. crassa* at the exponential growth phase.

MATERIALS AND METHODS

N. crassa wild-type 74A strain (FGSC No. 987) was obtained from the Fungal Genetics Stock Center (FGSC), Humboldt, California. Culturing of mycelial cells, procedures for isolation of unlabeled and ^{32}P-labeled mycelial DNA, tests for purity of isolated DNA, and techniques for shearing of ^{32}P-labeled DNA and for DNA·DNA reaction have been described by Dutta and

Ojha (4). Unlabeled whole RNA (unfractionated) was prepared by a modification of the hot-phenol method of Scherrer and Darnell (5). Isolation was done in the presence of diethyl pyrocarbonate to inhibit nucleases, and the RNA solution was passed through a bed of Dowex-50 resin to remove traces of basic proteins. These modifications ensured the stability of the whole RNA preparations during incubation. In our RNA preparation, the presence of DNA was not detected, as measured by lack of influence on the reassociation of trace amounts of ^{32}P-labeled homologous DNA.

Since measurement of the transcription of only the unique sequences was desired, repeated DNA segments were removed from unfractionated *Neurospora* DNA before the DNA was used for the hybridization experiments. To do this, ^{32}P-labeled sheared DNA was denatured by heating at 100°C for 3 min in a medium containing 0.14 M phosphate buffer (PB), 0.4% sodium laurylsulfate (SLS), and 10^{-4} M disodium ethylenediaminetetraacetate (EDTA). After denaturation, the DNA solution was rapidly cooled at 60°C and incubated at 60°C for sufficient time to obtain a $C_0 t$ of 2($C_0 t$ = OD at 260 nm/2 times incubation in hours). The mixture was then passed through a HA column equilibrated at 60°C with 0.14 M PB and 0.4% SLS. Approximately 90% of the DNA did not bind to HA and was found to represent nonrepeated DNA.

DNA·RNA hybridization experiments were done by incubating ^{32}P-labeled DNA and unlabeled whole RNA in PB-SLS-EDTA mixture at 60°C. The RNA concentration in the mixture varied, while the DNA $C_0 t$ was kept the same (between 0.005 and 0.008) so that very little DNA·DNA reassociation could occur. The incubation mixture was then passed through a HA column equilibrated with the same buffer at 60°C and washed with the same buffer until all the unhybridized single-stranded DNA was eluted. The column was then washed with 0.14 M PB to remove any SLS in the column. The material that remained adsorbed to the column represented DNA·RNA and DNA·DNA hybrids, which were eluted with 0.48 M PB. To determine the actual amount of ^{32}P] DNA hybridized with RNA, the procedures developed by D. E. Kohne, as described recently by Hough and Davidson (6), were followed. Samples of this fraction were digested with ribonuclease to remove RNA in DNA·RNA hybrids and excess RNA in the mixture. The digested materials were exhaustively dialyzed to remove nucleotides. The dialyzed materials were adjusted to PB-SLS and passed through HA columns equilibrated with PB-SLS at 60°C. The single-stranded ^{32}P] DNA eluted represented the amount of DNA hybridized with RNA, while DNA·DNA duplexes remained adsorbed to the column. The single-stranded DNA material that came out of the column was reacted with whole RNA from *Escherichia coli* under identical conditions. No appreciable DNA·RNA hybridization was obtained, suggesting that the reaction between *N. crassa* mycelial DNA and whole RNA was specific. Furthermore, ^{32}P] DNA that failed to react with *N. crassa* mycelial RNA in initial incubation did not hybridize in a subsequent incubation with *N. crassa* RNA, indicating that the initial DNA·RNA reaction was essentially complete. [^{32}P]DNA that did not react with whole RNA shows nearly complete reaction with unlabeled DNA of *N. crassa*.

RESULTS AND CONCLUSIONS

Table I summarizes results on saturation studies for DNA·RNA hybridization. At a DNA $C_0 t$ of 0.008, the minimum RNA $C_0 t$ that is necessary for maximum reaction is approximately 100,000. The maximum transcription of nonrepeated DNA is 30%. DNA sequences that code for rRNA and tRNA in *N. crassa* are repeated and represent 1% and 0.3%, respectively, of the total *N. crassa* genome (2,7,8). Ninety-eight percent DNA·DNA reactions and no reaction with *E. coli* RNA served as excellent control reactions to show the sensitivity of our procedures.

Estimates on the transcription of genetic information from eukaryotic nonrepeated DNA of mouse cells have been reported by Gelderman *et al.* (9). They have shown that about 6% of the single-copy DNA sequences are represented in the RNA of newborn mice. Hahn and Laird (10) have reported different estimates of transcription in mouse brain (10.8-12.4%), liver (3-5.2%), and kidney (2.7-4.8%) for single-copy DNAs. This compares with the 30% found for *N. crassa*. DNA transcription reported in this chapter was observed in exponen-

Table I. Summary of Estimates of Transcriptions of Nonrepeated ^{32}P-Labeled Mycelial DNA of *Neurospora crassa*[a]

[^{32}P]DNA	DNA $C_0 t$	RNA $C_0 t$	Percent hybridization
N. crassa	1500.00	0.000	98.00
	0.0054	1,168	0.00
	0.0054	6,132	6.00
	0.0054	12,250	10.36
	0.008	24,675	16.48
	"	50,400	20.70
	"	84,720	27.00
	"	96,000	28.7
	"	99,666	30.30
E. coli	0.005	90,000	00.90

[a]The [^{32}P]DNA $C_0 t$ was kept very small, which ensured negligible self-reaction. $C_0 t$ = optical density at 260 nm/2 × incubation in hours. DNA · RNA hybridization values given here are net; i.e., estimates of true DNA · RNA hybridization are given.

tially growing mycelial cells of *N. crassa*, where the transcriptional diversity of the genome is supposed to be at a maximum in order to meet the requirements of cell growth and differentiation. *N. crassa* information content has a mass of 2.2×10^{10} daltons (7), and 30% of this genome is expressed in mycelial cells of 16 hr growth. In prokaryotic cells of *E. coli,* McCarthy and Bolton (11) reported 50% DNA·RNA hybridization by using different DNA-agar procedures. Such high level of transcription in eukaryotic cells has not been reported yet, to the best of our knowledge.

ACKNOWLEDGMENTS

This study was supported in part by U.S. National Science Foundation grant No. GY-10452 and U.S. Atomic Energy Commission contract No. AT(40-1)-4182. We thank Dr. Bill H. Hoyer of Carnegie Institution of Washington, D.C., for his helpful suggestions and Mr. Theodore Osgood for laboratory assistance.

REFERENCES

1. R. J. Britten and D. E. Kohne. *Science* **161:**529 (1968).
2. R. R. Brooks and P. C. Huang. *Biochem. Genet.* **6:**41 (1972).
3. S. K. Dutta, W. P. McWhorter, M. Mandel, and V. W. Woodward. *Genetics* **57:**719 (1967).
4. S. K. Dutta and M. Ojha. *Mol. Gen. Genet.* **114:**232 (1972).
5. K. M. Scherrer and J. K. Darnell. *Biochem. Biophys. Res. Commun.* **7:**486 (1962).
6. B. R. Hough and E. H. Davidson. *J. Mol. Biol.* **70:**491-509 (1972).
7. S. K. Chattopadhyay, D. E. Kohne, and S. K. Dutta. *Proc. Natl. Acad. Sci. (USA)* **69:**No. 11 (1972).
8. R. Ray and S. K. Dutta. *Biochem. Biophys. Res. Commun.* **47:**1458-1463 (1972).
9. A. H. Gelderman, A. V. Rake, and R. J. Britten. *Proc. Natl. Acad. Sci. (USA)* **68:**172 (1971).
10. W. E. Hahn and C. D. Laird. *Science* **173:**158 (1971).
11. D. J. McCarthy and E. T. Bolton. *J. Mol. Biol.* **8:**184 (1964).

DISCUSSION

Question (Chakravorty): Why do you label DNA for DNA·RNA hybridization studies? You could label RNA. That would take care of your DNA·DNA hybrid that you are so worried about.

Answer: DNA is labeled so that we can isolate the DNA segments which code for RNAs. The transcribed DNA sequences, which are complementary to the specific RNA used, are trapped as DNA·RNA hybrids, which are then purified using hydroxylapatite chromatography. It is not possible to do this by labeling RNA.

Question (Chakravorty): I presume you shear DNA for your DNA·RNA hybrids?
Answer: Yes, we do shear DNA to 400-500 nucleotide pieces.

Question (Mishra): What are the points of similarity between the wild-type and the mutant slime?

Answer: Approximately 90% of the DNA sequences are common between the wild-type 74A strain and the mutant slime. My colleague, Dr. R. K. Chaudhuri, has measured almost the same DNA·RNA hybridizations at the saturation point between the wild-type and the mutant slime using ^{32}P-labeled DNA of the wild type. His observations indicate that even though the quantitative difference is not detectable, differential gene expression is responsible for altered phenotype.

Index